Clinical Biochemistry

AN ILLUSTRATED COLOUR TEXT

SEVENTH EDITION

Michael Murphy MA MD FRCP FRCPath
Reader in Biochemical Medicine
University of Dundee
Dundee, United Kingdom

Rajeev Srivastava MS FRCS FRCPath
Consultant Clinical Biochemist
NHS Greater Glasgow and Clyde
Glasgow, United Kingdom

Kevin Deans PhD FRCP FRCPath
Consultant Clinical Biochemist
NHS Grampian
Aberdeen, United Kingdom

For additional online content visit eBooks+.com.

ELSEVIER

First edition 1995
Second edition 1999
Third edition 2004
Fourth edition 2008
Fifth edition 2013
Sixth edition 2019

Notices

Practitioners and researchers must always rely on their own experience and knowledge in evaluating and using any information, methods, compounds or experiments described herein. Because of rapid advances in the medical sciences, in particular, independent verification of diagnoses and drug dosages should be made. To the fullest extent of the law, no responsibility is assumed by Elsevier, authors, editors or contributors for any injury and/or damage to persons or property as a matter of products liability, negligence or otherwise, or from any use or operation of any methods, products, instructions, or ideas contained in the material herein.

ISBN: 978-0-323-88057-2

Content Strategist: Trinity Hutton
Content Project Manager: Tapajyoti Chaudhuri
Cover Designer: Miles Hitchen
Marketing Manager: Deborah Watkins

Printed in India.

Last digit is the print number: 9 8 7 6 5 4 3 2 1

Working together
to grow libraries in
developing countries

www.elsevier.com • www.bookaid.org

Contents

Preface to the sixth edition

Clinical Biochemistry: An Illustrated Colour Text has been successful by any reasonable measure, with multiple editions and translations, and estimated total sales now in excess of 70,000. It has global reach, with readers in many countries across the world. As we embark on the latest edition, it is pertinent to examine why it has been so well received. Globalisation of higher education has played its part; fragmentation of the undergraduate curriculum across health science disciplines has drastically reduced the systematic teaching of many subjects, including clinical biochemistry. Our book – unashamedly introductory and laid out in richly illustrated two-page chapters (or 'spreads') – is ideally placed to cater for contemporary students, expected to acquire 'boluses' of subjects relevant to specific clinical topics and core problems. In it they find an accessible and practical source. Crucially, they can be confident that all essential information is covered; there is no 'dumbing-down'. The text has been refined over successive editions into a distillation of what students need to know.

What's new? The sixth edition represents the most radical revision since the book was first published in 1995. New 'Want to know more?' links throughout the book point interested readers to further information, and there are now multiple-choice questions for readers to test their knowledge. (We have, however, retained the popular clinical notes and case histories.) The entire content of the book has been reviewed, and every spread, table and illustration examined afresh to see if it merits inclusion or amendment. The first section has been comprehensively revamped, with a series of new spreads on interpretation.

The sixth edition marks a milestone as the first edition not to feature any of the original authors. We thank Allan Gaw, Bob Cowan and Denis O'Reilly as they step down; each has contributed decisively to the enduring success of the book. We welcome our colleague Kevin Deans, a consultant chemical pathologist in Aberdeen, to the writing team, and hope that the book does as well in the future as it has in the past.

Michael Murphy
Rajeev Srivastava
Kevin Deans

Preface to the seventh edition

Whenever a new edition of this book is commissioned, we inevitably wonder whether it will be as popular as previous ones, and find ourselves asking the same questions each time: what needs to be changed and what should we retain? Since *Clinical Biochemistry: An Illustrated Colour Text* was first published in 1995, it has proved enduringly popular across the world. Sales of the sixth edition – a very healthy 10,000 or so – have brought total global sales across all editions and translations to well over 80,000, and confirm the ongoing reach of the book. Feedback from educators and readers across the world likewise testifies to its appeal. So we should start by reassuring everyone that the seventh edition retains the same practical and patient-centred approach that has made previous editions so popular. Despite its accessibility, there is no 'dumbing-down': all essential information has been distilled in the updated text.

So: what have we changed? First, the illustrations, which are a major part of the visual appeal of the book, have been revisited and updated – some were 'showing their age'. In addition, the accompanying e-book now contains animations that facilitate understanding of the volume changes that accompany disturbances of sodium and water balance. We have also included a new chapter on the pancreas. Two additional chapters at the end of the book explain how some analyses are done; we think that readers will like the complementary insights that these provide. However, the emphasis remains firmly practical and clinical. The background to biochemical tests and how they should be interpreted are explained and applied, as before, through case histories and clinical notes. We have also retained multiple-choice questions for readers to test their knowledge, as well as 'Want to know more?' links which point interested readers to further information. We hope that, once again, the changes will ensure that the book remains as relevant and accessible as before.

Michael Murphy
Rajeev Srivastava
Kevin Deans

Acknowledgements

We would like to thank the following colleagues, who have helped us in many different ways in the preparation of the various editions of this book:

Bryan Adamson
Bill Bartlett
Sally Beard
Graham Beastall
Katie Booth
Iain Boyle
Sharon Boyle
Fiona Brandie
Kimberley Brown
Louise Brown
Ryan Carbone
John Card
Sam Chakraverty
Brian Cook
Christopher Dawson
Ellie Dow
Frances Dryburgh
Andy Duncan
Gordon Fell
Roy Fisher
Alan Foulis

Callum Fraser
Moira Gaw
Dairena Gaffney
Peter Galloway
Brian Gordon
Christina Gray
Helen Gray
David Halls
Sava Handjiev
John Hinnie
Fiona Jenkinson
Jennie Johnston
Jennifer Johnstone
Charlene Junkin
Anastasiya Kret
Witsanu Kumthornthip
Sara Laverton
Kim Lim
Grace Lindsay
Greig Louden
Tom MacDonald
Jean McAllister
Neil McConnell
Derek McLean
Jane McNeilly

Ellen Malcolm
Hazel Miller
Heather Murray
Brian Neilly
Jenny Nobes
Maurice O'Kane
John Paterson
Nigel Rabie
Margaret Rudge
Naveed Sattar
Peter Schwartz
Heather Stevenson
Ian Stewart
Judith Strachan
Mike Wallace
Janet Warren
Philip Welsby
Thomas Whitelaw
Peter H. Wise
Helen Wright
Alesha Zeschke

We would also like to thank our editorial and design team at Elsevier for their encouragement and patience during the preparation of this book.

Clinical biochemistry

1

Introducing clinical biochemistry

1 | The clinical biochemistry laboratory

This book is about clinical biochemistry. This term conveys two things: first, that the subject is about patients and patient care, and second, that it uses chemical or biochemical methods to investigate disease (Fig. 1.1). Other labels, such as clinical chemistry, chemical pathology, pathological biochemistry and biochemical medicine, also all attempt in different ways to convey this. The vast majority of patient samples sent for biochemical analysis are blood and urine, largely reflecting the relative ease with which they can be collected. Clinical biochemistry is a 'high-throughput' laboratory specialty – it accounts for approximately one-third of all hospital laboratory investigations.

The use of biochemical tests

Biochemical tests are widely used to diagnose disease and monitor treatment, so if a patient is having a blood test done, there is a good chance that at least one of the specimens collected will be sent for biochemical analysis. For example, someone with suspected viral hepatitis will likely have blood sent (to a virology laboratory) for viral serology but will also have blood sent to the clinical biochemistry laboratory to assess the degree of liver damage caused by the virus. Less common uses for biochemical tests include screening for disease and assessing prognosis (Fig. 1.2).

Core biochemistry

Even fairly small hospitals usually have a biochemistry laboratory facility, reflecting the widespread use of biochemical tests. Some tests are more commonly requested than others and are sometimes referred to as 'core analyses', reflecting the fact that the provision of these tests is seen as a core function of the clinical biochemistry laboratory. Table 1.1 lists some of these tests. Examples include creatinine, electrolytes, liver function tests and arterial blood gases.

Specialised tests

Other tests are less commonly requested, or more difficult to measure, or both, and are not performed in every biochemistry laboratory. Such specialised tests are usually sent to larger departments which may handle specimens from an entire region or even country. These tests are often grouped together. For example, hormones – substances produced by one part of the body that act on another part – are usually grouped together in laboratories. This is partly because the methods used to measure them are similar.

Urgent samples

Some biochemical tests are considered so important for diagnosis and management that they are provided at all times, including

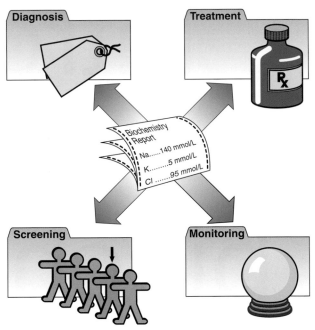

Fig. 1.2 How biochemical tests are used.

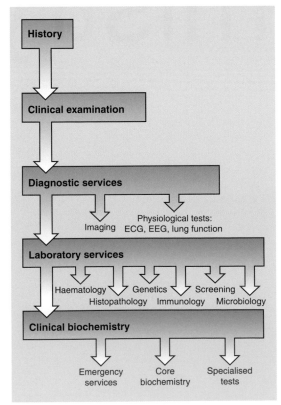

Fig. 1.1 The place of clinical biochemistry in medicine. *ECG,* electrocardiogram; *EEG,* electroencephalogram.

Table 1.1 The clinical biochemistry repertoire
Core Biochemical Tests
• Sodium and potassium
• Creatinine
• Calcium and phosphate
• Total protein and albumin
• Bilirubin and alkaline phosphatase
• Alanine aminotransferase (ALT)
• Free thyroxine and thyroid-stimulating hormone (TSH)
• Creatine kinase (CK)
• H^+, PCO_2 and PO_2 (blood gases)
• Glucose
• Amylase
Specialised Tests
• Hormones
• Specific proteins
• Trace elements
• Vitamins
• Drugs
• Lipids and lipoproteins
• Intermediary metabolites

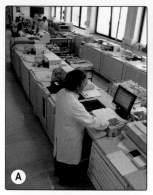
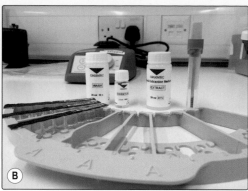
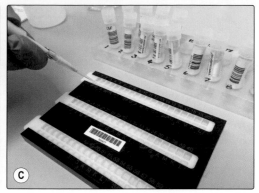

Fig. 1.3 Analysing the samples. (A) The automated analyser, **(B)** 'kit' analysis and **(C)** manual methods.

at night and at weekends, as well as during 'routine' hours. These tests sometimes need to be performed urgently, so all clinical biochemistry laboratories provide facilities or processes that allow for this, e.g. larger hospitals may have laboratory facilities away from the main laboratory, such as in surgical theatre suites.

Automation and computerisation

Once a sample is received in the laboratory, nearly all of the steps involved in processing it involve some degree of automation or computerisation. For example, the request form may be a simple barcode on the specimen that contains all of the necessary information. After that, the sample may be put onto a 'train-track', which conveys it to the centrifuge (where the heavier cells are separated from the lighter plasma), and then to the analyser, which will perform all of the requested tests. The results produced at the end of this process are then usually communicated electronically to the requesting clinician.

> ### Clinical note
>
> The clinical biochemistry laboratory plays only one part in the overall assessment and management of the patient. For some patients, biochemical analyses may play little or no part in their diagnosis or the management of their illness. For others, many tests may be needed before a diagnosis is made, and repeated analyses may be required to monitor treatment over a long period.

Test repertoire

Hundreds of different tests are carried out in clinical biochemistry laboratories. The technology involved varies in complexity, as shown in Fig. 1.3. Tests such as sodium and potassium are easily automated and are performed in high volume on automated analysers. Others, such as screening for drugs, identification of intermediary metabolites or differentiation of lipoprotein variants, involve technology that cannot be easily automated and require a high degree of staff involvement in the measurement process. Some tests are measured using commercially prepared reagents packaged in 'kit' form. Rarely, analyses are carried out manually.

This edition includes a small number of new chapters that aim to convey an understanding of some of the more widely used measurement techniques. However, this does not alter the primary focus of this book: how the results of biochemistry analyses are interpreted. Advances in analytical methodology and in our understanding of disease continue to change the test repertoire of the biochemistry department as the value of new tests is appreciated.

Laboratory personnel

As well as performing the analyses, the clinical biochemistry laboratory also provides advice to clinicians on how to make best use of the service. Medical and scientific personnel are familiar with the clinical significance and the analytical performance of the test procedures and will readily advise on the interpretation of the results. Do not be hesitant to take advantage of this advice, especially where a case is not straightforward.

> ### The clinical biochemistry laboratory
>
> - Biochemical tests are used in diagnosis, monitoring, screening and prognosis.
> - Core biochemical tests are carried out in every biochemistry laboratory. Specialised tests may be referred to larger departments. All hospitals provide for urgent tests in the 'emergency laboratory'.
> - Laboratory personnel will readily give advice, based on their knowledge and experience, on the use of the biochemistry laboratory, on the appropriate selection of tests and about the interpretation of results.

> ### Want to know more?
>
> Lab Tests Online UK: http://labtestsonline.org.uk/
>
> Written primarily for patients, this website provides a very useful database of laboratory tests, explaining why each test is carried out and what the result means. Laboratory tests from all of the main laboratory disciplines (including clinical biochemistry) are included. A mobile app is also available.
>
> http://acb.sagepub.com/content/50/3/285.full.pdf+html
>
> A personal look at the impact of automation on clinical biochemistry. It gives a glimpse into how hospital laboratories worked before the era of automation.

2 | The use of the laboratory

Specimen collection

In order to carry out biochemical analyses, the laboratory must have the correct specimen for the requested test and also enough information to ensure that the right test is performed and the result returned to the right person with a minimum of delay. As a starting point, there must be enough information to allow the patient to be identified uniquely, and the requested analyses must be clearly indicated. In addition, the request should include some indication of the suspected pathology, or at least the reason for the request. Such 'clinical information' helps laboratory and clinical staff interpret the results. Request forms differ in design, and paper forms are increasingly being replaced by electronic versions. In Europe, clinical biochemistry forms are conventionally coloured green.

A variety of specimens are used in biochemical analysis, and these are shown in Table 2.1.

Blood specimens

For many biochemical analyses, *serum* is the required specimen. Serum is obtained in two steps. First, the blood that has been collected from the patient ('whole blood') must be allowed to clot. Second, the heavier blood cells are 'spun down' during centrifugation, leaving a supernatant of serum (Fig. 2.1). The time it takes for specimens to clot can be an issue if the analyte (the substance to be measured) is unstable, or if the result is needed urgently. In this situation, speed is of the essence, and the time from collection to the availability of supernatant after centrifugation is shortened if the specimen contains *anticoagulant* (something to prevent clotting); the specimen can be centrifuged immediately on receipt in the

laboratory rather than having to wait until clotting has occurred. Commonly used anticoagulants include lithium heparin and potassium ethylene diamine tetra acetic acid (EDTA). The supernatant obtained after centrifugation of anticoagulated blood is called *plasma*. Plasma differs from serum in that it contains fibrinogen (a protein that is used up in the clotting process), as well as anticoagulant.

Urine specimens

For 24-hour urine collections, specimen bottles usually have a capacity of at least a litre and may include a preservative to inhibit bacterial growth, or acid to stabilise certain metabolites. By contrast, 'spot', or random, urine samples are collected into 'universal' containers with a much smaller capacity, e.g. 50 mL.

High-risk specimens

Specimens from patients with serious transmissible infections should be labelled as such so that laboratory staff can take appropriate precautions. Common examples include hepatitis B and C and HIV.

Sampling errors

Several potential errors may hinder the ability of the laboratory to provide the correct answers to the clinician's questions. Most of these arise at the point of specimen collection.
- *Blood sampling technique.* Difficulty in obtaining a blood specimen may lead to haemolysis (break-up of red blood cells), with consequent release of potassium and other red cell constituents.

- *Prolonged stasis during venepuncture.* When this occurs, plasma water diffuses from the vascular compartment into the interstitial space that separates it from the intracellular compartment. As a result of this loss of water, the serum (or plasma) sample obtained will be more concentrated. Proteins and protein-bound components of plasma, such as calcium or thyroxine, will be falsely elevated.
- *Insufficient specimen.* It may prove to be impossible for the laboratory to measure everything requested on a small volume. This is a common problem in neonates.
- *Errors in timing.* For 24-hour urine collections, patients may not accurately record the length of time during which the urine has been collected (duration of the collection) – this is a major source of error.
- *Incorrect specimen container.* For many analyses the blood must be collected into a container with anticoagulant and/or preservative. For example, samples for glucose should be collected into a special container containing fluoride, which inhibits glycolysis; otherwise, the time taken to deliver the sample to the laboratory can affect the result due to the metabolism of glucose. If a sample is collected into the wrong container, it should never be decanted into another type of tube. For example, blood that has been exposed, even briefly, to EDTA (an anticoagulant used in the sample container for full blood count) will have a markedly reduced calcium concentration, approaching zero, along with an artefactually high potassium concentration. This is because

Table 2.1 Specimens used for biochemical analyses

- Venous blood, serum or plasma
- Arterial blood
- Capillary blood
- Blood spot on a filter paper (Guthrie card)
- Urine
- Faeces
- Cerebrospinal fluid (CSF)
- Saliva
- Tissue and cells
- Aspirates, e.g.
  pleural fluid
  ascites
  joint (synovial) fluid
  intestinal (duodenal)
  pancreatic pseudocysts
- Calculi (stones)

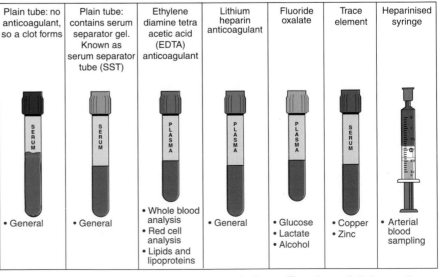

Plain tube: no anticoagulant, so a clot forms	Plain tube: contains serum separator gel. Known as serum separator tube (SST)	Ethylene diamine tetra acetic acid (EDTA) anticoagulant	Lithium heparin anticoagulant	Fluoride oxalate	Trace element	Heparinised syringe
SERUM	SERUM	PLASMA	PLASMA	PLASMA	SERUM	
• General	• General	• Whole blood analysis • Red cell analysis • Lipids and lipoproteins	• General	• Glucose • Lactate • Alcohol	• Copper • Zinc	• Arterial blood sampling

Fig. 2.1 Blood specimen tubes for specific biochemical tests. The colour-coded tubes are the Vacutainers in use in the authors' hospital laboratories.

EDTA is a chelator of calcium (which is necessary for clotting) and is present as its potassium salt.

- *Inappropriate sampling site.* Blood samples should not be taken 'downstream' from an intravenous drip. Occasionally the laboratory receives a blood glucose request on a specimen taken from the same arm into which 5% dextrose (glucose) is being infused, resulting in a 'drip arm' artefact. Usually the results are biochemically incredible, but it is just possible they may be acted upon with disastrous consequences for the patient. Whenever there is any possibility this might occur, the best course of action is to repeat to confirm the results.
- *Incorrect specimen storage.* A whole blood sample refrigerated overnight before being sent to the laboratory will show falsely high potassium, phosphate and red cell enzymes, such as lactate dehydrogenase, because of leakage into the extracellular fluid from the cells.

Analysing the specimen

The average biochemistry laboratory receives thousands of requests and samples each day. Samples proceed through the laboratory as shown in Fig. 2.2. It is essential that all are clearly identified so that 'mix-ups' do not occur. All analytical procedures are quality controlled, and the laboratory strives very hard for reliability.

Once the results are available, they are collated and a report is issued – usually electronically, with or without a paper report form. Cumulative reports allow the clinician to see at a glance how the most recent result(s) compare with those tests performed previously, providing an aid to the monitoring of treatment.

Timing

The main reason for asking for an analysis to be performed on an urgent basis is that immediate treatment depends on the result.

Many biochemical tests are repeated. How often depends on how quickly significant changes are liable to occur; there is little point in requesting repeat tests if a numerical change will not influence treatment.

Unnecessary testing

A request for a biochemical test is, de facto, a question to the laboratory. This is an important point for clinicians to reflect on, in order to avoid, or at least minimise, 'mindless' requesting where no real question is being posed. There are no general rules about the appropriateness, or otherwise, of laboratory testing, because of the huge variety of clinical circumstances that may arise.

The use of the laboratory

- Each biochemistry test request should be thought of as a question about the patient and each biochemical result as an answer.
- Request forms and specimens must be correctly labelled to ensure the correct results for the correct patient can be communicated quickly to the clinician.
- Many biochemical tests are performed on serum, the supernatant obtained from centrifugation of clotted blood collected into a plain container. Others require plasma, the supernatant obtained when blood is prevented from clotting by an anticoagulant.
- Various sampling errors may invalidate results.

Case history 1

A blood specimen was taken from a 65-year-old woman to check her serum potassium concentration because she had been on thiazide diuretics for some time. The general practitioner left the specimen in his car and dropped it off at the laboratory on the way to the surgery the next morning.

Immediately after analysing the sample, the biochemist was on the phone to the general practitioner. Why?

Comment in Case history comments.

Want to know more?

National Minimum Retesting Interval Project: https://www.rcpath.org/static/253e8950-3721-4aa2-8ddd4bd94f73040e/g147_national-minimum retesting intervals in pathology.pdf

Consensus recommendations for the minimum time before each biochemical test is repeated.

Choosing Wisely UK: http://www.choosing-wisely.co.uk/

Provides guidance about investigations/treatments which are not recommended in specific clinical situations. Links to relevant clinical guidelines.

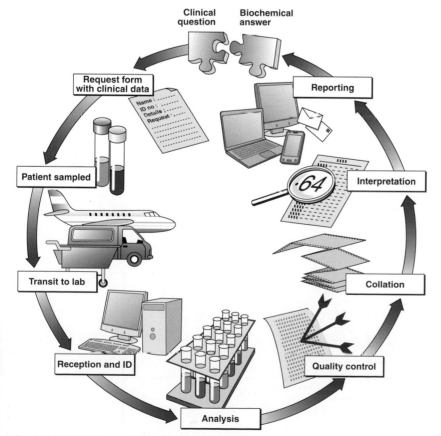

Fig. 2.2 Circuit diagram of the clinical biochemistry process.

Clinical question / Biochemical answer

Request form with clinical data — Name : / ID no : / Details : / Request :

Reporting

Patient sampled

·64· Interpretation

Transit to lab

Collation

Reception and ID

Quality control

Analysis

3 | Interpretation of results: general

The vast majority of biochemical analyses are quantitative (i.e. numerical). Most tests measure the amount of the analyte in a small volume of plasma, serum or other body fluid, and the end result of the analytical process is a number, whether it be on a computer, tablet, smartphone screen, or paper report. The numerical result is nearly always expressed in units of one kind or another, and usually a reference interval is included beside it to allow comparison. Often 'flags' are used to highlight unusual results. We will deal in turn with each of these.

How biochemical results are expressed

Units

Many biochemical results are reported as concentrations, usually in terms of the number of moles in one litre of fluid (mol/L) (Table 3.1). The concept of concentration is illustrated in Fig. 3.1. The concentration of any analyte in a body compartment expresses the amount of the substance dissolved in a known volume of fluid. (The fluid, whether it be whole blood, plasma, serum, urine or other bodily fluid, is always aqueous, and thus often referred

to generically as 'water'.) Changes in concentration can occur for two reasons:
- The amount of the analyte can increase or decrease.
- The volume of fluid in which the analyte is dissolved can similarly change.

Although this may seem obvious, many students struggle to understand that, for example hyponatraemia (a low serum concentration of sodium) develops because of either too little sodium or too much water. We will return to this in a later chapter (Chapter 9).

Some analytes are not readily measured in this way. For example, enzymes are not usually expressed in molar units but rather in units of enzyme activity. Enzyme assays are carried out in such a way that the activity measured is directly proportional to the amount of enzyme present. Similarly, some hormones are reported in units that involve comparison with standard reference preparations of known biological potency. Other biochemical measurements that are not expressed as concentrations include large molecules such as proteins that are not dissolved in the aqueous phase; these are reported in mass units (grams or milligrams) per litre. Finally, blood gas results (PCO_2 or PO_2) are expressed in kilopascals (kPa), the unit in which partial pressures are measured.

Reference intervals

The first thing a requesting clinician does after looking at a result is to compare it with the reference interval alongside. This immediately begs the question of the source of the reference interval. In theory, every

hospital laboratory should generate its own reference intervals, for all of its analytes, by measuring them in a population sample of, say, blood donors or laboratory or hospital staff. However, doing this takes considerable time and effort and is beyond the resources of many laboratories. In this circumstance, it is reasonable instead to use reference intervals generated by other laboratories using the same analytical method, or the available literature, looking particularly for reference intervals, published in peer-reviewed journals, that use the same method of measurement as the laboratory. In some groups, such as neonates, it is difficult or impossible for the average hospital laboratory to generate its own reference intervals; a few books address this issue, publishing reference intervals in well-characterised groups. If all else fails, the reference intervals supplied by the manufacturer of the assay may be used, particularly for unusual or novel assays for which there are no other sources of data.

By convention, reference intervals are chosen arbitrarily to include 95% of the values found in the population (Fig. 3.2). This means that, by definition, 5% of any population will have a result outside the reference interval; 2.5% will have higher values and 2.5% lower values. In general, the further a result is from the limits of the reference interval, the more likely it is to indicate pathology.

Biological factors affecting 'normality'

Distinguishing between 'normal' and 'abnormal' results is affected by various

Table 3.1 **Molar units**		
Mole	**Abbreviation**	**Definition**
Millimole	mmol	$\times 10^{-3}$ of a mole
Micromole	μmol	$\times 10^{-6}$
Nanomole	nmol	$\times 10^{-9}$
Picomole	pmol	$\times 10^{-12}$
Femtomole	fmol	$\times 10^{-15}$

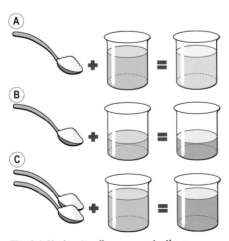

Fig. 3.1 Understanding concentrations. Concentration is always dependent on two factors: the amount of solute and the amount of solvent. The concentration of the sugar solution in the beaker can be increased from 1 spoon/beaker **(A)** to 2 spoons/beaker by either decreasing the volume of solvent **(B)** or increasing the amount of solute **(C)**.

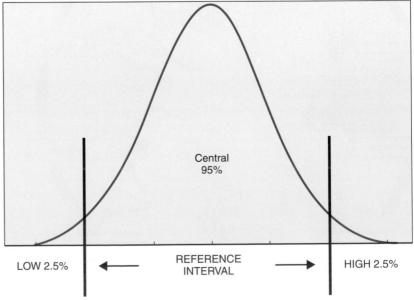

Fig. 3.2 Reference intervals.

physiological factors that must be considered when interpreting a result. These include:

- *Sex.* Reference intervals for some analytes such as serum creatinine are different for males and females.
- *Age.* There may be different reference intervals for neonates, children, adults and the elderly.
- *Diet.* The reference interval may depend on fasting status.
- *Timing.* There may be variations during the day and night.
- *Stress and anxiety.* These may affect the analyte of interest.
- *Posture of the patient.* Redistribution of fluid may affect the result.
- *Effects of exercise.* Strenuous exercise can release enzymes from tissues.
- *Medical history.* Infection and/or tissue injury can affect biochemical values independently of the disease process being investigated.
- *Pregnancy.* This alters some reference intervals.
- *Menstrual cycle.* Some hormone measurements vary throughout the menstrual cycle.
- *Drug history.* Drugs may have specific effects on the plasma concentration of some analytes.

Health versus disease

In reality, reference intervals are merely a guide to whether a patient has a disease. There are usually no rigid limits demarcating the diseased population from the healthy, and often there is a degree of overlap in the distribution of results between the population with the disease and the healthy population. This makes things a bit complicated and introduces a number of concepts and terms that are central to understanding the uses and limitations of biochemical (and other) tests in the diagnosis of disease (Fig. 3.3). A *diagnostic cut-off*, which might be a reference limit (but does not have to be), is a way of separating healthy and diseased populations. Usually this approach is less than perfect; some healthy subjects will

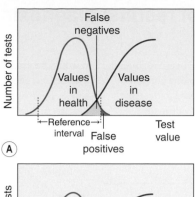

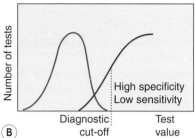

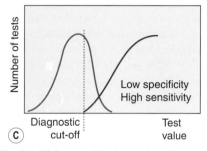

Fig. 3.3 (A) Overlap of biochemical results in health and disease. **(B)** and **(C)** The effect of changing the diagnostic cut-off on test specificity and sensitivity.

be incorrectly identified as having the disease (*false positives*) and some patients with the disease incorrectly identified as healthy (*false negatives*), because they have results on the 'wrong' side of the diagnostic cut-off. Other widely used terms to express this are sensitivity and specificity. *Sensitivity* indicates how often patients with the disease are correctly identified, and *specificity* how often healthy subjects are correctly identified. An ideal diagnostic test would be 100% sensitive, showing positive results in all diseased subjects, and 100% specific, showing negative results in all healthy subjects. These and other terms used to describe how good or bad a diagnostic test is (its *clinical utility*) are explored in more detail in the next chapter.

Clinical note

An abnormal result does not always indicate that a disease is present, nor a normal result that it is not. Reference intervals are merely a guide to whether a patient has a disease.

The interpretation of results: general

- Biochemistry results are often reported as concentrations. Concentrations change if the amount of the analyte changes or if the volume of water changes.
- The reference interval supplied with the test result gives only the probability of the results being 'normal' or 'abnormal'.
- Reference intervals may vary according to the age or sex of the patient.
- If a result does not accord with that expected for the patient, the finding should be discussed with a professional in laboratory medicine and a repeat test arranged.

Want to know more?

https://www.ncbi.nlm.nih.gov/pmc/articles/PMC3428257/

https://www.acb.org.uk

Historically, many hospital laboratories had different reference ranges for the same analyte even when they used the same analytical method. The first of the links above explains the rationale behind the UK-based Pathology Harmony initiative, which set out to establish whether these differences were well-founded, and the second provides a summary of harmonised ranges.

4 | Interpretation of results: diagnosis

The correct use of biochemistry tests to diagnose disease requires a detailed understanding of their clinical utility. In the previous chapter we introduced some of the terminology used to describe how good or bad a diagnostic test is. Here, we provide a more comprehensive summary of terms commonly used to evaluate test performance.

Diagnostic test outcomes

There are four possible outcomes of any diagnostic test. These can be tabulated as shown in Fig. 4.1. We defined false positives and false negatives in the previous chapter. The other two possibilities are that the patients with disease and the healthy subjects without disease have been correctly identified by the test (*true positives* and *true negatives*, respectively). The rows and columns can be totalled as shown. Using this diagnostic table, we can define various quantitative measures of test performance.

Sensitivity is the proportion of patients with disease correctly identified by the test result (in terms of the table, A/A+C). *Specificity* is the proportion of people without disease correctly identified (D/B+D). The problem with sensitivity and specificity is that you have to know who has and does not have the disease to be able to calculate them. If you have a patient in front of you, you do not know that; indeed, that is precisely why you are doing the test.

It would be much more useful to know what the probability of disease is in people with a positive test result. This is known as the *positive predictive value* (PPV) of a test, or the posttest probability of disease. In terms of the table, PPV is the proportion of those with a positive test result who have the disease (A/A+B). By analogy, the *negative predictive value* (NPV) is the probability of absence of the disease in someone with a negative (normal) test result, or posttest probability of health (D/C+D).

The impact of prevalence on test utility

Suppose that the same diagnostic test is applied to two separate groups of people with different prevalences of the disease. (The *prevalence* or pretest probability of disease is a measure of how common the disease is in the population being tested: A+C/A+B+C+D.) Fig. 4.2 shows how this affects the PPV and NPV. The first key point is that the sensitivity and specificity of the test – its ability to correctly identify disease and health – are the same in both groups. However, the probability of disease in people with a positive test result – PPV (A/A+B) – is much lower in the larger group with lower prevalence. This is because the number of false positives in box B is much larger compared with the number of true positives in box A than in the smaller group with higher prevalence. In a similar way, the probability of the absence of disease in a patient with a negative test result – NPV

		DISEASE		
		PRESENT	ABSENT	
TEST RESULT	POSITIVE	A TRUE POSITIVES	B FALSE POSITIVES	A+B TOTAL POSITIVES
	NEGATIVE	C FALSE NEGATIVES	D TRUE NEGATIVES	C+D TOTAL NEGATIVES
		A+C TOTAL DISEASE PRESENT	B+D TOTAL DISEASE ABSENT	A+B+C+D TOTAL TESTED

Fig. 4.1 The four possible outcomes of a diagnostic test.

	PRESENT	ABSENT
POSITIVE	80	10
NEGATIVE	20	90

	PRESENT	ABSENT
POSITIVE	80	100
NEGATIVE	20	900

PREVALENCE = A+C/A+B+C+D = 50%

Sensitivity = A/A+C = 80%
Specificity = D/B+D = 90%
PPV = A/A+B = 88.9%
(A) NPV = D/C+D = 81.8%

PREVALENCE = A+C/A+B+C+D = 9.1%

Sensitivity = A/A+C = 80%
Specificity = D/B+D = 90%
PPV = A/A+B = 44.4%
(B) NPV = D/C+D = 97.8%

Fig. 4.2 The effect of prevalence on the usefulness of a diagnostic test. *NPV*, Negative predictive value; *PPV*, positive predictive value.

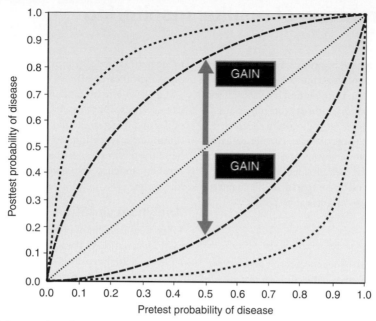

Fig. 4.3 Posttest probability of disease plotted against pretest probability for two separate diagnostic tests. The test with the bigger excursion from the diagonal is superior – it is associated with a bigger gain (change in the probability of disease).

(D/C+D) – is much higher, because the number of true negatives in box D is much bigger compared with the number of false negatives in box C than in the smaller group.

This concept – of how the prevalence or pretest probability of disease in the tested population affects the usefulness of the test – is easily understood with reference to extremes of prevalence. Consider, for example, doing a test to diagnose myocardial infarction in a population of young children, or, at the opposite end of the probability spectrum, diagnosing pregnancy by pregnancy testing in an antenatal clinic. Most people know intuitively that diagnostic testing in either of these scenarios would be pointless. The probability of what is being tested for is in the one case very low and in the other very high; in each case, doing the diagnostic test result will merely confirm what you already know.

Finally, we introduce one last concept. The PPV gives the probability of disease when you have a positive test result. In contrast, the NPV tells you the probability of the *absence* of disease when the test result is negative. What you really want to know is the probability of the *presence* of disease in someone with a negative result. Fortunately this is easily calculated: 1 minus the NPV. It is complementary to the PPV, whereas the NPV is the mirror image. With PPV and [1 minus NPV], you now have covered both bases – the probability of disease when the test result is positive and when it is negative.

We can now put this section together and plot the probability of disease after the test result is available (the posttest probability) against the pretest probability or prevalence (Fig. 4.3). Both possible test outcomes (positive and negative results) are taken into account by plotting both PPV and [1 minus NPV] against prevalence. There are several points to note. First, at the far left and right of the x axis – the extremes of prevalence – the pre- and posttest probability of disease hardly differ, no matter how good the test is, confirming intuition. Second, the biggest change from pre- to posttest probability is in the middle of the figure, where prevalence is 50%. This is where a diagnostic test is most useful. Third, the best test is one which gives the greatest gain (change in probability), whereas the worst test is the one which is nearest to the diagonal line.

Final thoughts

You might wonder how a clinician requesting diagnostic investigations can be expected to know where each investigation

lies in Fig. 4.3 – is it in the middle, or towards one or other end? It is true that most could not put an exact figure on the pretest probability of a disease. But most would be able to say if they thought it was one of the following: not likely; do not know; likely. Don't forget that diagnostic tests are not requested in a vacuum; they complement the information already obtained from history and examination, which will have led the requesting clinician to form an opinion about the probability of each of the possible specific differential diagnoses. It is when they simply do not know whether a patient has the suspected disease that the test has the most potential value – this is closest to the 50% optimum.

Clinical note

The test performance parameters described here apply to *all* information collected about a patient – symptoms and signs as well as diagnostic investigations of all kinds.

Interpretation of results: diagnosis

- Sensitivity is the proportion of patients with disease correctly identified by a test; specificity is the proportion of people without the disease correctly identified.

- PPV is the proportion with a positive test who have the disease. NPV is the proportion of people without the disease with a negative result. [1 minus NPV] is the proportion with a negative test result who do have the disease.

- A test is least useful when it confirms what you already know or strongly suspect and most useful when you do not know what the test result is likely to tell you.

Want to know more?

Sackett DL, Haynes BR, Tugwell P, Guyatt GH. *Clinical Epidemiology: A Basic Science for Clinical Medicine.* 2nd ed. Philadelphia: Lippincott Williams & Wilkins; 1991.

The first and second editions of this book provide an invaluable insight into how to use information in medicine. They are extremely readable and require little or no background medical knowledge.

5 | Interpretation of results: monitoring

We have seen already that biochemical investigations can be requested for various reasons. Diagnosis accounts for many requests. Another, commoner, reason why clinicians request biochemical tests is to monitor their patients. For example, primary care physicians often request the same panel of tests in periodic health checks in patients with chronic conditions such as diabetes. Equally, patients who are admitted to hospital will routinely have tests done, often on a daily basis, in order to monitor their progress. This raises the question of how serial results should be compared. In this chapter, we consider how to evaluate changes in consecutive results.

Sources of variation

When a biochemical test is repeated, the repeat result may be very similar to the previous one, in which case the clinician may decide to do nothing further. On the other hand, if the result is markedly different, further investigations may be requested to find out why. The size of the change may fall somewhere in between – large enough to make the clinician wonder whether it is significant, but not so large that it clearly needs follow-up. In general, the question being asked is: 'could the change just be due to random variation?' In order to answer this, the clinician needs to consider all of the possible sources of random variation in a laboratory test result. Broadly these can be divided into preanalytical variation, analytical variation and intrinsic biological variation (Fig. 5.1). The term used in Fig. 5.1 – the coefficient of variation (CV) – is a function of the standard deviation: $CV = (SD/mean) \times 100$.

Preanalytical variation

In Chapter 3 (Biological factors affecting 'normality') we saw that consideration of various physiological factors, including age and sex, help to distinguish 'normal' from 'abnormal' results. Many of the same factors also may contribute to preanalytical variation. Clearly some, such as sex, will be the same for an individual patient, but others, such as the time of day when the sample is collected or the posture of the patient, may vary from one occasion

to the next. Table 5.1 summarises some of the main contributors to preanalytical variation.

It makes sense to standardise preanalytical sources of variation whenever possible – e.g. by collecting blood at the same time of day and using standard procedures for sample types and tourniquet application, as well as for transport and subsequent handling of samples, such as centrifugation. Such standardisation is routine practice, so preanalytical variation is kept to a minimum.

Analytical variation

Every measurement of every test is associated with at least some random variation in the analysis. For measurements done on automated analysers, this random *analytical variation* is small, but it cannot be eliminated entirely, and not all measurements are automated. Although it is not feasible to analyse every sample repeatedly in order to establish analytical variation for that particular test, laboratory staff do measure internal quality control (IQC) samples repeatedly (see Chapter 6) and so have good information on the analytical variation for each test. In addition to random variation, measurements also may vary in a systematic way (called *bias*), which is important when comparing results against a reference interval or decision level. However, if the repeated measurements in samples from an individual are done over a short time, with a single operator, set of reagents and calibrator, any systematic bias will probably apply in a similar way to all of the measurements, so the observed spread of results is likely to reflect mostly random variation. Factors that contribute to random analytical variation include fluctuations in temperature in the laboratory, or (particularly for manual analyses) small differences in the pipetted volume of reagent or sample.

Biological variation

If preanalytical variation is minimised as outlined previously, and the magnitude of the analytical variation is established by replicate IQC measurements, it is possible to calculate the additional variation within the subject or patient that is not due to random preanalytical or analytical factors – we call this *within-subject biological variation*. This can be done by taking samples from the same individual over several consecutive days. There are detailed protocols about how to collect the data needed to establish the components of biological variation; these are beyond the scope of this chapter. Suffice to say that expert investigators have done this work for many tests, and the within- and between-subject biological variation is known. With this information, clinicians have data at their disposal which can guide them as to the amount of change between serial results which can reasonably be attributed to the total random variation. When the change exceeds this amount (the *reference change value*, or RCV, sometimes called the *critical difference*), it can be inferred that it is significant, i.e. unlikely to have arisen by chance, in which case further investigation may be appropriate.

Table 5.2 summarises typical analytical variation and within-subject biological variation associated with some commonly measured analytes.

Other biological variation

The biological variation discussed earlier refers to random fluctuation around a homeostatic set point. Some tests vary in nonrandom ways as well. For example, cortisol has a marked

$$CV_T = [CV_P^2 + CV_A^2 + CV_B^2]^{1/2}$$

Total Variation	Preanalytical Variation	Analytical Variation	Biological Variation
	Minimised by standardisation of sample collection, transport and handling	Established by replicate analysis of quality control samples	Estimates of within-subject biological variation obtained from the published literature

Fig. 5.1 Components of random variation between serial test results. The coefficient of variation *(CV)* is a function of the standard deviation. See text for details.

Table 5.1 Some contributors to preanalytical variation
• Time of day
• Posture
• Fasting status
• Recent exercise
• Time in transit to laboratory
• Temperature during transit
• Anticoagulant or preservative used
• Centrifugation time and force

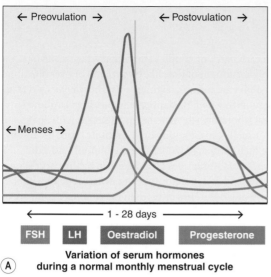

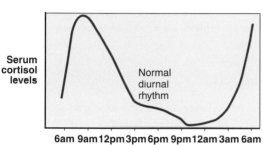

Fig. 5.2 (A–C) Examples of nonrandom biological variation. Note the different timescales over which the variation occurs. *FSH,* Follicle-stimulating hormone; *GFR,* glomerular filtration rate; *LH,* luteinising hormone.

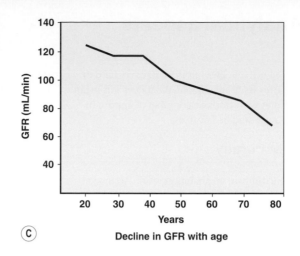

Table 5.2 Analytical and biological variation

Representative figures for analytical [CV_A (%)] and within-subject biological variation [CV_B (%)] of some commonly measured serum biochemical tests.

Test	CV_A (%)	CV_B (%)
Sodium	0.9	0.6
Potassium	1.1	4.6
Creatinine	1.6	6.0
ALT	1.0	19.4
Bilirubins	1.3	21.8
Albumin	0.8	3.2
Cholesterol	0.8	6.0
Glucose (fasting)	0.6	5.6

ALT, Alanine aminotransferase; *CV,* coefficient of variation.

circadian rhythm, so the time of collection has a crucial bearing on interpretation. Similarly, the hormones involved in controlling ovulation vary according to the point in the monthly cycle. Other analytes vary over a much longer timescale. For example, glomerular function declines gradually with age so plasma creatinine and urea rise. Fig. 5.2 shows some examples of nonrandom biological variation.

Clinical note

Many laboratories routinely flag up changes in serial results that exceed the reference change value, helping clinicians to make better decisions about their patients.

Interpretation of results: monitoring

- Understanding whether changes between serial results are significant requires knowledge of the different types of variation and the factors that contribute to them.

- Preanalytical variation can be minimised by standardising sampling procedures and transport and handling of samples as far as possible.

- Analytical variation of tests can be established by measuring samples repeatedly.

- Biological variation within an individual can be random or nonrandom, but random within-subject variation is most relevant to monitoring of results over time.

- Reference change values are used to decide whether differences between serial results can or cannot entirely be attributed to intrinsic random variation.

Want to know more?

Fraser CG. *Biological Variation: From Principles to Practice.* Washington, DC: AACC Press; 2001.

This text is only for the mathematically minded student, but is surprisingly accessible. It has become the 'bible' of biological variation in many parts of the world.

6 | Analytical aspects

We have already pointed out that laboratories strive very hard to ensure that the results they issue are reliable. What does this mean in practice? In this chapter we introduce a number of important concepts with which you should be familiar.

Precision and accuracy

Precision is the reproducibility of an analytical result. Accuracy defines how close the measured value is to the actual ('true') value. These concepts are often explained by analogy with a shooting target, shown in Fig. 6.1. Let's say that an analyser measures an analyte on the same sample ten times. Ideally, the results obtained should be both precise and accurate (see Fig. 6.1A). Sometimes results are produced that are not totally accurate but are nevertheless closely grouped together (precise) (see Fig. 6.1B). This is preferable to the situation in which the results are both inaccurate and imprecise (see Fig. 6.1C). Why? Because precision implies a degree of predictability in the result that is likely to be obtained; if a laboratory knows that its results are consistently different from the 'true' result, this allows for the possibility of adjusting the results obtained (a bit like adjusting the sights on a telescopic rifle). One important practical point: automation of analyses has improved precision in most cases, simply because steps which were previously manual are done in exactly the same way (i.e. more precisely) by automated machines.

Analytical sensitivity and specificity

These terms should not be confused with 'test' specificity and sensitivity, the test performance parameters discussed in previous chapters. Analytical sensitivity of an assay is a measure of how little of the analyte the method can detect. Analytical specificity of an assay relates to how good the assay is at discriminating between the requested analyte and potentially interfering substances.

Quality assurance

Laboratory staff continually monitor the performance of assays using quality control (QC) samples to reassure themselves that the methods are performing satisfactorily with the patients' specimens. There are, broadly, two kinds of QC sample. The expected values of *internal QC* (IQC) samples are known, and the actual results obtained on each batch of samples are compared with previous values. For high-throughput tests like electrolytes or liver function tests, IQC samples are run several times a day. In *external QC* (EQC) or quality assurance schemes, identical samples are distributed from a central laboratory (the scheme organiser) to participating laboratories, usually on a monthly or bi-monthly basis; the results obtained are then compared with each other. Importantly, the expected values of EQC samples are not known by the participating laboratories. Individual laboratories realise where they sit with reference to other laboratories only when the summary comparison is subsequently issued.

The results of IQC and EQC analyses can be presented serially, allowing laboratory staff to judge whether assays are performing to an acceptable standard. Such *Levey-Jennings charts* are widely used; an example is shown in Fig. 6.2. Decisions can be made with reference to various sets of rules, the most famous of which – the Westgard rules – are named after the person who first devised them.

Analytical aspects

- Accuracy defines how close the measured value is to the actual ('true') value. Precision is the reproducibility of an analytical method, i.e. how close together replicate results are.

- Analytical sensitivity is a measure of how little of the analyte an assay can detect. Analytical specificity relates to how good the assay is at distinguishing the analyte of interest from similar substances.

- QC samples are 'cross-checks' that allow laboratory staff to judge how well assays are performing.

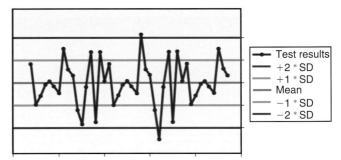

Fig. 6.2 Plot of serial measurements of a quality control sample. The 'true' result is represented by the mean.

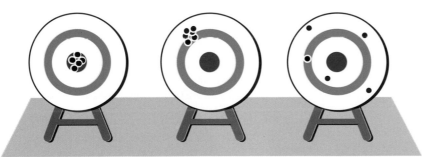

(A) Precise and accurate (B) Inaccurate but precise (C) Inaccurate and imprecise

Fig. 6.1 Accuracy and precision. See text for details.

2

Core biochemistry

7 | Fluid and electrolytes: basic concepts

The most commonly requested biochemical profile consists of serum sodium, potassium and creatinine, often also with urea and, less commonly, bicarbonate and chloride. In this chapter we consider some of the concepts that underpin sodium and water balance. These play a critical role in the well-being of patients and are central to the management of any patient who is seriously ill.

Body fluid compartments

The first key concept in considering sodium and water balance is the subdivision of body fluid (water) into different compartments, and their relative size (Fig. 7.1). Thus, someone who weighs 70 kg contains approximately 42 L of water. Two-thirds (28 L) of this is intracellular fluid (ICF) and one-third (14 L) is extracellular fluid (ECF). The ECF can be further subdivided into blood (3.5 L) and interstitial fluid (10.5 L).

The second key concept is that water is not confined to a particular body compartment, whereas sodium is largely confined to the extracellular compartment. A molecular 'pump' located in the plasma membrane of every cell maintains the relative concentrations of sodium in ECF and ICF shown in Fig. 7.1. (The same pump – known as the Na^+/K^+-ATPase – also pumps potassium in the opposite direction.) This pump has the effect of stopping sodium from 'leaking' out of the ECF, as it were.

The third key concept is that water follows sodium, so that, for example, sodium loss from the ECF is accompanied

by water loss, giving rise to the clinical signs of dehydration. Indeed, the kidneys use this property to regulate ECF volume, excreting sodium and water when the ECF volume is inappropriately increased, and retaining both in response to reduced ECF volume (see Chapter 8).

Changes in volume of body fluid compartments

Why are these concepts important? Let us return to the subject who weighs 70 kg. Imagine the loss or gain of a fixed amount of water, say 5 L, either alone (i.e. pure water) or accompanying sodium loss or gain. Fig. 7.2A,B and Vid. 7.1A,B show the *exact* changes in volume of body fluid compartments that would occur if 5 L of pure water

were lost or gained. Since water loss or gain is distributed evenly across all body compartments, it is clinically quite subtle, because the change in volume of individual body compartments is modest; this can readily be appreciated visually from Fig. 7.2A,B and Vid. 7.1A,B.

In contrast, if a patient lost enough sodium from the ECF to cause associated loss of 5 L water, this would give rise to clinically obvious dehydration, since the water would be lost exclusively from the ECF (in a 70-kg patient, the ECF volume is 14 L – loss of 5 L amounts to more than one-third of the total ECF volume). Similarly, if gain of sodium was associated with 5 L water gain, the increase in ECF volume would be obvious for a similar reason. Again, this can be readily be

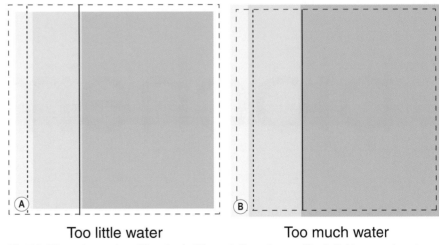

Too little water   Too much water

Fig. 7.2 Effect of water loss (A) and gain (B) on relative volumes of body fluid compartments. The *dotted lines* indicate in each case the normal size of the compartments. The figures show the changes in volume associated with loss or gain of 5 L pure water in someone who weighs 70 kg. See text for details. Readers are referred to the animated versions of these figures in Vid. 7.1 in the e-book on Elsevier eBooks+.

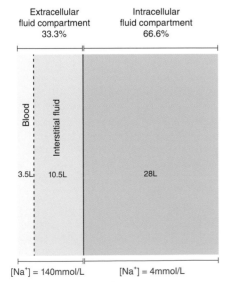

Extracellular fluid compartment 33.3%	Intracellular fluid compartment 66.6%

Blood | Interstitial fluid | 28L
3.5L | 10.5L |

$[Na^+]$ = 140mmol/L $[Na^+]$ = 4mmol/L

Fig. 7.1 Relative volumes of body fluid compartments and the concentration of sodium in each.

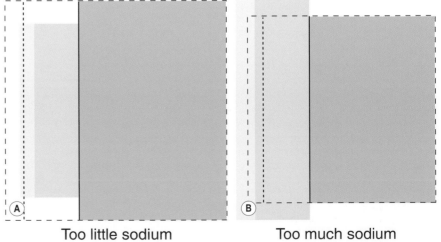

Too little sodium   Too much sodium

Fig. 7.3 Effect of sodium loss (A) and gain (B) on relative volumes of body fluid compartments. The *dotted lines* indicate in each case the normal size of the compartments. The figures show the changes in volume associated with loss or gain of 5 L water accompanying sodium in someone who weighs 70 kg. See text for details. (For simplicity these figures ignore the osmotic effect of altered ectracellular fluid tonicity on intracellular fluid volume – cells expand or shrink in response to lower or higher than normal tonicity.) Readers are referred to the animated versions of these figures in Vid. 7.2 in the e-book on Elsevier eBooks+.

appreciated visually from Fig. 7.3A,B and Vid. 7.2A,B, which show the *exact* changes in volume of ECF that occur with loss or gain of 5 L water accompanying changes in sodium status.

The relative volumes of ICF and ECF (see Fig. 7.1) also help to explain why, for example, loss of water (accompanying sodium) from ECF alone will be much more clinically obvious than loss of the same amount of pure water from [ICF + ECF], since the combined volume of [ICF + ECF] is three times the volume of the ECF alone.

Loss of fluid from individual body compartments gives rise to distinct signs and symptoms. ICF loss causes cellular dysfunction, which may present as lethargy, confusion and coma. Loss of ECF produces the signs of dehydration summarised in Table 7.1 and discussed in more detail in Chapter 10. Loss of blood, an ECF fluid, leads to circulatory collapse, shutdown of the kidneys and other organs, and clinical shock.

The principal features of disordered hydration are shown in Table 7.1. An additional clinical sign of disordered hydration is oedema. This is commonly

Table 7.1 **The principal clinical features of severe hydration disorders**		
Feature	**Dehydration**	**Overhydration**
Pulse	Increased	Normal
Blood pressure	Decreased	Normal or increased
Skin turgor	Decreased	Increased
Eyeballs	Soft/sunken	Normal
Mucous membranes	Dry	Normal
Urine output	Decreased	May be normal or decreased
Consciousness	Decreased	Decreased

observed and clinically useful. Its significance is considered in more detail in Chapter 10.

Osmolality

Body fluids vary greatly in their composition. However, whereas the concentration of substances may vary in the different body fluids, the overall number of solute particles — the osmolality — is the same. Body compartments are separated by semipermeable membranes through which water moves freely, in order to keep the osmolality the same, even if this water movement causes cells to shrink or expand in volume (Fig. 7.4). Thus the osmolality of the ICF is *normally the same as the ECF*.

The osmolality of a solution is expressed in millimoles (mmol) of solute per kilogram (kg) of solvent, which is aqueous, i.e. water-based. In humans, the osmolality of serum is approximately 285 mmol/kg. This can be measured directly, or may be calculated if the concentrations of the major solutes are already known. There are many formulae used to calculate the serum osmolality. Clinically, the simplest is:

$$\text{Serum osmolality [mmol/kg]} = 2 \times \text{serum [sodium] [mmol/L]}$$

This formula holds only if the serum concentration of urea and glucose is within the reference intervals. If either or both are abnormally high, the concentration of either or both (in mmol/L) must be added in to give the calculated osmolality. Sometimes there is an apparent difference between the

measured and calculated osmolality. This is known as the *osmolal gap*.

Oncotic pressure

The capillary membrane separates the intravascular and interstitial compartments. Small molecules move freely across this membrane, but plasma proteins do not. Thus, they exert a colloid osmotic (oncotic) pressure, since the protein concentration of interstitial fluid is much less than that of blood. The balance of oncotic and hydrostatic forces across the capillary membrane may be disturbed if the plasma protein concentration changes significantly (Chapter 25).

Clinical note

When water moves across cell membranes, the cells may shrink or expand. When this happens in the brain, neurological signs and symptoms may result. These include seizures, coma and death.

Fluid and electrolyte balance: concepts and vocabulary

- The body has two main fluid compartments: the ICF and the ECF.
- The volume of the ICF is twice as large as that of the ECF.
- Water retention will cause an increase in the volume of both ECF and ICF.
- Water loss will result in a decreased volume of both ECF and ICF.
- Sodium ions are the main ECF cations.
- Potassium ions are the main ICF cations.
- The volumes of the ECF and ICF are estimated from knowledge of the patient's history and by clinical examination.
- Serum osmolality can be measured directly or calculated from the serum sodium, urea and glucose concentrations.

Want to know more?

https://www.youtube.com/watch?v=xjNW6LgPJVY

This helpful animation illustrates how the Na+/K+-ATPase pump works. Note that three sodiums are exchanged for two potassiums. The concentration gradients and the positive charge that this creates outside the cell are used to drive other transport processes, including nerve conduction.

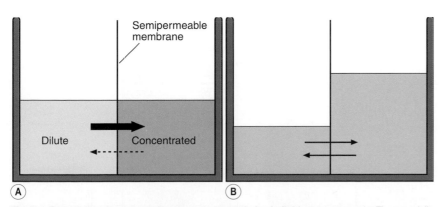

Fig. 7.4 Osmolality changes and water movement in body fluid compartments. The osmolality in different body compartments must be equal. This is achieved by the movement of water across semipermeable membranes in response to concentration changes. **(A)** Before water movement; **(B)** after water movement.

8 | Water and sodium balance: physiological mechanisms

Body water and sodium are in a state of flux. We are vulnerable to changes in our fluid compartments, and a number of important homeostatic mechanisms exist to prevent or minimise these. Key to survival and well-being is maintenance of the extracellular fluid (ECF) volume. Humans deprived of fluids die after a few days from circulatory collapse as a result of the reduction in the total body water. Failure to maintain ECF volume and its impact on impaired blood circulation rapidly lead to tissue death due to lack of oxygen and nutrients and failure to remove waste products.

Water

Normal water balance is illustrated in Fig. 8.1.

Water intake is very variable. Some people drink less than half a litre each day, and others more than 5 L in 24 hours, without harm. Thirst is rarely an overriding factor in determining intake.

Water losses vary in tandem with intake and are reflected in the volume of urine produced. The kidneys respond quickly to meet the body's need to excrete water. However, even when there is need to conserve water, humans cannot completely shut down urine production. Total body water remains remarkably constant in health despite massive fluctuations in intake. This is because water excretion by the kidney is very tightly controlled by arginine vasopressin (AVP).

The body also loses water through the skin and from the lungs. This 'insensible' loss is obligatory and amounts to between 500 and 850 mL/day. Water also may be lost in disease, e.g. from fistulae, in diarrhoea or because of prolonged vomiting.

AVP and the regulation of osmolality

Specialised cells in the hypothalamus sense differences between their intracellular osmolality and that of the ECF and adjust the secretion of AVP from the posterior pituitary gland accordingly. A high osmolality promotes secretion of AVP, whereas a low osmolality switches secretion off (Fig. 8.2). AVP causes renal water retention. Fluid deprivation stimulates endogenous AVP secretion, which reduces the urine flow rate to as little as 0.5 mL/min in order to conserve body water. However, within an hour of drinking 2 L of water, the urine flow rate may rise to 15 mL/min as AVP secretion is shut down.

The mechanism by which AVP causes renal water retention is complex, and reflects the anatomical arrangement of part of the renal tubule (the loop of Henle), as well as the movement of solute and water between renal tubule and surrounding medullary interstitium. (The functional anatomy of the kidney and nephron is described in Chapter 15, Functions of the kidney). This mechanism produces concentrated medullary blood surrounding the filtrate in the loop of Henle. AVP makes the walls of the loop permeable to water, which moves out of the tubules and down the concentration gradient, leaving behind a small volume of concentrated urine. Hence the alternative name for AVP: *antidiuretic hormone* (ADH).

Sodium

The total body sodium of the average 70-kg subject is approximately 3700 mmol, of which approximately 75% is exchangeable (Fig. 8.3). The remainder is incorporated into tissues such as bone. Most exchangeable sodium is in the ECF, where the sodium concentration is tightly regulated at approximately 140 mmol/L.

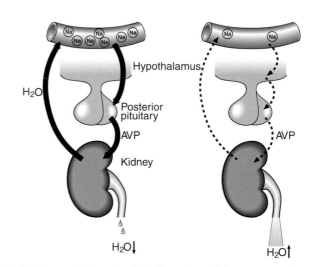

Fig. 8.2 The regulation of water balance by arginine vasopressin (AVP) and osmolality.

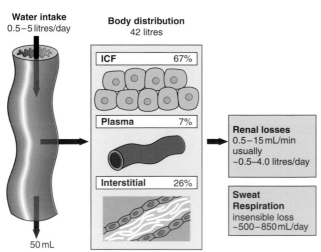

Fig. 8.1 Normal water balance. *ICF*, Intracellular fluid.

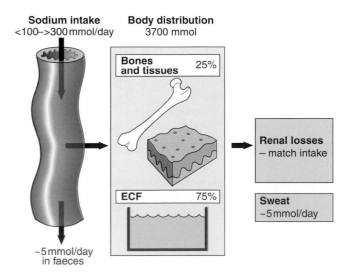

Fig. 8.3 Normal sodium balance. *ECF*, Extracellular fluid.

Sodium intake varies from less than 100 mmol/day to more than 300 mmol/day. In health, total body sodium does not change even if intake falls to as little as 5 mmol/day or is greater than 750 mmol/day.

Sodium losses – mostly in the form of urinary sodium excretion – vary with sodium intake. Some sodium is lost in sweat (~5 mmol/day) and in faeces (~5 mmol/day). However, in disease the gastrointestinal tract is often the major route of sodium loss. This is a very important clinical point, especially in paediatric practice, because infantile diarrhoea may result in death from salt and water depletion.

Urinary sodium output is regulated by two hormones:
- aldosterone
- atrial natriuretic peptide (ANP).

Aldosterone

Aldosterone is a steroid hormone secreted by the zona glomerulosa of the adrenal cortex. It decreases urinary sodium excretion by increasing sodium reabsorption in the renal tubules at the expense of potassium and hydrogen ions (Fig. 8.4); this action is known as *mineralocorticoid activity*. Water is reabsorbed along with sodium. Indeed, reduced ECF volume is the major stimulus to aldosterone secretion, since it helps to restore volume. Specialised cells in the juxtaglomerular apparatus of the nephron sense a decrease in blood pressure and secrete renin, the first step in a sequence of events that leads to the secretion of aldosterone by the glomerular zone of the adrenal cortex.

Atrial natriuretic peptide

ANP is a polypeptide hormone predominantly secreted by the right atrium of the heart. The physiological role of this hormone, in terms of sodium balance and ECF volume, is the exact opposite of that of aldosterone. Whereas aldosterone decreases urine sodium excretion in response to reduced ECF volume, ANP – as you might expect from its name – increases urine sodium excretion in response to increased ECF volume. Its physiological effect is replicated in the pharmacological effect of loop diuretics, which play a central role in the treatment of heart failure; these drugs

greatly increase urine sodium excretion (i.e. cause natriuresis), thereby reducing the ECF volume and hence strain on myocardial pump function.

Regulation of volume

As we have alluded to in Chapter 7, water will remain in the extracellular compartment only if it is held there by the osmotic effect of ions. Sodium is largely restricted to the extracellular compartment, and the amount of sodium in the ECF determines the ECF volume. Aldosterone and AVP interact to maintain normal volume and concentration of the ECF. Consider a patient who has been vomiting and has diarrhoea from a gastrointestinal infection. Sodium and water are lost from the gut, and, with no oral intake, fluid depletion occurs. The resulting low ECF volume stimulates aldosterone secretion and AVP secretion. As the patient begins to take fluids orally, any salt ingested is maximally retained. This raises the ECF osmolality, further stimulating AVP secretion and water retention.

Clinical note

Assessment of volume status (hydration) provides critically important information in the evaluation of water and sodium balance. This complements the information provided by measurement of electrolytes and creatinine.

Water and sodium balance

- AVP regulates renal water loss and thus causes changes in the osmolality of body fluid compartments.
- Water is lost from the body as urine and as obligatory 'insensible' losses from the skin and lungs.
- Aldosterone and ANP exert opposite effects on renal sodium loss and control the sodium content of the ECF.
- Changes in sodium content of the ECF cause changes in volume of this compartment, because water follows sodium.
- Sodium may be lost from the body in urine or from the gut, e.g. prolonged vomiting, diarrhoea, intestinal fistulae.

Case history 2

A man is trapped in a collapsed building after an earthquake. He has sustained no serious injuries or blood loss. He has no access to food or water until he is rescued after 72 hours.

- What will have happened to his body fluid compartments?

Comment in Case history comments.

Want to know more?

https://www.youtube.com/watch?v=hjQd9nWAxQk

The mechanism that produces concentrated renal medullary blood involves countercurrent multiplication and exchange. This is one of various online sources that explain it in more detail.

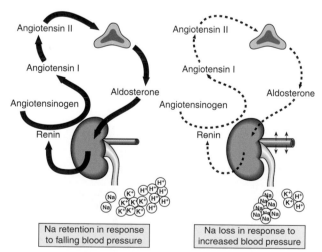

Fig. 8.4 **The regulation of sodium balance by aldosterone.**

9 | Hyponatraemia: pathophysiology

Hyponatraemia is defined as a serum sodium concentration below the reference interval of 133 to 146 mmol/L. It is the electrolyte abnormality most frequently seen in clinical biochemistry.

Mechanisms of hyponatraemia

The serum concentration of sodium is simply a ratio of sodium (in millimoles) to water (in litres), and hyponatraemia is either due to too little sodium or too much water. In practice it arises either because of loss of sodium ions or retention of water.

- *Loss of sodium.* Sodium is the main extracellular cation and plays a critical role in the maintenance of blood volume and pressure by osmotically regulating the passive movement of water ('water follows sodium'). Thus, when significant sodium depletion occurs, water is lost with it, giving rise to the characteristic clinical signs associated with extracellular fluid (ECF) volume reduction. Primary sodium depletion *always* should be actively considered in hyponatraemic patients, even if only to be excluded; failure to do so can have fatal consequences.
- *Water retention.* Retention of water in the body compartments dilutes the constituents of the extracellular space, including sodium, causing hyponatraemia. Water retention occurs much more frequently than sodium loss, and where there is no evidence of fluid loss from history or examination, water retention as the mechanism becomes a near-certainty.

Water retention

Mechanisms of hyponatraemia are summarised in Fig. 9.1. Water retention usually results from impaired water excretion; increased intake (compulsive water drinking) is rare. Most patients who are hyponatraemic due to water retention have the so-called syndrome of inappropriate antidiuresis (SIAD). The term *inappropriate* here is used specifically to indicate that the secretion of arginine vasopressin (AVP) is inappropriate *for the serum osmolality*. Its secretion in this context occurs in response to powerful *nonosmotic* stimuli. These include hypovolaemia and/or hypotension, nausea and vomiting, hypoglycaemia, and pain. (It should be stressed that the increase in AVP secretion induced by, e.g. hypovolaemia, is an entirely appropriate mechanism to try to restore blood volume to normal.) To give an idea of the relative concentrations of AVP in response to osmotic and nonosmotic stimuli, respectively: whereas in health, AVP fluctuates between 0 and 5 pmol/L due to changes in osmolality, in SIAD huge increases (up to 500 pmol/L) may be seen due to nonosmotic stimuli.

SIAD is seen in many conditions (Box 9.1); the frequency with which it occurs in clinical practice mirrors their prevalence. Clinicians consider it in most hyponatraemic patients. A list of criteria and associated laboratory investigations is shown in Box 9.2.

Sodium loss

Sodium depletion occurs when there is pathological sodium loss, either from the gastrointestinal tract or in urine (see Fig. 9.1). Vomiting, diarrhoea and fistulae are often implicated in gut losses. Less obvious are urinary losses resulting from mineralocorticoid deficiency or from aldosterone antagonists, e.g. spironolactone.

Initially, in all of these situations, sodium loss is accompanied by water loss and the serum sodium concentration remains normal. As sodium and water loss continue, the reduction in ECF and blood volume stimulates AVP secretion nonosmotically, overriding the

---

Box 9.1 Causes of SIAD

- Central nervous system pathology, e.g. stroke, infection, trauma
- Chest pathology, e.g. pneumonia, some lung tumours
- Long list of drugs: centrally acting drugs, e.g. anticonvulsants, selective serotonin reuptake inhibitors, antipsychotics; drugs used in chemotherapy; nonsteroidal antiinflammatory drugs; amiodarone; interferons
- Surgery: probably pain-driven (see text); especially common after pituitary surgery
- Malignancies: lung, especially small cell lung cancer; gastrointestinal cancers; genitourinary cancers; head and neck cancers
- Other: human immunodeficiency virus infection; acute intermittent porphyria; hereditary (gain-of-function mutations in renal AVP receptors).

AVP, Arginine vasopressin; *SIAD,* syndrome of inappropriate antidiuresis.

Box 9.2 Criteria for SIAD, and associated laboratory investigations

- Hyponatraemia with corresponding hypoosmolality (serum osmolality usually <280 mosmol/kg)
- Continued renal excretion of sodium (spot urine sodium typically >30 mmol/L)
- Urine less than maximally dilute (urine osmolality typically >100 mosmol/kg, where 40 mosmol/kg represents maximal dilution)
- No clinical evidence of volume depletion (patient typically euvolaemic)
- Other causes of hyponatraemia ruled out (in practice, cortisol and thyroid-stimulating hormone commonly used to rule out adrenal and thyroid disease)

SIAD, Syndrome of inappropriate antidiuresis.

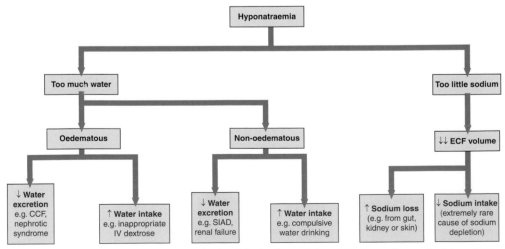

Fig. 9.1 Mechanisms of hyponatraemia according to the patient's clinical volume status. *CCF,* Congestive cardiac failure; *ECF,* extracellular fluid; *SIAD,* syndrome of inappropriate antidiuresis.

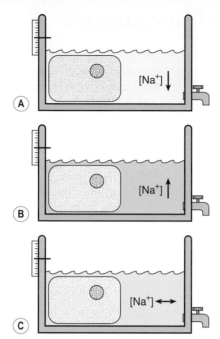

Fig. 9.2 Water tank models showing that reduced ECF volume may be associated with reduced (A), increased (B) or normal (C) serum [Na⁺]. *ECF*, extracellular fluid.

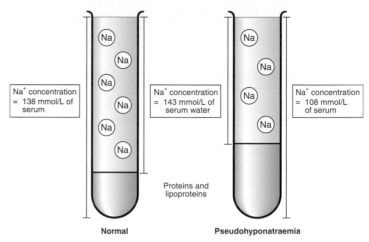

Fig. 9.3 Pseudohyponatraemia.

osmotic control mechanism. The increase in AVP secretion causes pure water retention, and thus patients become hyponatraemic.

Sodium depletion – a word of caution

Not all patients with sodium depletion are hyponatraemic (Fig. 9.2). As pointed out in the previous paragraph, the sodium concentration in, for example, adrenal insufficiency remains normal until hypovolaemia stimulates compensatory AVP-mediated retention of pure water. Patients with sodium loss due to osmotic diuresis may even become hypernatraemic if water is lost with, for example, glucose, resulting in greater loss of water than sodium. So the serum sodium concentration does not of itself provide any information about the presence or severity of sodium depletion. History and examination are much more useful, especially the patient's volume status (see Clinical note).

Pseudohyponatraemia

The total plasma volume consists of an aqueous phase, in which electrolytes are dissolved, contributing to the serum osmolality, and a nonaqueous phase consisting mostly of proteins and lipids, which are not dissolved in the water and do not contribute to the osmolality. Normally the aqueous phase occupies approximately 95% of the total plasma volume, with proteins and lipids occupying the remainder. Rarely, patients develop gross increases in either proteins or lipids. When this happens, the nonaqueous fraction occupies much more of the total plasma volume than usual, e.g. 20%, and the water phase correspondingly less (Fig. 9.3). Clinically, this is not of itself problematic (although the underlying problem causing the increase in proteins or lipids clearly is), since these patients have a normal sodium concentration in their plasma water. The problem is that many widely used analytical instruments measure the sodium concentration in the total plasma volume and take no account of a water fraction that occupies less of the plasma volume than usual. In these circumstances, an artefactually low sodium result may thus be obtained. Such *pseudohyponatraemia* should be suspected in a patient who has no symptoms of hyponatraemia, despite what appears to be a dangerously low serum sodium, e.g. 110 mmol/L. It can be easily diagnosed by measuring the serum osmolality. A normal serum osmolality in

> ### Clinical note
>
> In a patient with hyponatraemia, hypovolaemia is diagnostic of sodium depletion, since the clinical findings are evidence of reduced ECF volume, i.e. fluid (water) depletion, whilst the hyponatraemia (reduced ratio of sodium to water) indicates that there is even less sodium than water.

> ### Hyponatraemia: pathophysiology
>
> - Water retention is a nonspecific feature of illness, and hyponatraemia due to water retention is the commonest biochemical disturbance encountered in clinical practice.
> - In SIAD, nonosmotic stimuli of AVP secretion override its osmotic regulation. High AVP drives the serum osmolality down and the urine osmolality up; the patient is usually euvolaemic.
> - Sodium depletion is associated with clinical signs of dehydration due to loss of sodium and water from ECF.
> - Gut loss of sodium and water is usually obvious. Renal loss may be missed if it is not suspected, e.g. in undiagnosed adrenal insufficiency.

> ### Case history 3
>
> A 64-year-old woman was admitted with anorexia, weight loss and anaemia. Carcinoma of the colon was diagnosed. She was normotensive and did not have oedema. The following biochemical results were obtained shortly after admission:
>
> | Na⁺ | K⁺ | Cl⁻ | HCO₃⁻ | Urea | Creatinine |
> |-----|-----|-----|-----|-----|-----|
> | | | mmol/L | | | μmol/L |
> | 123 | 3.9 | 86 | 22 | 6.2 | 115 |
>
> Serum osmolality was measured as 247 mmol/kg; urine osmolality was 178 mmol/kg.
>
> - How may this patient's hyponatraemia be explained?
> - What contribution does the urine osmolality make to the diagnosis? *Comment in Case history comments.*

> ### Want to know more?
>
> http://mjmbiochem.com/evaluation-hyponatraemia-too-much-water-too-little-sodium/
>
> This blog post covers the evaluation of hyponatraemia in more detail. The figures illustrating water gain and loss of sodium (and water) are animated.

an asymptomatic patient with severe hyponatraemia is strongly suggestive of pseudohyponatraemia. Osmolality is unaffected by changes in proteins or lipids, since they are not dissolved in water and therefore do not contribute to the osmolality.

10 | Hyponatraemia: assessment and management

Clinical assessment

Clinicians assessing a patient with hyponatraemia should ask themselves several questions:

- Am I dealing with dangerous (life-threatening) hyponatraemia?
- Am I dealing with too much water or too little sodium?
- How should I treat this patient?

To answer these questions, they must use the patient's history, the findings from clinical examination and the results of laboratory investigations. Each of these may provide valuable clues.

Severity

In assessing the risk of serious morbidity or mortality in the patient with hyponatraemia, several pieces of information should be used:

- the presence of signs or symptoms attributable to hyponatraemia
- evidence of sodium depletion
- the serum sodium concentration
- how quickly the sodium concentration has fallen from normal to its current level.

The serum sodium concentration itself gives some indication of dangerous or life-threatening hyponatraemia. Many experienced clinicians use a concentration of 120 mmol/L as a threshold in trying to assess risk (the risk declines at concentrations significantly greater than 120 mmol/L and rises steeply at concentrations less than 120 mmol/L). However, this arbitrary cut-off should be applied with caution, particularly if it is not known how quickly the sodium concentration has fallen from normal to its current level. A patient whose serum sodium falls from 145 to 125 mmol/L in 24 hours may be at great risk.

Often, the clinician must rely exclusively on history and clinical examination to assess the risk. Symptoms due to hyponatraemia reflect neurological dysfunction resulting from cerebral overhydration induced by hypoosmolality. They are nonspecific, e.g. nausea, malaise, headache, lethargy, reduced level of consciousness or cognition. Seizures, coma and focal neurological signs are not usually seen until the sodium concentration is less than approximately 115 mmol/L.

If clinical evidence of sodium depletion (see later) is present, there is a high risk of mortality if treatment is not instituted quickly.

Mechanism

History

Fluid loss, e.g. from gut or kidney, should be sought as a possible pointer towards primary sodium loss. Even if there is no readily identifiable source of loss, the patient should be asked about symptoms that may reflect sodium depletion, e.g. dizziness, weakness, light-headedness.

If there is no history of fluid loss, water retention is likely. Few patients will give a history of water retention as such; history taking should instead be aimed at identifying possible causes of syndrome of inappropriate antidiuresis (SIAD). For example, rigors may point towards infection or weight loss towards malignancy.

Clinical examination

The clinical signs characteristic of extracellular fluid (ECF) and blood volume depletion are shown in Fig. 10.1. As pointed out in the Clinical note from Chapter 9, in hyponatraemic patients these are diagnostic of sodium depletion, and their presence or absence always should be determined. If they are present in the recumbent state, severe life-threatening sodium depletion is present and urgent treatment is needed. In the early phases of sodium depletion, postural hypotension may be the only sign.

By contrast, even when water retention is strongly suspected, there may be no clinical evidence of water overload. There are two reasons for this. First, water retention due to SIAD occurs gradually, often over weeks or even months. Second, as we have seen (see Fig. 7.2B), the retained water is distributed evenly over all body compartments, minimising the increase in the ECF volume.

Biochemistry

Sodium depletion is diagnosed largely on clinical grounds, whereas in patients with suspected water retention, history and examination may be unremarkable. However, sodium depletion and SIAD produce a similar biochemical picture: reduced serum sodium and osmolality, high urine osmolality reflecting arginine vasopressin (AVP) secretion. AVP secretion is, in both cases, 'inappropriate' for the hypoosmolal state. In sodium depletion, it is secreted in response to a powerful *non*osmotic stimulus, the hypovolaemia resulting from sodium and water loss; in SIAD it is responding to other *non*osmotic stimuli). Urinary sodium excretion is usually increased in SIAD (a hypervolaemic state). In sodium depletion, it is low if the loss is from the gut. It may not be low if the loss is renal due to failure or antagonism of aldosterone.

When clinicians are phoned with a very low sodium result, they need rapid answers to several important questions. These are summarised in Table 10.1.

Oedema

Oedema (Fig. 10.2) refers to accumulation of fluid in the interstitial compartment. It arises from a reduced effective circulating

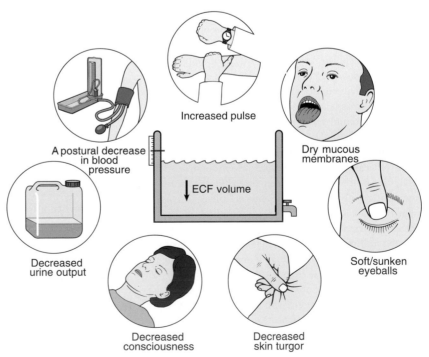

Fig. 10.1 The clinical features of extracellular fluid (ECF) compartment depletion.

Increased pulse

A postural decrease in blood pressure

Dry mucous membranes

ECF volume

Decreased urine output

Soft/sunken eyeballs

Decreased consciousness

Decreased skin turgor

Table 10.1 **Initial approach to severe hyponatraemia: what to ask and why**

Does patient have symptoms of hyponatraemia?	If present, they indicate the need for urgent correction. It may be appropriate to give sodium (saline), even if the mechanism is water retention, just to restore the ratio of sodium to water.
Is patient clinically dehydrated?	Dehydration (or, in its absence, postural hypotension) indicates sodium depletion, and the need for urgent sodium replacement.
Is patient oedematous?	Oedema indicates an excess of total body water and sodium. Usual treatment is with loop diuretics, which cause natriuresis, reducing both.
Is this a genuinely hypoosmolal state or pseudohyponatraemia?	Measured and calculated serum osmolality should be roughly equal. In severe hyponatraemia, a normal osmolality in an asymptomatic patient indicates pseudohyponatraemia.
Does patient have adrenal insufficiency?	Most physicians seek to exclude this even if index of suspicion is low, because they do not want to miss it. Random cortisol is helpful if high, e.g. >600 nmol/L, or low, e.g. <100 nmol/L.

The first two questions are the most important and, crucially, can be answered by clinical examination alone. The list of questions above is not exhaustive.

Clinical note

Correction of severe hyponatraemia must be closely monitored. Over-rapid correction produces severe osmotic shifts and, rarely, a devastating neurological complication called *central pontine myelinolysis*. In a patient with symptomatic hyponatraemia, balancing the relative risks of under- and over-rapid correction requires considerable experience.

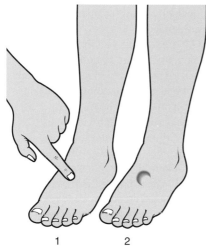

Fig 10.2 Pitting oedema. After depressing the skin firmly for a few seconds *(1)*, an indentation, or pit, is seen *(2)*.

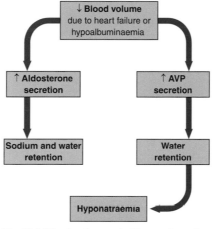

Fig. 10.3 The development of hyponatraemia in the oedematous patient. Note that it is the retention of pure water in response to arginine vasopressin (AVP) that causes hyponatraemia. The sodium retained due to aldosterone is accompanied by water; their equimolar reabsorption does not contribute to hyponatraemia.

Hyponatraemia: clinical assessment and management

- Patients with hyponatraemia because of sodium depletion show clinical signs of fluid loss such as hypotension. They do not have oedema.

- Treatment of hyponatraemia due to sodium depletion should be with sodium replacement.

- Hyponatraemic patients without oedema, who have normal serum urea and creatinine and blood pressure, have water overload. This may be treated initially by fluid restriction.

- Hyponatraemic patients with oedema are likely to have both water and sodium overload. These patients may be treated initially with loop diuretics.

blood volume, due either to heart failure or hypoalbuminaemia. The response to this is secondary hyperaldosteronism, causing sodium (and water) retention, thus expanding the ECF volume. Patients with oedema become hyponatraemic despite sodium retention because the hypovolaemia also stimulates AVP secretion, resulting in additional pure water retention (Fig. 10.3).

Treatment

Treatment follows logically from clinical assessment, especially the volume status. Hypovolaemic patients are sodium-depleted and should be given sodium. Normovolaemic patients are likely to be retaining water and should be fluid restricted. Oedematous patients have an excess of both total body sodium and water; they should be given a diuretic to induce natriuresis. More aggressive treatment (usually requiring hypertonic saline) may be indicated if symptoms attributable to hyponatraemia are present or the sodium concentration is less than 110 mmol/L. This should only be administered under senior supervision.

Case history 4

A 42-year-old man was admitted with a 2-day history of severe diarrhoea with some nausea and vomiting. During this period his only intake was water. He was weak and unable to stand; when he was recumbent, his pulse was 104/min and blood pressure was 100/55 mmHg. On admission, his biochemistry results were:

Na^+	K^+	Cl^-	HCO_3^-	Urea	Creatinine
		mmol/L			µmol/L
131	3.0	86	19	17.8	150

- What is the most appropriate treatment for this patient? *Comment in Case history comments.*

Want to know more?

http://www.medscape.org/viewarticle/736415_5

The most exciting development in recent times has been the advent of vaptans, a class of drugs that block AVP receptors. The attached link summarises quite a detailed article on these by Gary Robertson, a world expert on AVP. (In order to access the above link – and one or two other 'Want to know more' links in this book – registration is required. It is worth the effort – overall this is a very useful resource. All content is available free of charge).

11 | Hypernatraemia

Hypernatraemia is an increase in the serum sodium concentration above the reference interval of 133 to 146 mmol/L. It develops because of water loss or sodium gain. The mechanisms of hypernatraemia are summarised in Fig. 11.1.

Water loss

Pure water loss may arise from decreased intake or excessive loss. Severe hypernatraemia due to poor intake is most often seen in elderly patients who stop eating and drinking voluntarily, or who cannot drink, e.g. an unconscious patient after a stroke. The mechanism of hypernatraemia is simple – failure of intake to match ongoing insensible water loss. Hypernatraemia due to water loss can also result from failure of arginine vasopressin (AVP) secretion or action. This is called *diabetes insipidus – central* or *cranial* if it results from failure of AVP secretion, or *nephrogenic* if the renal tubules do not respond to AVP. Fig. 7.2A in Chapter 7 illustrates the effect of pure water loss on the size of different body compartments.

Combined loss of both water and sodium can result in hypernatraemia if water loss exceeds the sodium loss. This can happen in osmotic diuresis, e.g. poorly controlled diabetes mellitus, or due to excessive sweating or diarrhoea, especially in children (although, as discussed in Chapter 9 under 'Sodium loss,' loss of body fluids because of vomiting or diarrhoea usually results in hyponatraemia). The

effect of combined water and sodium loss on the size of different body compartments is shown in Fig. 11.2.

Sodium gain

Hypernatraemia due to sodium gain is much less common than water loss and is easily missed if it is not suspected. It can occur in several different clinical contexts. First, sodium bicarbonate is occasionally given to correct life-threatening acidosis. However, the sodium concentration in 8.4% sodium bicarbonate is 1000 mmol/L. A 1.26% solution is preferred. Second, near-drowning in the sea may result in ingestion of significant amounts of seawater, the sodium concentration of which is vastly in excess of physiological. Third, infants are susceptible to hypernatraemia if given high-sodium feeds either accidentally or on purpose. For example, the administration of 1 tablespoon of NaCl to a newborn baby can raise the plasma sodium by as much as 70 mmol/L. Fig. 7.3B in Chapter 7 illustrates the effect of sodium gain on the size of the extracellular fluid (ECF).

In primary hyperaldosteronism (Conn's syndrome), excessive aldosterone secretion causes sodium retention by the renal tubules. Cushing's syndrome (excess cortisol) has a similar effect, as cortisol has some mineralocorticoid activity. Interestingly, in both of these conditions, sodium rarely rises above 150 mmol/L, as rising osmolality stimulates AVP secretion.

Clinical features

Hypernatraemia may be associated with normal sodium balance (e.g. diabetes insipidus), sodium gain (e.g. sodium bicarbonate administration) or sodium depletion (e.g. osmotic diuresis). As you might expect, the sodium balance helps determine the ECF volume, but so too does the amount of pure water lost. Thus, for example, in severe cranial diabetes insipidus due to head injury, the loss of pure water, although distributed throughout all body compartments, may be so great that there is a significant reduction in ECF volume despite normal sodium balance. By contrast, osmotic diuresis is associated with loss of sodium and greater loss of water; their combined impact on ECF volume is substantial.

It may be more helpful to use the serum sodium concentration as the starting point, since this is often how the problem (or at least the extent of the problem) comes to light. With mild hypernatraemia (sodium <150 mmol/L), if the patient is clearly dehydrated (Fig. 11.3), then it is likely that the ECF volume is reduced and that one is dealing with loss of both water and sodium. With more severe hypernatraemia (sodium 150–170 mmol/L), pure water loss is likely if the clinical signs of dehydration are mild in relation to the severity of the hypernatraemia, because pure water loss is distributed evenly throughout all body compartments. With gross hypernatraemia (sodium >180 mmol/L), one should

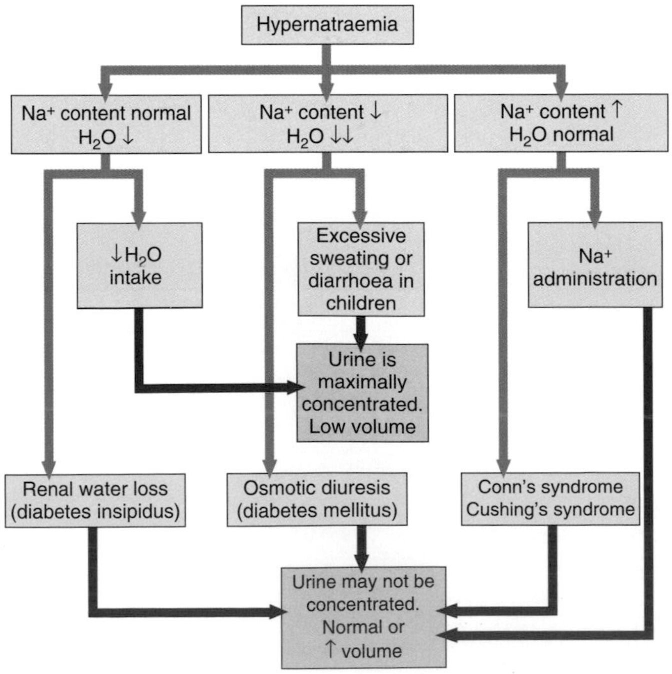

Fig. 11.1 Mechanisms of hypernatraemia.

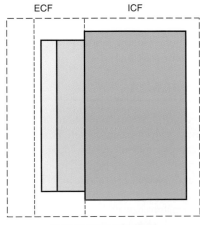

Water loss > sodium loss

Fig. 11.2 Combined water and sodium loss. Pure water is lost evenly from all body compartments. Sodium loss (and associated further obligatory water loss) is confined to the extracellular fluid (*ECF*). Thus the ECF is more reduced than the intracellular fluid (*ICF*). (The *dotted rectangle/lines* indicate the normal size of the compartments.)

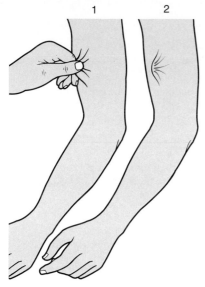

Fig. 11.3 Decreased skin turgor.

calculated osmolality (osmolal gap) (see Chapter 7, Osmolality), this suggests the presence of a significant contributor to the measured osmolality, unaccounted for in the calculated osmolality. This is most often due to the presence of ethanol in the blood. Occasionally, however, it may be due to other substances, such as methanol or ethylene glycol (also known as *toxic alcohols*). Thus calculation of the osmolal gap can be clinically useful in the assessment of comatose patients.

The consequences of disordered osmolality are due to the changes in volume that arise as water moves in or out of cells to maintain osmotic balance. Of the previous three examples, only glucose causes significant fluid movement. Glucose cannot freely enter cells, and by increasing ECF concentration, it causes water to move out of cells, leading to intracellular dehydration. Urea and ethanol permeate cells and do not cause such large fluid shifts, as long as concentration changes occur slowly.

> **Clinical note**
>
> Patients often become hypernatraemic because they are unable to complain of being thirsty. Comatose patients are a good example – they are unable to communicate their needs, yet insensible losses of water will continue from lung and skin.

suspect sodium gain if there is little or no clinical evidence of dehydration; the amount of water that would need to be lost to elevate the sodium to this degree should be clinically obvious, irrespective of whether there has been concomitant sodium loss. Salt (sodium) gain is more likely to present with clinical evidence of overload, such as raised jugular venous pressure or pulmonary oedema.

Treatment

Patients with hypernatraemia due to pure water loss should be given water; this may be given orally, or intravenously as 5% dextrose. If there is clinical evidence of dehydration indicating probable loss of sodium as well, sodium should be administered. Salt poisoning is a difficult clinical problem to manage. The sodium overload can be treated with diuretics and the natriuresis replaced with water. Caution must be exercised with the use of intravenous dextrose in salt-poisoned patients, however – they are volume-expanded already and susceptible to pulmonary oedema.

High osmolality: other causes

Other causes of high serum osmolality include increased urea, hyperglycaemia or the presence of ethanol or some other ingested substance. If there is a difference between measured and

> **Hypernatraemia**
>
> - Hypernatraemia is most commonly due to water loss (e.g. continuing insensible losses in the patient who is unable to drink).
> - Failure to retain water as a result of impaired AVP secretion or action may cause hypernatraemia.
> - Hypernatraemia may be the result of a loss of both sodium and water as a consequence of an osmotic diuresis, e.g. in diabetic ketoacidosis.
> - Excessive sodium intake, particularly from the use of intravenous solutions, may cause hypernatraemia. Rarely, primary hyperaldosteronism (Conn's syndrome) may be the cause.
> - A high plasma osmolality may be due to the presence of glucose, urea or ethanol, rather than sodium.

> **Case history 5**
>
> A 76-year-old man with depression and very severe incapacitating disease was admitted as an acute emergency. He was clinically dehydrated. His skin was lax, and his lips and tongue appeared dry and shrivelled. His pulse was 104 beats per minute, and his blood pressure was 95/65 mmHg. The following biochemical results were obtained on admission:
>
> | Na^+ | K^+ | Cl^- | HCO_3^- | Urea | Creatinine |
> |---|---|---|---|---|---|
> | | | mmol/L | | | μmol/L |
> | 172 | 3.6 | 140 | 18 | 22.9 | 155 |
>
> - Comment on these biochemical findings.
> - What is the diagnosis?
>   *Comment in Case history comments.*

> **Want to know more?**
>
> https://en.wikipedia.org/wiki/Fractional_sodium_excretion
>
> Fractional excretion of sodium may help distinguish sodium excess from water loss as the mechanism of hypernatraemia. It is high in the former and low in the latter. It also may be used to distinguish different causes of renal impairment. This wiki link outlines how it is calculated.

12 | Hyperkalaemia

Potassium disorders are commonly encountered in clinical practice. They are important because of the role potassium plays in determining the resting membrane potential of cells. Changes in plasma potassium mean that the response to stimuli of 'excitable' cells, such as nerve and muscle, may be affected. In the heart (which is largely composed of muscle and nerve), the consequences, e.g. arrhythmias, can be fatal.

Serum potassium and potassium balance

Serum potassium concentration is normally kept within a tight range (3.5–5.3 mmol/L). *Potassium intake* is variable (30–100 mmol/day), and *potassium losses* (through the kidneys) usually mirror intake. The two most important factors that determine potassium excretion are the glomerular filtration rate (GFR) and the plasma potassium concentration. A small amount (~5 mmol/day) is lost in the gut. Potassium balance can be disturbed if any of these fluxes is altered (Fig. 12.1). Also, nearly all of the total body potassium (98%) is inside cells. If there is significant tissue damage, the contents of cells, including potassium, leak out into the extracellular compartment, causing potentially dangerous increases in serum potassium (see later).

Hyperkalaemia

Severe hyperkalaemia (>7.0 mmol/L) is immediately life-threatening and must be dealt with as an absolute priority; cardiac arrest may be the first manifestation. Electrocardiogram (ECG) changes seen in hyperkalaemia (Fig. 12.2) include the classic tall 'tented' T-waves and widening of the QRS complex, reflecting altered myocardial contractility. Other symptoms include muscle weakness and paraesthesiae.

Decreased excretion

- *Renal failure*. Hyperkalaemia is a central feature of reduced glomerular function. It is exacerbated by the associated metabolic acidosis, due to the accumulation of organic ions that would normally be excreted; potassium and hydrogen share an excretory pathway (see under Redistribution out of cells).
- *Hypoaldosteronism*. Aldosterone deficiency, antagonism or resistance results in loss of sodium and water, reducing the GFR. In clinical practice, hyperkalaemia due to hypoaldosteronism is most often seen

with angiotensin-converting enzyme (ACE) inhibitors, angiotensin receptor blockers (ARBs) and the aldosterone antagonist spironolactone, all of which are used to treat hypertension. Primary adrenal insufficiency is not common, but potentially fatal if missed (see Chapter 48).

Redistribution out of cells

- *Metabolic acidosis*. As the concentration of hydrogen ions increases with the development of metabolic acidosis, so

potassium ions inside cells are displaced from the cell by hydrogen ions in order to maintain electrochemical neutrality (Fig. 12.3).
- *Potassium release from damaged cells*. Cell damage occurs in rhabdomyolysis (in which skeletal muscle is broken down), extensive trauma or, rarely, tumour lysis syndrome, in which malignant cells break down.
- *Insulin deficiency*. Insulin stimulates cellular uptake of potassium. Where there is insulin deficiency or severe

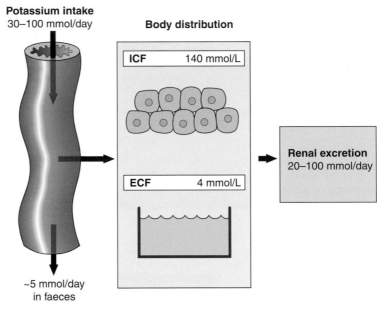

Fig. 12.1 **Potassium balance and distribution.** *ECF*, Extracellular fluid; *ICF*, intracellular fluid.

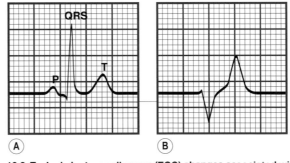

Fig. 12.2 **Typical electrocardiogram (ECG) changes associated with hyperkalaemia. (A)** Normal ECG. **(B)** Patient with hyperkalaemia: note peaked T-wave and widening of the QRS complex.

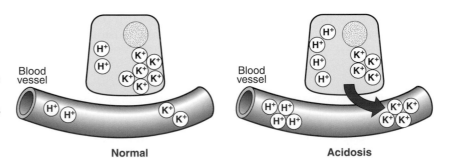

Fig. 12.3 **Hyperkalaemia is associated with acidosis.**

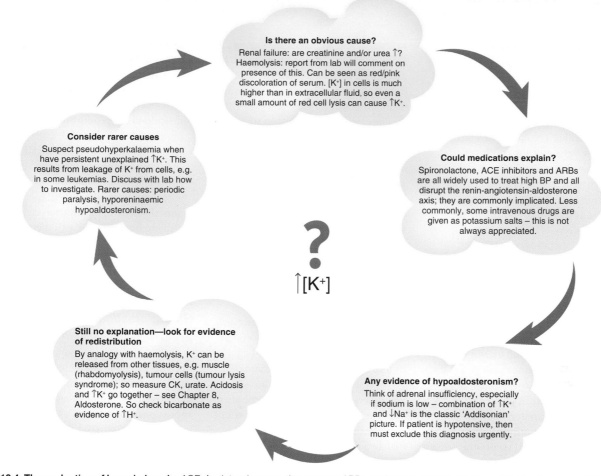

Is there an obvious cause?
Renal failure: are creatinine and/or urea ↑?
Haemolysis: report from lab will comment on
presence of this. Can be seen as red/pink
discoloration of serum. [K⁺] in cells is much
higher than in extracellular fluid, so even a
small amount of red cell lysis can cause ↑K⁺.

Consider rarer causes
Suspect pseudohyperkalaemia when
have persistent unexplained ↑K⁺. This
results from leakage of K⁺ from cells, e.g.
in some leukemias. Discuss with lab how
to investigate. Rarer causes: periodic
paralysis, hyporeninaemic
hypoaldosteronism.

Could medications explain?
Spironolactone, ACE inhibitors and ARBs
are all widely used to treat high BP and all
disrupt the renin-angiotensin-aldosterone
axis; they are commonly implicated. Less
commonly, some intravenous drugs are
given as potassium salts – this is not
always appreciated.

?
↑[K⁺]

**Still no explanation—look for evidence
of redistribution**
By analogy with haemolysis, K⁺ can be
released from other tissues, e.g. muscle
(rhabdomyolysis), tumour cells (tumour lysis
syndrome); so measure CK, urate. Acidosis
and ↑K⁺ go together – see Chapter 8,
Aldosterone. So check bicarbonate as
evidence of ↑H⁺.

Any evidence of hypoaldosteronism?
Think of adrenal insufficiency, especially
if sodium is low – combination of ↑K⁺
and ↓Na⁺ is the classic 'Addisonian'
picture. If patient is hypotensive, then
must exclude this diagnosis urgently.

Fig. 12.4 The evaluation of hyperkalaemia. *ACE*, Angiotensin-converting enzyme; *ARBs*, angiotensin receptor blockers; *BP*, blood pressure; *CK*, creatine kinase.

resistance to the actions of insulin, as in diabetic ketoacidosis (see Chapter 33), hyperkalaemia is an associated feature.

- *Pseudohyperkalaemia.* This should be considered when hyperkalaemia is otherwise unexplained (see later).
- *Hyperkalaemic periodic paralysis.* In this rare autosomal dominant disorder, paralysis occurs classically after exercise.

Increased intake

Unrecognised potassium intake may result in dangerous hyperkalaemia, particularly in patients with impaired renal function. For example, some oral drugs are administered as potassium salts. Potassium also may be given intravenously. *Intravenous potassium should not be given faster than 20 mmol/hour except in extreme cases.* Occasionally, blood products may cause hyperkalaemia (as stored red blood cells release potassium). The risk of this is reduced by using relatively fresh blood and/or by 'washing' units prior to transfusing.

Treatment

- Calcium counteracts the effects of hyperkalaemia on the resting membrane potential of cells.

- Insulin causes potassium to move into cells along with glucose. Glucose is also given to prevent hypoglycaemia.
- Dialysis may be required for refractory hyperkalaemia.

> **Clinical note**
>
> Some oral and intravenous drugs are administered as potassium salts. Unexplained, persistent hyperkalaemia should always prompt review of the drug history.

Pseudohyperkalaemia

Pseudohyperkalaemia refers to an increase in the concentration of potassium due to its movement out of cells during or after venesection. The commonest causes are: (1) delay in centrifugation separating plasma/serum from the cells/clot, especially if the specimen is chilled. This is very common in specimens from primary care. (2) *In vitro* haemolysis. (3) An increase in the platelet and/or white cell count.

Formal investigation of suspected pseudohyperkalaemia should include simultaneous collection and processing of serum and plasma specimens (the anticoagulant in plasma specimens

prevents clotting). Varying the time to sample centrifugation also may provide evidence, in the form of a progressive steep rise in serum potassium seen with delayed centrifugation.

Fig. 12.4 provides a practical approach to the assessment of hyperkalaemia.

> **Hyperkalaemia**
>
> - Most potassium in the body is intracellular.
> - The commonest cause of hyperkalaemia is renal impairment.
> - Severe hyperkalaemia is immediately life-threatening, and death may occur with no clinical warning signs.
> - Sometimes hyperkalaemia is artefactual – this is called pseudohyperkalaemia.

> **Want to know more?**
>
> https://www.scribd.com/
> document/253568590/
> VS7048-Troubleshooting-Erroneous-
> Potasslums-Poster
>
> This poster was produced by Becton Dickinson, one of the major manufacturers of blood collection tubes. It provides a detailed approach to artefactual hyperkalaemia and how it can be minimised.

13 | Hypokalaemia

Factors affecting potassium balance have been described in Chapter 12. Hypokalaemia frequently results from increased losses or redistribution of potassium into cells. Reduced intake is relatively uncommon except in anorexia nervosa and will not be considered further. As with hyperkalaemia, the clinical effects of hypokalaemia are seen in 'excitable' tissues such as nerve and muscle. Symptoms include muscle weakness, hyporeflexia and cardiac arrhythmias. Subtle cognitive impairment is an early feature. Fig. 13.1 shows the electrocardiogram (ECG) changes associated with hypokalaemia.

Diagnosis

The cause of hypokalaemia can usually be determined from the history. Common causes include vomiting and diarrhoea, and diuretic use. Where the cause is not immediately obvious, urine potassium measurement may help. Increased urinary potassium excretion despite hypokalaemia suggests urinary loss rather than redistribution or gut loss; low or undetectable urinary potassium indicates renal retention of potassium.

Redistribution into cells

- *Metabolic alkalosis*. The reciprocal relationship between potassium and hydrogen ions means that just as metabolic acidosis is associated with hyperkalaemia, so metabolic alkalosis is associated with hypokalaemia. As [H+] decreases, potassium ions move inside cells in order to maintain electrochemical neutrality (Fig. 13.2).
- *Treatment with insulin*. Insulin stimulates cellular uptake of potassium and plays a central role in treatment of severe hyperkalaemia (see Chapter 12, Treatment). Thus, when it is given in treatment of diabetic ketoacidosis (DKA) (see Chapter 33), the risk of hypokalaemia is predictable and well-recognised; DKA treatment protocols take this into account.
- *Refeeding*. The so-called 'refeeding syndrome' occurs when previously malnourished patients are fed with high-carbohydrate loads. Refeeding is associated with rapid falls in phosphate, magnesium and potassium, mediated by insulin as it moves glucose into cells. Postoperative patients and those with anorexia nervosa, cancer and alcoholism are all at risk. Many of the complications result from hypophosphataemia rather than hypokalaemia.
- *β-agonism*. Acute physiological stress can cause potassium to move into cells, an effect mediated by catecholamine action on β2-receptors. β-agonists such as salbutamol (used to treat asthma) or dobutamine (used in heart failure) induce a similar effect.
- *Treatment of anaemia*. Folic acid or vitamin B12 for megaloblastic anaemia often produces hypokalaemia in the first couple of days of treatment, due to increased uptake of potassium by the new blood cells. Treatment of irondeficiency anaemia results in a much slower rate of new blood cell production and is rarely implicated.
- *Hypokalaemic periodic paralysis*. Like its hyperkalaemic counterpart, hypokalaemic periodic paralysis has autosomal dominant inheritance and typically occurs at rest after exercise. It also can be associated with thyrotoxicosis (possibly due to increased sensitivity to catecholamines), especially in Chinese males.

Increased losses
Gastrointestinal

Diarrhoea and vomiting are obvious, and the risk of hypokalaemia is well-recognised. In cholera (in which fluid loss from the gut is massive), daily potassium losses may exceed 100 mmol, compared with approximately 5 mmol normally. Less frequently, chronic laxative abuse may be responsible. However, this normally should be considered only when more likely causes of hypokalaemia have been excluded.

Urinary

- *Diuretics*. Both loop diuretics and thiazide diuretics produce hypokalaemia. Various mechanisms are implicated, including increased flow of water and sodium to the site of distal potassium secretion, and secondary hyperaldosteronism induced by the loss of volume. Loop diuretics also interfere with potassium reabsorption in the loop of Henle.
- *Mineralocorticoid excess*. Aldosterone increases sodium reabsorption in the renal tubules at the expense of potassium and hydrogen ions (Chapter 8, Aldosterone). This *mineralocorticoid* effect is shared by many steroids, and hypokalaemia is a predictable consequence of mineralocorticoid excess. Overproduction of steroid hormones is dealt with in more detail in Chapter 49. Less frequently, renal artery stenosis drives the renin–angiotensin–aldosterone axis, resulting in hypokalaemia associated with severe, refractory hypertension.
- *Hypomagnesaemia*. Hypomagnesaemia from any cause may lead to hypokalaemia due to impaired renal tubular absorption. Hypomagnesaemia due to proton pump inhibitors is an increasingly common cause of hypokalaemia.

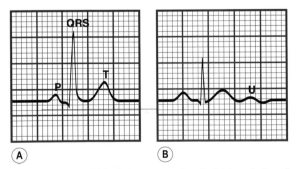

Fig. 13.1 Typical ECG changes associated with hypokalaemia. (A) Normal ECG. (B) Patient with hypokalaemia: note flattened T wave. U waves are prominent in all leads.

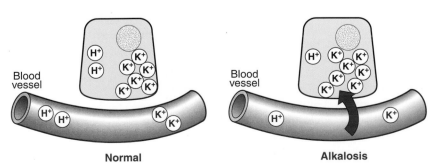

Fig. 13.2 Hypokalaemia is associated with alkalosis.

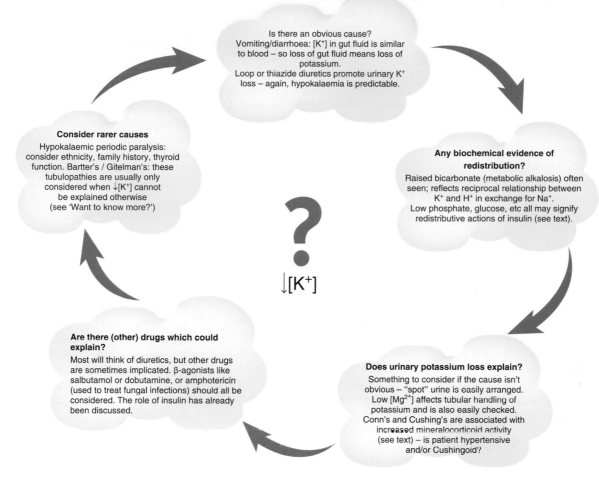

Fig. 13.3 The evaluation of hypokalaemia.

- *Tubulopathies*. The commonest causes of tubular dysfunction are chemotherapeutic agents, especially platinum-containing drugs. Rarely, inherited defects in tubular function produce hypokalaemia, by various mechanisms.

Investigation

Fig. 13.3 provides a framework for investigation of hypokalaemia. Often the cause is obvious, e.g. vomiting, diarrhoea, and further investigations are not required. Some of the causes of hypokalaemia listed previously, e.g. diuretics, gut loss and insulin treatment, are well-recognised by clinicians. Other causes are infrequently implicated (treatment of anaemia) or very rare (hypokalaemic periodic paralysis) and may not be considered. Where the cause is not immediately evident, it may help to go back to first principles by classifying potential causes into the three broad categories outlined earlier: increased loss, redistribution and reduced intake. Measurement of urinary potassium excretion may help identify (or exclude) renal loss as the likely mechanism. Diagnoses which can be difficult to pin down include laxative abuse (may be intermittent and usually undeclared) and tubulopathies (rare, and phenotypic expression varies).

Treatment

Potassium salts are unpleasant to take orally and are usually given in an enteric coating. Severe potassium depletion usually requires intravenous potassium, which should not be given faster than 20 mmol/hour except in extreme cases and under ECG monitoring.

Clinical note

Alcoholic patients are especially prone to hypokalaemia through various mechanisms.

Hypokalaemia

- Hypokalaemia rarely results from decreased intake.
- Bicarbonate always should be measured in unexplained hypokalaemia.
- Increased mineralocorticoid activity leads to hypokalaemia.
- Low magnesium should be suspected in persistent hypokalaemia.

Case history 6

Mrs MM, a 67-year-old patient with extensive vascular disease, attends the hypertension clinic and is on five different antihypertensive drugs. At her most recent clinic visit, blood pressure was 220/110 mmHg, and a set of urine and electrolyte studies showed the following:

Na^+	K^+	Cl^-	HCO_3^-	Urea	Creatinine
		mmol/L			μmol/L
139	2.7	106	33	21.7	254

- What would explain the coexistent hypertension and hypokalaemia in this patient? *Comment in Case history comments.*

Want to know more?

http://mjmbiochem.com/bartter&gitelman

Inherited tubulopathies are daunting to the unfamiliar. This account attempts to demystify them and to put them in their proper context.

14 | Intravenous fluid therapy

Intravenous (IV) fluid therapy is an integral part of clinical practice in hospitals. Every hospital doctor should be familiar with the principles underlying the appropriate administration of IV fluids. Each time fluids are prescribed, the following questions should be addressed:

- Does the patient need IV fluids?
- Which fluids should be given?
- How much fluid should be given?
- How quickly should the fluids be given?
- How should the fluid therapy be monitored?

Does this patient need IV fluids?

The easiest and best way to give fluids is orally. For example, oral rehydration solutions are the least expensive and most effective way to manage dehydration caused by infective diarrhoea. However, patients may be unable to take fluids orally. Often the reason for this is self-evident, e.g. because the patient is comatose, has undergone major surgery or is vomiting. Sometimes fluids are given intravenously even if the patient is able to tolerate oral fluids, e.g. because there is clinical evidence of fluid depletion, or biochemical evidence of electrolyte disturbance that is severe enough to require immediate correction.

Which IV fluids should be given?

The list of IV fluids available for prescription in many hospital formularies is long and potentially bewildering. However, with a few exceptions, many of these fluids are variations on the three basic types of fluid shown in Fig. 14.1. Their administration requires an understanding of the concepts outlined in Chapter 7.

- *Plasma, whole blood or plasma expanders.* These replace deficits in the vascular compartment only. They are indicated where there is a reduction in the blood volume due to blood loss from whatever cause. Such solutions are sometimes referred to as 'colloids' to distinguish them from 'crystalloids' Colloidal particles in solution cannot pass through the (semipermeable) capillary membrane, in contrast with crystalloid particles such as sodium and chloride ions, which can. This is why they are confined to the vascular compartment, whereas sodium chloride ('saline')

solutions are distributed throughout the entire extracellular fluid (ECF).

- *Isotonic sodium chloride (0.9% NaCl).* It is called *isotonic* because its effective osmolality, or tonicity, is similar to that of the ECF. Once it is administered, it is confined to the ECF and is indicated where there is a reduced ECF volume, e.g. in sodium depletion.

- *Water.* If pure water (severely hypotonic) were infused, it would rapidly shift into blood cells as it entered the vein, causing them to lyse, causing gross intravascular haemolysis. For this reason, 'water' is instead given as 5% dextrose (glucose), which, like 0.9% saline, is isotonic with plasma initially. The dextrose is rapidly metabolised. The water that remains is distributed evenly through all body compartments and contributes to both ECF and intracellular fluid (ICF). Therefore 5% dextrose is designed to replace deficits in total body water, e.g. in most hypernatraemic patients, rather than those specifically with reduced ECF volume.

How much fluid should be given?

The amount of fluid given depends on the extent of the losses that have already occurred of both fluid and electrolytes, and on the losses/requirements anticipated over the next 24 hours. The latter depends, in turn, on both insensible losses and measured losses.

Existing losses

It may not be possible to calculate the exact deficit of water or electrolytes. This is not as critical as one might expect. Even where there is a severe deficit of water or sodium, it is important not to replace too quickly if complications of over-rapid correction are to be avoided. Unless there are severe ongoing losses, it is the duration rather than the rate of fluid replacement that varies.

Anticipated losses

It is useful to know what 'normality' is, i.e. what the fluid and electrolyte requirements would be for a healthy subject if for some reason the person were unable to eat or drink orally. Most textbooks quote a water throughput of 2 to 3 L/day, a sodium throughput of 100 to 200 mmol/day, and a potassium throughput of 20 to 200 mmol/day. Insensible water loss from skin and breathing amounts to about 800 mL/day. On the other hand, metabolism accounts for about 400 mL of water production. In clinical practice, since neither of these can be accurately accounted for, they are often not used to calculate fluid balance.

How quickly should the fluids be given?

The appropriate rate of fluid replacement varies enormously according to the clinical situation. The following example illustrates what must be considered in prescribing IV fluids to a patient undergoing elective surgery.

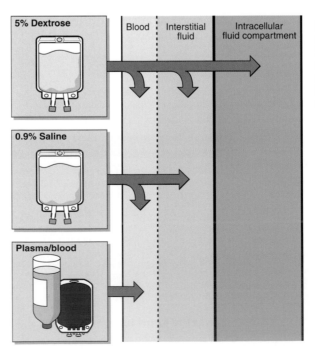

5% Dextrose

Blood | Interstitial fluid | Intracellular fluid compartment

0.9% Saline

Plasma/blood

Fig. 14.1 The three types of fluid normally used in intravenous fluid therapy are shown with the different contributions they make to the body fluid compartments.

Fluid balance chart

Hospital: _____	Reason for fluid balance chart ___NBM___	Does patient require thickened fluids?	**NHS** Greater Glasgow and Clyde
Ward: __11B__	Is patient fluid restricted? Yes ☐ No ☐	Yes ☐ No ☐ Stage _____	
Date: __1/1/17__	If yes how many mL in 24 hours? _____	Is the patient on an oral supplement? Yes ☐ No ☑	
		If yes please indicate:	
		1. Type _____ circle how many daily 1 2 3	
	Fluid balance from previous 24 hours	2. Type _____ circle how many daily 1 2 3	
	+/− __+80__	Signature: _____ Designation: _____	

ONLY RECORD INTAKE CONSUMED NOT WHAT IS GIVEN TO PATIENT

Time	Input Oral Fluids Type	Volume	Enteral Type	Volume	IV/Other Type	Volume	Type	Volume	Running total Input	Output Urine	Gastric/ vomit	Bowel	Type	Type	Type	Running total Output	Initials
00:00					IV	100	TPN	78									
01:00					Fluids	100		78									
02:00						100		78									
03:00						100		78		500	(e)						
04:00						100		78									
05:00						100		78									
06:00						100		78									
07:00						100		78									
08:00						100		78									
09:00						100		78		900	(e)						
10:00						100		78									
11:00						100		78									
12:00						100		78									
13:00			meds	420 200		100		78		500	(e)					1900	
14:00						100		78									
15:00								78									
16:00								78									
17:00								78									
18:00			meds	150 + 420				78	2592								
19:00								78									
20:00								78		1000						2900	
21:00								78									
22:00			meds +	Flush 120				78									
23:00								78									
							*Total intake	3102						*Total output	2900	

*Transfer total intake/total output/24hours fluid balance to cumulative fluid balance on back of food, fluid and nutrition profile.

*24 hours fluid Balance+/− +202

Fig. 14.2 A completed fluid balance chart of a patient in the early postoperative period.

Perioperative patient

Based on normality, IV fluid therapy for a patient undergoing elective surgery might be expected to include between 2.0 and 3.0 L isotonic fluids, of which 1.0 L should be 0.9% saline (which will provide ~155 mmol sodium), with potassium supplementation. However: (1) the metabolic response to trauma/surgery stimulates arginine vasopressin secretion with resultant water retention; (2) physiological stress both reduces sodium excretion and increases potassium excretion; (3) redistribution of potassium occurs as a result of tissue damage. In the immediate postoperative period, 1.0 to 1.5 L IV fluid containing 30 to 50 mmol sodium and no potassium will often meet baseline requirements; additional requirements will be based on continuing losses, e.g. from large open wounds or nasogastric tube aspirates. Fig. 14.2 shows the completed fluid balance chart for the previous 24 hours of a patient in the postoperative period.

How should the fluid therapy be monitored?

The best place to study monitoring of IV fluid replacement in practice is in the intensive care setting. Here, comprehensive monitoring of a patient's fluid and electrolyte balance, along with vital signs, allows the prescribed fluid regimen to be tailored to the patient's individual requirement.

Clinical note

In hyponatraemia, it is recommended that sodium be raised by not more than 10–12 mmol/L/day. At faster rates, central pontine myelinolysis may rarely occur, due to osmotic shrinkage of axons leading to severing of their myelin sheaths. It is not entirely clear why the pons is especially vulnerable to this complication.

Want to know more?

https://www.nice.org.uk/guidance/cg174?u nlid=5626372362015113012362

National Institute for Health and Care Excellence (NICE) guidelines on intravenous fluid therapy in adults in hospitals are pitched at doctors but may be of interest. It would be a useful exercise to see what level of evidence there is to support specific recommendations.

Intravenous fluid therapy

- IV fluid therapy is commonly used to correct fluid and electrolyte imbalance.

- The simple guidelines for IV fluid therapy are:

  - first assess the patient clinically, then biochemically, paying particular attention to cardiac and renal function

  - use simple solutions

  - in prescribing fluids, attempt to make up deficits and anticipate future losses

  - monitor the patient closely at all times during fluid therapy

Case history 7

Postoperatively, a 62-year-old woman was noted to be getting progressively weaker. There was no evidence of fever, bleeding or infection. Blood pressure was 120/80 mmHg. Before the operation her serum electrolytes were normal, as were her renal function and cardiovascular system. Three days after the operation, her electrolytes were retested.

Na^+	K^+	Cl^-	HCO_3^-	Urea	Creatinine
		mmol/L			µmol/L
125	4.2	77	32	21.4	145

- Random urine osmolality = 920 mmol/kg
- Urine [Na^+] <10 mmol/L
- Urine [K^+] = 15 mmol/L
  - What is the pathophysiology behind these findings?
  - What other information do you require in order to prescribe the appropriate fluid therapy?
  Comment in Case history comments.

15 | Investigation of renal function (1)

Functions of the kidney

The functional unit of the kidney is the nephron, shown in Fig. 15.1. The functions of the kidneys include regulation of water, electrolyte and acid–base balance and excretion of the products of protein and nucleic acid metabolism: e.g. urea, creatinine and uric acid. It is convenient to discuss renal function in terms of *glomerular* and *tubular* function.

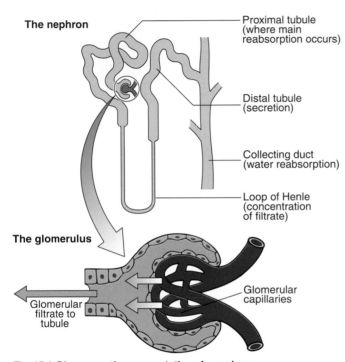

The nephron

Proximal tubule (where main reabsorption occurs)

Distal tubule (secretion)

Collecting duct (water reabsorption)

Loop of Henle (concentration of filtrate)

The glomerulus

Glomerular capillaries

Glomerular filtrate to tubule

Fig. 15.1 Diagrammatic representation of a nephron.

Glomerular function

The rate at which plasma is filtered at the glomeruli – the glomerular filtration rate (GFR) – is defined as the volume of plasma from which a given substance is completely cleared by glomerular filtration per unit time. This is approximately 140 mL/min in a healthy adult but varies enormously with body size. Conventionally, it is corrected to a body surface area of 1.73 m^2 (so units are mL/min/1.73 m^2).

Serum creatinine

Measurement of creatinine in serum is still widely used in the assessment of glomerular function. Although convenient, it is an imperfect measure of glomerular function. This is illustrated in Fig. 15.2, which shows that GFR has to halve before a significant increase in serum creatinine becomes apparent.

Estimated GFR (eGFR)

The relatively poor inverse correlation between serum creatinine and GFR shown in Fig. 15.2 can be improved by taking into account some of the confounding variables, such as age, sex, race and body weight. The formula developed by Cockcroft and Gault in the 1970s, the four-variable equation derived more recently from the Modification of Diet in Renal Disease (MDRD) Study and the Chronic Kidney Disease Epidemiology Collaboration (CKD-EPI) creatinine equation are the most widely used of these prediction equations. These are compared in Table 15.1.

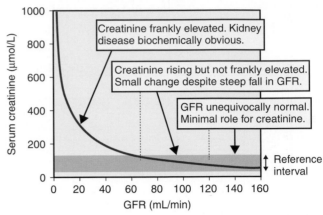

Creatinine frankly elevated. Kidney disease biochemically obvious.

Creatinine rising but not frankly elevated. Small change despite steep fall in GFR.

GFR unequivocally normal. Minimal role for creatinine.

Reference interval

Fig. 15.2 The relationship between glomerular filtration rate (GFR) and serum creatinine concentration. GFR has to fall considerably before serum creatinine is obviously increased.

Estimates of GFR should be interpreted with caution. They are more likely to be inaccurate in subjects with relatively normal GFR, and for this reason many hospital laboratories do not report a specific result when the GFR is greater than 60 mL/min/1.73 m^2. Other patient groups in whom eGFR is less accurate include those with abnormal body shape or mass, e.g. in people with muscle wasting or amputation. Finally, some estimates of GFR are affected by consumption of meat.

Despite these limitations, estimates of GFR are undoubtedly better than serum creatinine on its own at identifying reduced glomerular function, because they take some of the confounding variables into account (see Table 15.1). Reduced glomerular function, e.g. eGFR of 50–60 mL/min/1.73 m^2, is associated with cardiovascular risk and subsequent progression to more severe kidney disease, but much remains to be clarified about this group of patients, e.g. the time course of progression. This is an area of active research.

Other ways of measuring GFR

There are other ways of measuring GFR, but these are too costly and labour-intensive to be widely applied; their use is mainly limited to research or specialised nephrology settings such as screening potential kidney donors. They include clearance of

Table 15.1 Comparison of equations for estimated GFR (eGFR)		
Cockcroft–Gault	**Four-Variable ("Simplified") MDRD Equation**	**CKD-EPI Creatinine Equation**
Developed in the mid-1970s	Developed in the late 1990s	Developed in 2009; revised 2021
Incorporates age, sex and weight in addition to creatinine	Incorporates age, sex and race in addition to creatinine	Incorporates age and sex in addition to creatinine; initial version also included race
Widely used to calculate drug dosages	Widely used on biochemistry reports	Has now emerged as the recommended equation for estimating GFR
Developed in a population with reduced GFR	Developed in a population with reduced GFR[a]	Developed in diverse range of clinical and research populations

CKD-EPI, Chronic Kidney Disease Epidemiology Collaboration; *GFR,* glomerular filtration rate; *MDRD,* Modification of Diet in Renal Disease.
[a]But has only been validated in some ethnic groups, e.g. Caucasians, Afro-Caribbeans.

inulin, iothalamate, iohexol and radioisotopic markers such as ^{51}Cr-EDTA. The latter is, however, commonly used in oncology units for estimation of renal function prior to chemotherapy dose calculation.

More recently, cystatin C has emerged as an alternative to creatinine. Serum concentrations of this low-molecular-weight protein, like creatinine, correlate inversely with GFR. However, unlike creatinine, the concentration of cystatin C is independent of weight and height, muscle mass, age (>1 year) or sex and is largely unaffected by intake of meat or non–meat-containing foods.

Creatinine clearance

The volume of plasma from which a given substance is completely cleared by glomerular filtration per unit time (i.e. the GFR) can be estimated by measuring urinary excretion of creatinine. This *creatinine clearance* is calculated as follows:

- The amount of creatinine excreted in urine over a given interval is the volume of urine collected (say, V litres in 24 hours) multiplied by the urine creatinine concentration (U).
- The volume of plasma that would have contained this amount of creatinine is calculated by dividing the amount excreted ($U \times V$) by the plasma concentration of creatinine (P):

$$\text{Volume of plasma} = \frac{U \times V}{P}$$

In other words this is the theoretical volume of plasma that would be completely "cleared" of creatinine in order to give the amount seen in the urine during the time of collection. Urinary clearance of creatinine is more sensitive than serum creatinine in detecting reduced GFR. For example, a serum creatinine of 100 µmol/L can be associated with markedly different GFR depending on the age, sex and size of the patient (Fig. 15.3). Prediction equations which estimate GFR performance also take these confounders into account and have largely superseded creatinine clearance; it is inconvenient, and many patients struggle to perform a 24-hour urine collection accurately.

Creatinine clearance in practice

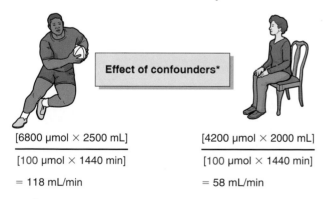

Effect of confounders*

[6800 µmol × 2500 mL] / [100 µmol × 1440 min] = 118 mL/min

[4200 µmol × 2000 mL] / [100 µmol × 1440 min] = 58 mL/min

<u>Same</u> serum [creatinine], but <u>two-fold</u> difference in GFR!

*Confounders include muscle mass and diet. Age, sex and ethnicity are proxies for these.

Fig. 15.3 Creatinine clearance results on two patients at opposite ends of the spectrum of muscle mass. Note that the serum creatinine concentration is the same despite grossly different glomerular filtration rates (GFRs).

Proteinuria

Another aspect of glomerular function is its "leakiness". This is dealt with separately in Chapter 18.

Endocrine aspects

The kidneys are also endocrine organs, producing a number of hormones, and are subject to control by others (Fig. 15.4). Arginine

vasopressin (AVP) acts to influence water balance, and aldosterone affects sodium and water reabsorption and, potassium excretion in the nephron. Parathyroid hormone promotes tubular reabsorption of calcium, phosphate excretion and the synthesis of 1,25-dihydrocholecalciferol (the active form of vitamin D). Renin is made by the juxtaglomerular cells and catalyses the formation of angiotensin I and ultimately aldosterone synthesis.

Clinical note

It is important to take the patient's age and sex into account when interpreting GFR results. For example, the GFR of 58 mL/min/1.73 m² seen in the elderly lady in Fig. 15.3 may simply reflect the physiological decline of GFR with age rather than renal pathology requiring investigation.

Investigation of renal function (1)

- Serum creatinine concentration is an insensitive index of renal function, as it may not appear to be elevated until the GFR has fallen below 50% of normal.
- eGFR is an improvement on serum creatinine but is an estimate and should be interpreted cautiously.
- Proteinuria may be used as a marker of renal damage and predicts its progression.

Case history 8

A 35-year-old man presenting with loin pain has a serum creatinine of 150 µmol/L. A 24-hour urine of 2160 mL is collected and found to have a creatinine concentration of 7.5 mmol/L.

- Calculate the creatinine clearance and comment on the results.
- An error in the timed collection was subsequently reported by the nursing staff, and collection time was reported to be 17 hours.
- How does this affect the result and its interpretation?
  Comment in Case history comments.

Want to know more?

Preiss DJ, Godber IM, Lamb EJ, et al. The influence of a cooked-meat meal on estimated glomerular filtration rate. *Ann Clin Biochem*. 2007;44: 35-42. Available online at http://journals.sagepub.com/doi/pdf/10.1258/000456307779595995.

This is a nice little study showing the effect on serum creatinine, and eGFR, of ingesting cooked meat. Median eGFR fell from 84.0 mL/min/1.73 m² to 59.5 mL/min/1.73 m² after consumption of cooked meat.

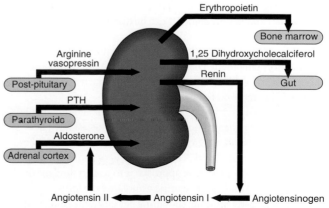

Fig. 15.4 Endocrine links in the kidney. *PTH*, Parathyroid hormone.

16 | Investigation of renal function (2)

Renal tubular function

The glomeruli provide an efficient filtration mechanism for ridding the body of waste products and toxic substances. To ensure that important constituents are not lost from the body, tubular reabsorption must be equally efficient. Approximately 180 L of fluid passes into the glomerular filtrate each day, and more than 99% of this is recovered. However, compared with glomerular filtration rate as a global assessment of glomerular function, there is no single measure of tubular function that plays a similar role, although urine osmolality is sometimes used as a crude proxy (see later).

Tubular dysfunction

Some disorders of tubular function are inherited, e.g. the ability of some patients to acidify urine is limited by a failure of hydrogen ion secretion. However, renal tubular damage is much more frequently secondary to other conditions or insults. Any cause of acute kidney injury may be associated with renal tubular failure.

Investigation of tubular function

Osmolality measurements in plasma and urine

Although the renal tubules perform a bewildering array of functions, urine osmolality serves as a useful general marker of tubular function. This is because, of all tubular functions, the one most frequently affected by disease is the ability to concentrate urine. If the tubules and collecting ducts are working efficiently, and if arginine vasopressin (AVP) is present, they will be able to reabsorb water. Just how well can be assessed by measuring urine concentration (osmolality) and *comparing this to the plasma (serum) osmolality*. If the urine osmolality is 600 mmol/kg or more, tubular function is usually regarded as intact. When the urine osmolality does not differ greatly from plasma (urine/plasma osmolality ratio ~1), the renal tubules are not reabsorbing water.

The water deprivation test

Where measurement of baseline urine osmolality is inconclusive, formal evaluation of tubular concentrating ability may be indicated. This is conventionally done by the *water deprivation test*. The body normally retains water in response to water deprivation, thereby minimising the rise in plasma osmolality that would otherwise be observed. It does this by secreting AVP, the action of which on the renal tubules may be inferred from a rising urine osmolality. In practice, if the urine osmolality rises to 600 mmol/kg or more in response to water deprivation, serious disruption of the water axis is effectively excluded. A flat urine osmolality response is characteristically seen in diabetes insipidus (DI) where AVP is lacking (central DI) or not working (nephrogenic DI). Central and nephrogenic DI can be distinguished by the urine osmolality response to the administration of exogenous AVP (desmopressin (DDAVP)). In central DI the renal tubules respond normally to the DDAVP and the urine osmolality rises. In nephrogenic DI the urine osmolality response remains flat (the tubules fail to respond to DDAVP).

Water deprivation is unpleasant for the patient and potentially dangerous if the patient cannot retain water. (The test must be terminated if more than 3 L of urine are passed or there is a fall of >3% in body weight.) For this reason, instead of a formal water deprivation test, an alternative approach is to restrict fluid overnight (8 p.m.–10 a.m.) and measure urine osmolality the following morning in an early morning spot urine. Recently, measurement of copeptin, a precursor of AVP, has been examined as an alternative to the water deprivation test (see 'Want to know more?').

Renal tubular dysfunction is one of several causes of disordered water homeostasis. The causes of polyuria are summarised in Table 16.1.

Renal tubular acidosis

Renal tubular acidosis (RTA) is simply a metabolic acidosis (low serum bicarbonate) resulting from defective renal tubular function, specifically relating to its ability to handle hydrogen and bicarbonate. The main subtypes involve either impaired hydrogen ion secretion in the distal tubule (inherited or acquired) or reduced capacity to reabsorb bicarbonate in the proximal tubule. In addition to these primary defects in renal tubular function, bicarbonate reabsorption by the renal tubule may be impaired by reduced renal action of aldosterone (due to deficiency, receptor defects or aldosterone antagonists).

RTA is usually suspected where a low bicarbonate cannot be explained by other means, particularly where the anion gap is normal (see Chapter 22, The anion gap). Measurement of urine pH can be helpful in securing – or excluding – the diagnosis. A *fresh* urine specimen should be collected. (If the specimen is not fresh, urease-splitting bacteria may alkalinise the specimen post-collection, giving a falsely high urine pH.) The normal response to metabolic acidosis is to increase acid excretion, and a urine pH of less than 5.3 makes RTA unlikely as the cause of the acidosis.

Where the baseline urine pH is not convincingly acidic, by analogy with the water deprivation test mentioned earlier, the renal tubular ability to handle hydrogen and bicarbonate may be stressed by making the blood more acidic (by giving ammonium chloride) and measuring the urine pH serially. This test is very unpleasant for the patient and may be associated with vomiting. A more acceptable alternative is to administer furosemide, which reduces reabsorption of chloride and sodium from the loop of Henle. This increases the delivery of sodium to the distal tubule, where it is normally reabsorbed in exchange for hydrogen ions, thereby producing acidic urine. Failure to produce at least one urine sample with a pH less than 5.3 in response to either ammonium chloride or furosemide is consistent with RTA.

Specific proteinuria

The appearance of abnormal amounts of protein in urine may indicate 'leaky' glomeruli. α_1-microglobulin and β_2-microglobulin are small proteins filtered at the glomeruli, but usually they are reabsorbed by the tubular cells. An increased concentration of these proteins in urine is a sensitive indicator of renal tubular cell damage. Proteinuria is discussed in detail in Chapter 18.

Glycosuria

The presence of glucose in urine when blood glucose is normal usually reflects the inability of the tubules to reabsorb glucose

Table 16.1 **Causes of polyuria**

Cause	Urine Osmolality	Plasma Osmolality
	mmol/kg	
Increased osmotic load, e.g. due to glucose	~500	~310
Increased water ingestion	<200	~280
Central (cranial) diabetes insipidus	<200	~300
Nephrogenic diabetes insipidus	<200	~300

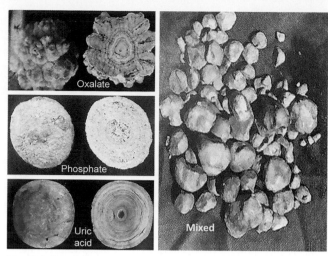

Fig. 16.1 Renal stones.

Investigation of renal function (2)

- Specific tests are available to measure urinary concentrating ability and the ability to excrete an acid load.
- A comparison of urine and serum osmolality measurements will indicate if a patient is able to concentrate urine.
- Chemical examination of urine is one aspect of urinalysis.
- The presence of specific small proteins in urine indicates tubular damage.
- Analysis of renal stones is important in the investigation of their aetiology.

Case history 9

A 30-year-old woman fractured her skull in an accident. She had no other major injuries, she had no significant blood loss, and her cardiovascular system was stable. She was unconscious for 2 days after the accident. On the fourth day of her admission to hospital, she was noted to be producing large volumes of urine and complaining of thirst. Biochemical findings were:

Na^+	K^+	Cl^-	HCO_3^-	Urea	Creatinine	Glucose
		mmol/L			μmol/L	mmol/L
150	3.6	106	25	5.5	80	5.4

Serum osmolality = 310 mmol/kg
Urine osmolality = 110 mmol/kg
Urine volume = 8 L/24 h

- Is a water deprivation test required to make the diagnosis in this patient?
Comment in Case history comments.

because of a specific tubular lesion. Here, the renal threshold (the capacity for the tubules to reabsorb the substance in question) has been exceeded. This is called *renal glycosuria* and is benign. Glycosuria also can present in association with other disorders of tubular function, e.g. the Fanconi syndrome.

Aminoaciduria

Normally, amino acids in the glomerular filtrate are reabsorbed in the proximal tubules. They may be present in urine in excessive amounts because either the plasma concentration exceeds the renal threshold or there is specific failure of normal tubular reabsorptive mechanisms. The latter may occur in the inherited metabolic disorder cystinuria or more commonly because of acquired renal tubular damage.

Specific tubular defects

The Fanconi syndrome

The Fanconi syndrome is a term used to describe the occurrence of generalised tubular defects and is generally characterised by glycosuria, phosphaturia and aminoaciduria. It can occur as a result of heavy metal poisoning or from the effects of toxins and inherited metabolic diseases such as cystinosis.

Renal stones

Renal stones (calculi) produce severe pain and discomfort and are common causes of obstruction in the urinary tract (Fig. 16.1). Analysis of renal stones (by infrared spectroscopy or X-ray diffraction) and biochemical analysis of urine is important in the investigation of why stones have formed. Types of stone include:

- *Calcium phosphate*: may be a consequence of primary hyperparathyroidism or RTA.
- *Magnesium, ammonium and phosphate*: are often associated with urinary tract infections.
- *Oxalate*: may be a consequence of hyperoxaluria.
- *Uric acid*: may be a consequence of hyperuricaemia (see Chapter 74).
- *Cystine*: are rare and a feature of the inherited metabolic disorder cystinuria (see Chapter 84).

Want to know more?

Penney MD, Oleesky DA. Renal tubular acidosis. *Ann Clin Biochem.* 1999;36:408-422. Available online at http://journals.sagepub.com/doi/pdf/10.1177/000456329903600403

This review, written some years ago, provides a very useful algorithm for investigation of suspected RTA, as well as a table comparing the key features of the different types of RTA.

European Association of Urology Guideline on Urolithiasis – http://uroweb.org/guideline/urolithiasis/

This guideline recommends which patients with renal stones should be further investigated for an underlying cause and discusses how to investigate them.

Refardt J, Winzeler B, Christ-Crain M. Copeptin and its role in the diagnosis of diabetes insipidus and the syndrome of inappropriate antidiuresis. *Clin Endocrinol.* 2019;91:22–32. doi:10.1111/cen.13991

AVP is difficult to measure, and is only available in a small number of specialised centres. Copeptin, its precursor, is easier to measure. This review provides a useful perspective on its potential role in the diagnosis of disorders of the water axis.

17 | Urinalysis

Urinalysis is so important in screening for disease that it is regarded as an integral part of the complete physical examination of every patient and not just in the investigation of renal disease. Urinalysis comprises a range of analyses that are usually performed at the point of care rather than in a central laboratory. Examination of a patient's urine should not be restricted to biochemical tests. Fig. 17.1 summarises the different ways urine may be examined.

Procedure

Biochemical testing of urine involves the use of commercially available disposable strips (Fig. 17.2). Each strip is impregnated with a number of coloured reagent "blocks" separated from each other by narrow bands. When the strip is manually immersed in the urine specimen, the reagents in each block react with a specific component of urine in such a way that (1) the block changes colour if the component is present and (2) the colour change produced is proportional to the concentration of the component being tested for.

To test a urine sample:
- fresh urine is collected into a clean, dry container
- the sample is not centrifuged
- the disposable strip is briefly immersed in the urine specimen; care must be taken to ensure that all reagent blocks are covered
- the edge of the strip is held against the rim of the urine container to remove any excess urine
- the strip is then held in a horizontal position for a fixed length of time that varies from 30 seconds to 2 minutes
- the colours of the test areas are compared with those provided on a colour chart (see Fig. 17.2). The strip is held close to the colour blocks on the chart, matched carefully and then discarded.

The range of components routinely tested for in commonly available commercial urinalysis strips is extensive and includes glucose, bilirubin, ketones, specific gravity, blood, pH (hydrogen ion concentration), protein, urobilinogen, nitrite and leucocytes (white blood cells).

Urinalysis is one of the commonest biochemical tests performed outside the laboratory. It is most commonly performed by non-laboratory staff. Although the test is simple, failure to follow the correct procedure may lead to inaccurate results. A frequent example of this is where test strips are read too quickly or left too long. Other potential errors may arise because test strips have been stored wrongly or are out of date. As an alternative to manual strip testing of urine, many areas now use automated point-of-care analysers for urinalysis, e.g. ketone meters.

Glucose

The presence of glucose in urine (glycosuria) indicates that the filtered load of glucose exceeds the ability of the renal tubules to reabsorb all of it. This usually reflects hyperglycaemia and, therefore, should prompt consideration of whether more formal testing for diabetes mellitus is appropriate, e.g. by measuring fasting blood glucose. However, glycosuria is not always due to diabetes. The renal threshold for glucose may be lowered, e.g. in pregnancy, and glucose may enter the filtrate even at normal plasma concentrations (renal glycosuria).

Blood glucose rises rapidly after a meal, overcoming the normal renal threshold temporarily (alimentary glycosuria). Both renal and alimentary glycosuria are unrelated to diabetes.

Bilirubin

Bilirubin exists in the blood in two forms: conjugated and unconjugated. Only the conjugated form is water-soluble, so bilirubinuria signifies the presence in urine of conjugated bilirubin. This is always pathological. Conjugated bilirubin is normally excreted through the biliary tree into the gut, where it is broken down; a small amount is reabsorbed into the portal circulation, taken up by the liver and reexcreted in bile. Interruption of this so-called enterohepatic circulation usually stems from mechanical obstruction and results in high levels of conjugated bilirubin in the systemic circulation, some of which spills over into the urine.

Urobilinogen

In the gut, conjugated bilirubin is broken down by bacteria to products known collectively as faecal urobilinogen or stercobilinogen. This too undergoes an enterohepatic circulation. However, unlike conjugated bilirubin, urobilinogen is found in the systemic circulation and is often detectable in the urine of normal subjects. Thus the finding of urobilinogen in urine is of less diagnostic significance than the finding of bilirubin. High levels are found in any condition in which bilirubin turnover is increased, e.g. haemolysis, or where its enterohepatic circulation is interrupted, e.g. by liver damage.

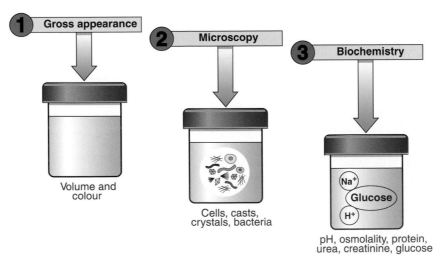

Fig. 17.1 The place of biochemical testing in urinalysis.

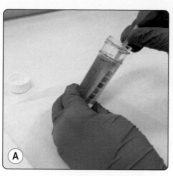 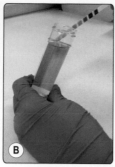 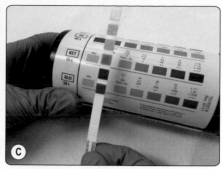

Fig. 17.2 Multistix testing of a urine sample. (A) Immersion of test strip in urine specimen. **(B)** Excess urine removed. **(C)** Test strip is compared with colour chart on bottle label.

Ketones

Ketones are products of fatty acid breakdown. Their presence usually indicates that the body is using fat to provide energy rather than storing it for later use. This can occur in uncontrolled diabetes, in which glucose is unable to enter cells (diabetic ketoacidosis), in alcoholism (alcoholic ketoacidosis) or in association with fasting or vomiting.

Specific gravity

This is a semi-quantitative measure of urinary density, which in turn reflects concentration. A higher specific gravity indicates a more concentrated urine. Assessment of urinary specific gravity usually just confirms the impression gained by visually inspecting the colour of the urine. When urine concentration needs to be quantitated, most people will request urine osmolality, which has a much wider working range.

pH (hydrogen ion concentration)

Urine is usually acidic (urine pH substantially less than 7.4 indicating a high concentration of hydrogen ions). Measurement of urine pH is useful either in cases of suspected adulteration, e.g. drug screens, or where there is an unexplained metabolic acidosis (low serum bicarbonate). The renal tubules normally excrete hydrogen ions by mechanisms that ensure tight regulation of the blood hydrogen ion concentration. Where one or more of these mechanisms fail, an acidosis results (see Chapter 16, Renal tubular acidosis). Measurement of urine pH, therefore, may be used to screen for RTA in unexplained metabolic acidosis; a pH less than 5.3 indicates that the renal tubules are able to acidify urine and, thus, are unlikely to be responsible for the metabolic acidosis.

Protein

Proteinuria may signify abnormal excretion of protein by the kidneys (due to abnormally "leaky" glomeruli or to the inability of the tubules to reabsorb protein normally), or it may simply reflect the presence in the urine of cells or blood. For this reason it is important to check that the dipstick test is not also positive for blood or leucocytes (white cells); it may also be appropriate to screen for a urinary tract infection by sending urine for microbiological investigation. Proteinuria and its causes are discussed in detail in Chapter 18.

Blood

The presence of blood in the urine (haematuria) is consistent with various possibilities ranging from malignancy through urinary tract infection to contamination from menstruation. Dipstick tests for blood are able to detect haemoglobin and myoglobin in addition to red blood cells – the presence in the urine sediment of large numbers of red cells establishes the diagnosis of haematuria. The absence of red cells, despite a strongly positive dipstick test for blood, points towards myoglobinuria or haemoglobinuria.

Nitrite

This dipstick test depends on the conversion of nitrate (from the diet) to nitrite by the action in the urine of bacteria that contain the necessary reductase. A positive result points towards a urinary tract infection.

Leucocytes

The presence of leucocytes in the urine suggests acute inflammation and the presence of a urinary tract infection.

Clinical note

Microbiological testing of a urine specimen (usually a mid-stream specimen) is routinely performed to confirm the diagnosis of a urinary tract infection. These samples should be collected into sterile containers and sent to the laboratory without delay for analysis, which may include culture and antibiotic sensitivity tests.

Urinalysis

- Urinalysis should be part of the clinical examination of every patient.
- Chemical analysis of a urine specimen is carried out using commercially available disposable strips.
- The range of components routinely tested for includes glucose, bilirubin, ketones, specific gravity, blood, pH, protein, urobilinogen, nitrite and leucocytes.

Case history 10

A patient attending an obesity clinic is found to have ketonuria on urinalysis. There is no glycosuria, and point-of-care blood glucose measurement using a meter is 5.9 mmol/L.

- What might explain these findings?
  Comment in Case history comments.

Want to know more?

http://emedicine.medscape.com/article/2074001-overview

For those wanting more detail about urinalysis, the Medscape site provides a comprehensive but accessible account. (In order to access the above link – and one or two other "Want to know more" links in this book – registration is required. It is worth the effort – overall this is a very useful resource. All content is available free of charge.)

18 | Proteinuria

Proteinuria refers to abnormal urinary excretion of protein. Detection of proteinuria is important. It is associated with renal and cardiovascular disease; it identifies people with diabetes who are at risk of nephropathy and other microvascular complications; and it predicts end-organ damage in people with hypertension. Although proteinuria may arise through various mechanisms (see later), it is most often an indication of abnormal glomerular function. It can be measured and expressed in various ways.

Mechanisms of proteinuria

The mechanisms of proteinuria are shown in Fig. 18.1.

Glomerular proteinuria

The glomerular basement membrane through which blood is filtered does not usually allow passage of albumin and large proteins, and proteinuria is most often due to abnormally "leaky" glomeruli. The extent of this "leakiness" varies enormously. At its most extreme, the glomerulus allows large quantities of protein to escape. When this happens, the ability of the body to replace the lost protein is exceeded, and the protein concentration in the patient's blood falls. Protein is measured in blood either as total protein or albumin. When patients become hypoproteinaemic and hypoalbuminaemic due to excessive proteinuria, the normal balance of oncotic and hydrostatic forces at the capillary level is disturbed, leading to loss of fluid into the interstitial space (oedema). This is known as the *nephrotic syndrome* (defined in terms of protein excretion as >3 g/day) – see Fig. 18.2 for an example of pitting oedema in a patient with nephrotic syndrome.

Tubular proteinuria

Some proteins are so small that, unlike albumin and other larger proteins, they pass through the glomerulus freely. The best-known examples are α_1-microglobulin and β_2-microglobulin. Others include retinol-binding protein and N-acetyl-glucosaminidase. If these proteins are detected in excess in the urine, this reflects tubular rather than glomerular dysfunction, i.e. an inability of the renal tubules to reabsorb them. However, tubular function is normally investigated in other ways, and the measurement of these proteins in urine is normally confined to the screening and detection of chronic asymptomatic tubular dysfunction or to a small number of specific clinical scenarios, e.g. toxicity due to aminoglycosides, lithium or mercury.

Overflow proteinuria

Overflow proteinuria occurs when the ability of the glomeruli to hold back proteins is overwhelmed by the sheer quantity of protein. The best-characterised example of overflow proteinuria is seen in multiple myeloma. This condition involves malignant proliferation of a clone of plasma cells (a special kind of lymphocyte, the function of which is to produce immunoglobulins). This results in the production of vast amounts of the immunoglobulin produced by the malignant clone. In this kind of proteinuria, the glomeruli are normal (at least initially). Bence-Jones proteins are light chain fragments of immunoglobulin that can be detected in the urine – see Fig. 18.3

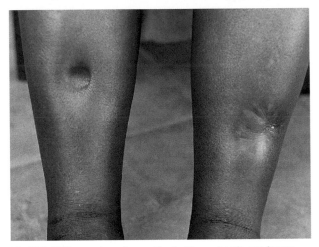

Fig 18.2 Pitting oedema in a patient with nephrotic syndrome.

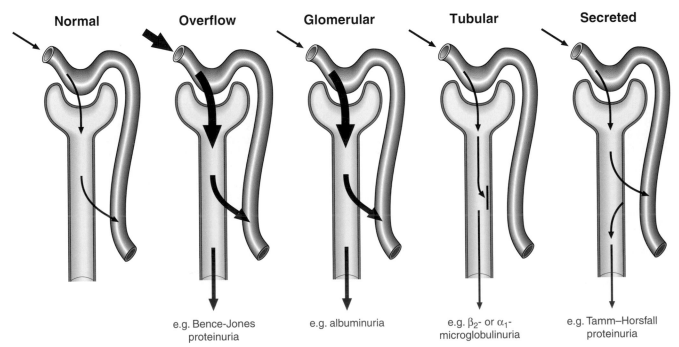

Fig. 18.1 Mechanisms of proteinuria.

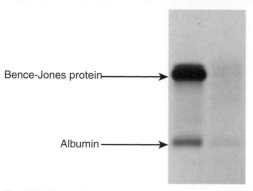

Bence-Jones protein

Albumin

Fig. 18.3 Bence-Jones protein detected by urine electrophoresis.

for an example of Bence-Jones protein being detected in urine by electrophoresis, a technique which is described in Chapter 26.

Tamm–Horsfall proteinuria

This glycoprotein gets its name from the authors of a 1952 paper describing its purification. It is one of the most abundant proteins in urine. Its significance lies in the fact that, unlike the other proteins mentioned earlier, it is not derived from the blood, but rather is produced and secreted into the filtrate by the thick ascending limb of the loop of Henle. It forms large aggregates that, when concentrated, can form urinary casts (gel-like cylindrical structures that reflect the shape of the renal tubules) that may get dislodged and pass into the urine.

Ways of measuring proteinuria

Proteinuria is detected and quantified in a variety of ways.

Dipstick urinalysis

The procedure for dipstick urine testing is shown in Fig. 17.2 in Chapter 17. Dipsticks are commercially available disposable strips, impregnated with coloured reagent blocks, which are immersed in urine. The reagents in each block react with a specific component of urine in such a way that the block changes colour if the component is present. Protein is just one of several components tested for; others include glucose, blood and bilirubin.

Dipstick testing is the most widely used method of screening for proteinuria. It is convenient for both patient and clinician and provides a near-instant result at the point of care. However, it gives only a rough indication of the presence or absence of pathological proteinuria and cannot be used alone to diagnose or exclude proteinuria. It must be used in conjunction with more reliable methods.

Protein/creatinine ratio

Quantitative measurement of protein in urine provides a much more reliable evaluation of proteinuria. Accuracy is further improved by measuring the urinary creatinine concentration as well and expressing the result as the protein/creatinine ratio (PCR); this corrects for variation in urine concentration. Dipstick urine testing and PCR both require a spot urine sample and so are equally convenient from a patient perspective. An early morning sample is preferred (because it correlates best with 24-hour protein excretion), but random samples are acceptable.

Urine protein excretion

A 24-hour timed urine collection for protein excretion is still sometimes used. However, timed urine collections are inconvenient and not always completely accurate. It has been suggested that

daily protein excretion (in mg/24 hours) can be 'guesstimated' by multiplying the PCR (in mg/mmol) by a factor of 10 (i.e. assuming average daily creatinine excretion of 10 mmol/day).

Albumin/creatinine ratio and 'microalbuminuria'

Methods for measuring albumin in urine are more accurate than methods for measuring protein in urine, especially at low concentrations. 'Microalbuminuria' refers to the excretion of albumin in urine in amounts that are abnormal, but not detectable by standard urine dipstick testing. (The term is misleading – the albumin excreted in microalbuminuria is exactly the same as in other proteinuric conditions.) If detected in a patient with diabetes, microalbuminuria signifies early diabetic nephropathy and therefore allows treatment with, for example, angiotensin-converting enzyme inhibitors or angiotensin receptor blockers that may help reduce the progression of kidney damage. Current guidance on classification of chronic kidney disease (CKD) places urine albumin/creatinine ratio (ACR) as a cornerstone of classification of CKD, being used in conjunction with glomerular filtration rate (GFR) to assess risk of adverse outcomes (e.g. cardiovascular events and progression of renal disease) and to guide frequency of monitoring of GFR. CKD is addressed further in Chapter 20.

Table 18.1 summarises how these different ways of expressing proteinuria relate to each other.

Table 18.1 How the different ways of expressing proteinuria relate to each other				
	Dipstick Reading	PCR (mg/ mmol)	Total Protein (g/24 h)	ACR (mg/ mmol)
Normal	Negative	<15	<0.150	<3
Microalbuminuria	Negative	<15	<0.150	3–30
Clinical proteinuria	1+	45–149	0.15–1.40	>30
	2+	150–449	1.50–4.49	
Nephrotic	3+	≥450	≥4.50	

ACR, Albumin/creatinine ratio; PCR, protein/creatinine ratio.

Clinical note

Orthostatic, or postural, proteinuria is common in teenagers. It is a benign condition in which proteinuria occurs only when the subjects are standing upright and is a result of an increase in the hydrostatic pressure in the renal veins.

Case history 11

A patient attending the hospital outpatient clinic is found to have proteinuria on dipstick testing. On examination he has pitting oedema of both ankles.

• What might explain these findings?
  Comment in Case history comments.

Want to know more?

https://www.nice.org.uk/guidance/ng203/resources/visual-summary-chronic-kidney-disease-g15-a13-managing-proteinuria-pdf-9206256495

Albumin/creatinine ratio is key to clinical decision making, especially in people with diabetes or hypertension. This visual summary from the NICE guideline on chronic kidney disease demonstrates how results influence decisions about treatment.

19 | Acute kidney injury

Acute kidney injury (AKI) refers to rapid deterioration in renal function. It is common, occurring in 13% to 18% of people admitted to hospital. In AKI, renal function deteriorates over a period of hours or days. Chronic kidney disease (CKD) develops over months or years and leads eventually to end-stage kidney disease.

Aetiology

AKI arises from a variety of problems affecting the kidneys and/or their circulation. It usually presents as a sudden deterioration of renal function indicated by rapidly rising serum creatinine and urea concentrations. As AKI is common in the severely ill, sequential monitoring of kidney function is important for early detection in this group of patients.

Fig. 19.1 summarises the causes of AKI. They may be:
- *Prerenal*. The kidney fails to receive a proper blood supply.
- *Postrenal*. The urinary drainage of the kidneys is impaired because of an obstruction.
- *Renal*. Intrinsic damage to the kidney tissue. This may be due to a variety of diseases, or the renal damage may be a consequence of prolonged prerenal or postrenal problems.

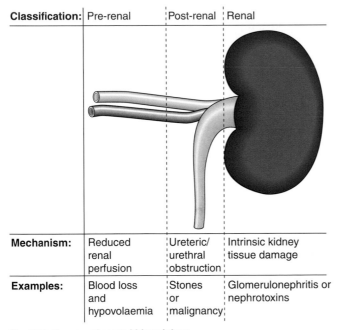

Classification:	Pre-renal	Post-renal	Renal
Mechanism:	Reduced renal perfusion	Ureteric/ urethral obstruction	Intrinsic kidney tissue damage
Examples:	Blood loss and hypovolaemia	Stones or malignancy	Glomerulonephritis or nephrotoxins

Fig. 19.1 Causes of acute kidney injury.

Definition of AKI

AKI is defined technically. A patient has AKI if any one of the following is noted:
- Serum creatinine increases by 26 µmol/L or more within 48 hours.
- Serum creatinine increases by 50% or more within the past 7 days (or is presumed to have occurred within the past 7 days).
- Urine output decreases to less than 0.5 mL/kg/hour for more than 6 hours in adults and more than 8 hours in children and young people.
- Estimated glomerular filtration rate (eGFR) decreases by 25% or more in children and young people in the past 7 days.

AKI can be staged as detailed in the Kidney Disease: Improving Global Outcomes (KDIGO) guidance (Table 19.1). Clinical biochemistry departments are increasingly implementing automated systems to alert clinicians to the presence of AKI. It is important that clinical pathways have been agreed upon beforehand with renal specialists and other clinicians so that it is clear what action should be taken when AKI is detected.

Identifying the cause of AKI

The first step in assessing the patient with AKI is to identify any pre- or postrenal factors that could be readily corrected and allow recovery of renal function. The history and examination of the patient, including the presence of other severe illness, drug history and time course of the onset of the AKI, may well provide important clues. Factors that precipitate prerenal uraemia are usually associated with a reduced effective extracellular fluid (ECF) volume and include:
- decreased plasma volume because of prolonged vomiting or diarrhoea, blood loss, or burns
- diminished cardiac output
- local factors, such as an occlusion of the renal artery.

Prerenal factors lead to decreased renal perfusion and reduction in GFR. Both arginine vasopressin and aldosterone are secreted maximally, and a small volume of concentrated urine is produced.

Biochemical findings in prerenal uraemia include the following:
- *Serum urea and creatinine are increased*. Urea is increased more than creatinine because of its reabsorption by the tubular cells, particularly at low urine flow rates. Creatinine is not so readily reabsorbed.
- *Metabolic acidosis*. Occurs because of the inability of the kidney to excrete hydrogen ions and acidic organic anions.
- *Hyperkalaemia*. Occurs because of the decreased GFR and acidosis.
- *A high urine osmolality*.

Postrenal factors cause decreased renal function because the effective filtration pressure at the glomeruli is reduced due to the back pressure caused by the blockage. Causes include:
- *Renal stones*.
- *Carcinoma of cervix, prostate or bladder*.

If these pre- or postrenal factors are not corrected, patients will develop intrinsic renal damage (acute tubular necrosis (ATN)).

Acute tubular necrosis

ATN may develop in the absence of preexisting prerenal or postrenal kidney disease. The causes include:
- acute blood loss in severe trauma
- septic shock
- specific renal disease, such as glomerulonephritis

Table 19.1 **Staging of Acute Kidney Injury (AKI)**		
Stage	**Serum Creatinine**	**Urine Output**
1	1.5–1.9 times baseline OR ≥26 µmol/L increase	<0.5 mL/kg/h for 6–12 h
2	2.0–2.9 times baseline	<0.5 mL/kg/h for ≥12 h
3	3.0 times baseline OR increase in serum creatinine to ≥354 µmol/L OR initiation of renal replacement therapy OR, in patients <18 y, decrease in eGFR to <35 mL/min/1.73 m²	<0.3 mL/kg/h for >24 h OR anuria for >12 h

eGFR, Estimated glomerular filtration rate.

- nephrotoxins, such as aminoglycosides, analgesics or herbal toxins.

Patients in the early stages of ATN may have only modestly increased serum urea and creatinine that then rise rapidly over a period of days, in contrast to the slow increase over months and years seen in CKD.

Management

Important issues in the management of the patient with AKI include:

- Correction of prerenal factors, if present, by replacement of any ECF volume deficit. Care should be taken that the patient does not become fluid overloaded.
- Treatment of the underlying disease (e.g. to control infection).
- Biochemical monitoring. Daily fluid balance charts provide an assessment of body fluid volume. Serum creatinine indicates the degree of impairment of the GFR and the rate of deterioration or improvement. Potassium should be monitored closely.
- Dialysis. Indications for dialysis include a rapidly rising serum potassium concentration, severe acidosis and fluid overload.

Recovery

There may be three distinct phases in the resolving clinical course of a patient with AKI (Fig. 19.2). An initial oliguric phase, in which glomerular impairment predominates, is followed by a diuretic phase when urine output is high, as glomerular function slowly improves but tubular function remains impaired. During a recovery phase, complete renal function may return. Careful clinical and biochemical monitoring is necessary throughout the course of the patient's illness.

It should be noted that initially the urea and creatinine may be normal in AKI. The serum potassium usually rises very quickly in catabolic patients, with or without tissue damage, and falls quickly once the urine flow rate increases. The urine volume cannot be related to the GFR. The serum urea and creatinine remain high during the diuretic phase because the GFR is still low and the large urine volumes reflect tubular damage. In the recovery phase the serum urea and creatinine fall as the GFR improves and the serum potassium concentration returns to normal as the tubular mechanisms recover.

Clinical note

Acute tubular necrosis (ATN) is the commonest cause of severe life-threatening hyperkalaemia. The rapidly increasing serum potassium is usually the indication to start the patient on dialysis.

Acute kidney injury

- Acute kidney injury (AKI) is characterised by an increase in serum creatinine and/or a decrease in urine output over a period of hours or days. AKI may be caused by prerenal, renal or postrenal factors.
- Prompt identification of pre- or postrenal factors may allow correction of the problem before damage to nephrons occurs.
- Management of a patient with intrinsic renal damage will include sequential measurement of creatinine, sodium, potassium, phosphate and bicarbonate in serum and may require measurement of urine sodium and potassium excretion and osmolality.
- Care should be taken to prevent fluid overload in the treatment of patients with renal disease.
- Life-threatening hyperkalaemia may be a consequence of AKI.

Case history 12

A 50-year-old man presented with pyrexia. He was clinically dehydrated and oliguric.

Na^+	K^+	Cl^-	HCO_3^-	Urea	Creatinine
		mmol/L			μmol/L
140	5.9	112	162	2.9	155

Serum osmolality = 305 mmol/kg
Urine osmolality = 629 mmol/kg

- What do these biochemistry results indicate about the patient's condition?
  Comment in Case history comments.

Want to know more?

https://www.nice.org.uk/guidance/ng148

Acute kidney injury: prevention, detection and management. National Institute for Health and Care Excellence (NICE) Guideline 148

https://kdigo.org/guidelines/acute-kidney-injury/

Kidney Disease: Improving Global Outcomes (KDIGO) Clinical Practice Guideline for Acute Kidney Injury.

These publications are two key sources of clinical guidance about how to prevent, detect and manage acute kidney injury (AKI).

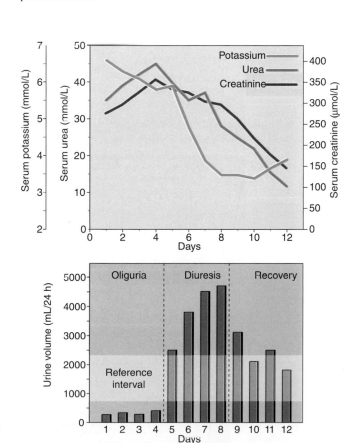

Fig. 19.2 The biochemical course of a typical patient with acute kidney injury.

20 | Chronic kidney disease

Chronic kidney disease (CKD) encompasses abnormalities of kidney function or structure which are present for more than 3 months and have adverse effects on health. Patients with CKD may have mild, nonspecific symptoms until the glomerular filtration rate (GFR) falls below 15 mL/min (i.e. to 10% of normal function) and the disease is far advanced.

Consequences of CKD

Sodium and water metabolism

Most patients with CKD retain the ability to reabsorb sodium ions, but the renal tubules may lose their ability to reabsorb water and so concentrate urine. The polyuria that would normally result may be partly masked because the GFR is so low. Because of their impaired ability to regulate water balance, patients with renal disease may become fluid overloaded or fluid depleted very easily.

Potassium metabolism

Hyperkalaemia is a feature of advanced CKD and poses a threat to life (Fig. 20.1). The ability to excrete potassium decreases as the GFR falls, but hyperkalaemia may not be a major problem in CKD until the GFR falls to very low levels. Then, a sudden deterioration of renal function may precipitate a rapid rise in serum potassium concentration. An unexpectedly high serum potassium concentration in an outpatient should always be investigated with urgency.

Acid–base balance

As CKD progresses, the ability of the kidneys to regenerate bicarbonate and excrete hydrogen ions in the urine becomes impaired. The retention of hydrogen ions causes metabolic acidosis.

Calcium and phosphate metabolism

The ability of the renal cells to make 1,25-dihydroxycholecalciferol (the active form of vitamin D) falls as the renal tubular damage progresses. Calcium absorption from the gut is reduced, and there is a tendency towards hypocalcaemia. Phosphate retention, along with low calcium, induces a rise in parathyroid hormone (PTH), and the latter may have adverse effects on bone if this is allowed to continue (Fig. 20.2).

Erythropoietin synthesis

Anaemia is often associated with CKD. The normochromic normocytic anaemia is due primarily to failure of renal production of erythropoietin. Recombinant human erythropoietin may be used to treat the anaemia of CKD.

Clinical features

These are illustrated in Fig. 20.3. Early in CKD, the normal reduction in urine formation when the patient is recumbent and

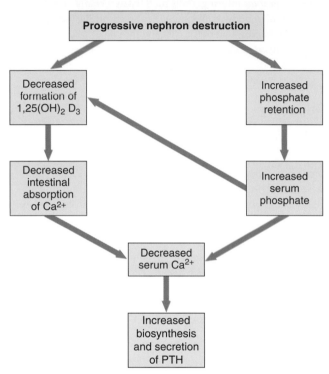

Fig. 20.2 How hypocalcaemia and secondary hyperparathyroidism develop in renal disease. *PTH*, Parathyroid hormone.

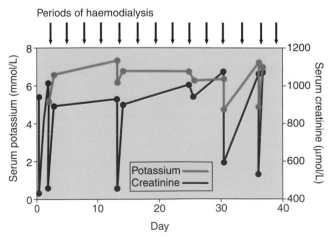

Fig. 20.1 The biochemical course of a typical patient with chronic kidney disease (CKD). Note that biochemical analyses have not been performed before and after all periods of dialysis.

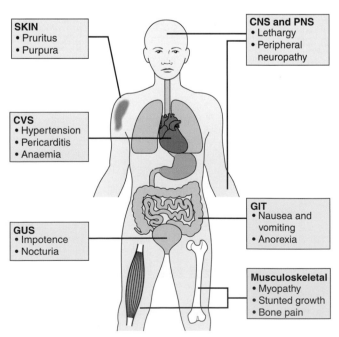

Fig. 20.3 The clinical consequences of chronic kidney disease (CKD). *CNS*, Central nervous system; *CVS*, cardiovascular system; *GIT*, gastrointestinal tract; *GUS*, genitourinary system; *PNS*, peripheral nervous system.

asleep is lost. Patients who do not experience daytime polyuria may nevertheless have nocturia as their presenting symptom.

Detection

It is important to identify CKD early so that measures can be taken to slow progression of CKD and treat other cardiovascular risk factors. Factors indicating increased risk of CKD include diabetes mellitus and hypertension, and people with these risk factors should have renal function monitored.

Classification

CKD is classified on the basis of GFR and proteinuria. The most widely used system is the Kidney Disease: Improving Global Outcomes (KDIGO) system, shown in Fig. 20.4. Proteinuria is expressed as the albumin/creatinine ratio (ACR) (Chapter 18). A patient with a GFR of 20 mL/min/1.73 m^2 and urine ACR of 20 mg/mmol, for example, would be classified as CKD G4A2. Increased ACR and decreased GFR are each associated with increased risk of adverse outcomes, and the combination of both multiplies the risk of adverse outcomes. Fig. 20.4 is colour-coded so that increased risk is easily visualised.

Management

In some cases it may be possible to treat the cause of the CKD and at least delay the progression of the disease. Important considerations are:

- Blood pressure should be aggressively controlled in order to slow deterioration of GFR and reduce proteinuria.
- People with CKD should receive dietary advice about potassium, phosphate, calorie and salt intake.
- The administration of hydroxylated vitamin D metabolites may be needed to prevent the development of CKD-related mineral and bone disorders. There is a risk of hypercalcaemia with this treatment.

Some patients with CKD will eventually require dialysis, in which case these conservative measures must be continued. In contrast, after a successful kidney transplant, normal renal function is reestablished.

Dialysis

Haemodialysis and peritoneal dialysis will sustain life when other measures can no longer maintain fluid, electrolyte and acid–base balance. The key to dialysis is the provision of a semipermeable membrane through which ions and small molecules, present in plasma at high concentration, can diffuse into the low concentrations of a rinsing fluid. In haemodialysis, an artificial membrane is used. In peritoneal dialysis, the dialysis fluid is placed in the peritoneal cavity, and molecules move out of the blood vessels of the peritoneal wall.

Note that haemodialysis and peritoneal dialysis may relieve many of the symptoms of end-stage kidney disease and rectify abnormal fluid and electrolyte and acid–base balance. These treatments do not, however, reverse the other metabolic, endocrine and haematological consequences of CKD.

Renal transplant

Although transplant of a kidney restores almost all of the renal functions, patients require long-term immunosuppression. Ciclosporin is an immunosuppressant which is nephrotoxic at high concentrations, and monitoring of both creatinine and ciclosporin is necessary to balance the fine line between rejection (due to too little ciclosporin) and renal damage (due to too much).

Clinical note

It is important to note that people who have chronic kidney disease (CKD) are at increased risk of cardiovascular disease, and other risk factors for cardiovascular disease should be managed appropriately.

Chronic kidney disease

- CKD is a long-term condition caused by usually irreversible damage to both kidneys and associated with ill health.
- Patients with CKD may be without symptoms until the glomerular filtration rate (GFR) falls to very low values.
- Consequences of CKD include disordered water and sodium metabolism, hyperkalaemia, abnormal calcium and phosphate metabolism and anaemia.

Case history 13

A 40-year-old woman with end-stage kidney disease is being treated by haemodialysis. Her serum biochemistry just prior to her last dialysis showed:

Na^+	K^+	Cl^-	HCO_3^-	Urea	Creatinine
		mmol/L			μmol/L
129	5.7	100	17	25.5	1430

- What is the significance of these results?
- What other biochemical tests should be performed, and how might the results influence treatment?
  Comment in Case history comments.

Prognosis of CKD by GFR and albuminuria categories				Albuminuria categories Description and range		
				A1	**A2**	**A3**
				Normal to mildly increased	Moderately increased	Severely increased
				<30 mg/g <3 mg/mmol	30–299 mg/g 3–29 mg/mmol	≥300 mg/g ≥30 mg/mmol
GFR categories (ml/min/1.73 m^2) Description and range	G1	Normal or high	≥90			
	G2	Mildly decreased	60–90			
	G3a	Mildly to moderately decreased	45–59			
	G3b	Moderately to severely decreased	30–44			
	G4	Severely decreased	15–29			
	G5	Kidney failure	<15			

Green: low risk (if no other markers of kidney disease, no CKD); Yellow: moderately increased risk; Orange: high risk; Red, very high risk. KDIGO 2012

Fig. 20.4 Classification of chronic kidney disease. *(With permission from Kidney Disease: Improving Global Outcomes (KDIGO) working group 2012. Available at: https://kdigo.org/guidelines/.)*

Want to know more?

https://www.nice.org.uk/guidance/ng203

Chronic kidney disease in adults: assessment and management. National Institute for Health and Care Excellence (NICE) Guideline NG203.

This guideline provides evidence-based recommendations to identify, classify and manage chronic kidney disease (CKD). It includes details of the Kidney Disease: Improving Global Outcomes (KDIGO) system for using glomerular filtration rate (GFR) and albumin/creatinine ratio (ACR) to classify the stage of chronic kidney disease (CKD).

21 | Acid–base: concepts and vocabulary

Hydrogen ion concentration [H⁺]

Blood [H⁺] is maintained within tight limits (35–45 nmol/L). Concentrations greater than 120 nmol/L or less than 20 nmol/L require urgent treatment; if sustained, they are incompatible with life.

[H⁺] is often expressed as pH, the negative logarithm of [H⁺]. This may be an appropriate way to express the [H⁺] of urine, which is normally profoundly acidic. However, blood is normally much less acidic than urine, and [H⁺] varies over a much narrower range. Where available, [H⁺] is preferred in the analysis of arterial blood gases. The relation between the direct linear scale of [H⁺] and the negative logarithmic scale of pH is shown in Fig. 21.1.

H⁺ production

Approximately 60 mmol H⁺ is produced by metabolism every day. If all of this were to be diluted in the extracellular fluid (ECF) ($\approx$14 L), [H⁺] would be 4 mmol/L, or 100,000 times more acidic than normal! Efficient urinary excretion of the H⁺ produced ensures that this does not happen; as a result, urine is profoundly acidic.

Metabolism also produces carbon dioxide (CO_2). In solution this converts to a weak acid (H_2CO_3, carbonic acid). The large amount of CO_2 produced by cellular activity each day could upset acid–base balance, but under normal circumstances this too is excreted, via the lungs. Only when respiratory function is impaired do problems occur.

Buffering

A buffer is a solution of a weak acid and its salt (or a weak base and its salt) that can bind H⁺ and therefore resist changes in [H⁺]. Buffering does not remove H⁺ from the body – it is a short-term solution to the problem of excess H⁺, mopping it up temporarily. Ultimately, the body must get rid of the H⁺ by renal excretion (see later). The body contains many buffers. Proteins can act as buffers; for example, haemoglobin in erythrocytes has a high capacity for binding H⁺. However, simple buffers become ineffective as the association of H⁺ and the anion of the weak acid reaches equilibrium.

In the ECF, the bicarbonate buffer system is the most important. In this system, bicarbonate (HCO_3^-) combines with H⁺ to form H_2CO_3. This dissociates almost completely to water and CO_2; the continual removal of CO_2 via the lungs means that in the bicarbonate buffer system, uniquely, equilibrium is never reached. As a result, the bicarbonate buffer system is much more effective than other buffers, being limited only by the initial concentration of bicarbonate. Only when all of the bicarbonate is used up does the system have no further buffering capacity. The ECF contains a large excess of bicarbonate, around 25 mmol/L, i.e. 25,000,000 nmol/L, relative to the normal blood [H⁺] (around 40 nmol/L).

The breakdown of carbonic acid to CO_2 and water happens relatively slowly. It is accelerated by carbonic anhydrase, which is present particularly where this reaction is most needed – in the kidneys and erythrocytes. The CO_2 that is formed can be breathed out, and the water mixes with the large body water pool.

Renal handling of H⁺ and HCO_3^-

Buffered H⁺ must eventually be excreted from the body via the kidneys. The process by which this occurs simultaneously regenerates the bicarbonate used up in buffering (Fig. 21.2). The starting point is either too much CO_2 in the blood or too little HCO_3^-, i.e. processes that would tend to increase H⁺. The finish points are (a) the excretion of H⁺ into the filtrate (urine) and (b) the simultaneous *regeneration* of bicarbonate which comes back into the blood. The reactions linking these are mediated by carbonic anhydrase and occur in distal renal tubular cells (see Fig. 21.2A). The excreted H⁺ is then buffered by, e.g. phosphate and ammonia and lost in urine (Fig. 21.3). This is the mechanism of *metabolic compensation* for a *respiratory acidosis* (see later for definitions of these terms).

The same reactions and enzyme (carbonic anhydrase) are involved in a completely separate mechanism which has a different purpose entirely, namely the reabsorption or *reclamation* of bicarbonate filtered at the glomerulus, which would otherwise be lost. The starting point here is the appearance of bicarbonate in the filtrate. Crucially, the reactions mediated by carbonic anhydrase occur in the renal tubular lumen as well as the proximal renal tubular cells (see Fig. 21.2B); as a result, the filtered bicarbonate can be 'captured' by

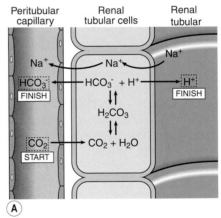

(A)

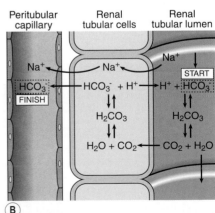

(B)

Fig. 21.2 The regeneration and reclamation of bicarbonate by the kidneys. (A) 'Regeneration' of bicarbonate – excretion of hydrogen ion. (B) 'Recovery' of bicarbonate. Note that in both processes, H⁺ is actively secreted into the urine while CO_2 diffuses along its concentration gradient.

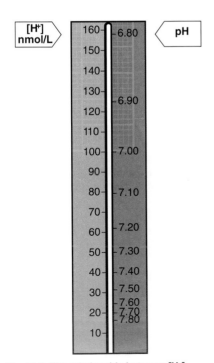

Fig. 21.1 The relationship between [H⁺] and pH.

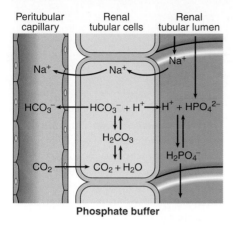

Phosphate buffer

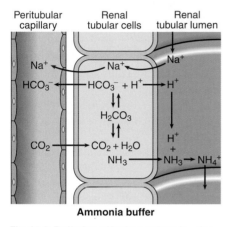

Ammonia buffer

Fig. 21.3 Buffering of hydrogen ions in urine.

secreted H⁺, forming carbonic acid and then CO_2 and water. The CO_2 diffuses back into the renal tubular cell, where bicarbonate is re-formed by the same reactions in reverse. The finish point is the return of bicarbonate to the blood from whence is came. H⁺, the other product of the cellular reactions, is recycled into the tubular lumen, meaning that there is no net loss.

Assessing status

In chemical terms, the bicarbonate buffer system can be considered in the same way as any other chemical dissociation.

$$[H^+] + [HCO_3^-] \Leftrightarrow [H_2CO_3]$$

By the law of mass action:

$$[H^+] = \frac{K[H_2CO_3]}{[HCO_3^-]}$$

where K is the first dissociation constant of carbonic acid. The carbonic acid (H_2CO_3) component is proportional to the dissolved CO_2, which is in turn proportional to the partial pressure of CO_2. [H_2CO_3] can, therefore, be replaced in the previous equation by PCO_2. In other words, the role of the bicarbonate buffer system in acid–base balance can be simply summarised thus:

$$[H^+] \propto \frac{PCO_2}{[HCO_3^-]}$$

If everything else remains constant:
- Adding H⁺, removing bicarbonate or increasing the PCO_2 will all have the same effect, i.e. an increase in [H⁺].
- Removing H⁺, adding bicarbonate or lowering PCO_2 will all cause the [H⁺] to fall.

Blood [H⁺] is controlled by our respiration and the functioning of our kidneys.

The acid–base status of the patient and the magnitude of the disturbance is usually assessed by measuring these components of the bicarbonate buffer system.

Acid–base disorders

Acid–base disorders that affect PCO_2 are termed 'respiratory' since CO_2 is exhaled by the lungs. Impaired respiratory function causes a build-up of CO_2 in blood; less commonly, hyperventilation can cause a decreased PCO_2. Acid–base disorders that cause a change in the bicarbonate concentration are termed *metabolic*. Examples include diabetes mellitus, in which altered intermediary metabolism in the absence of insulin causes a build-up of H⁺ from the ionisation of acetoacetic and β-hydroxybutyric acids (ketones), or loss of bicarbonate from the ECF, e.g. from a duodenal fistula.

Terminology

Acidosis and alkalosis are clinical terms that define the primary acid–base disturbance. They can be used even when the [H⁺] is within the normal range, i.e. when the disorders are fully compensated. The definitions are:
- *Metabolic acidosis.* The primary disorder is a decrease in bicarbonate concentration.
- *Metabolic alkalosis.* The primary disorder is an increased bicarbonate.
- *Respiratory acidosis.* The primary disorder is an increased PCO_2.

- *Respiratory alkalosis.* The primary disorder is a decreased PCO_2.

'Acidaemia' and 'alkalaemia' refer simply to whether the [H⁺] in blood is higher or lower than normal.

Compensation

The body has physiological mechanisms that try to return [H⁺] to normal when acid–base balance is deranged, termed *compensation*. Thus, where lung function is compromised, leading to a build-up of CO_2, H⁺ is excreted (and bicarbonate simultaneously regenerated) as shown in Fig. 21.2A. Such *metabolic compensation* for the primary respiratory disorder may take several days to take full effect.

In contrast, *respiratory compensation* for primary metabolic disorders occurs almost instantaneously – it takes the form of increased 'blowing off' of CO_2 by the lungs.

If compensation is complete, [H⁺] returns to normal, even though the PCO_2 and [HCO_3^-] may remain abnormal – it is their *ratio* that determines the [H⁺]; the acid–base disorder is described as *fully compensated*. A good example is stable chronic obstructive pulmonary disease. The primary problem here is inability to 'blow off' CO_2 due to the lung condition. Renal compensation ensures that the bicarbonate used up in buffering the retained CO_2 is regenerated, and eventually the ratio (and therefore [H⁺]) is restored to normal even though the CO_2 and HCO_3^- are both grossly increased. With *partial* compensation, the [H⁺] remains abnormal even though the process of restoring the ratio to normal has begun. The actual blood [H⁺] at any time in the course of an acid–base disorder is a consequence of the severity of the primary disturbance and the amount of compensation that has occurred.

Clinical note

Over-compensation cannot occur. This 'golden rule' allows clinicians to distinguish between primary and compensatory processes.

Acid–base: concepts and vocabulary

- Assessment of acid–base status involves measuring [H⁺], [HCO_3^-] and PCO_2, the components of the bicarbonate buffer system in blood.

- Adding H⁺, removing bicarbonate or increasing the PCO_2 all have the same effect – an increase in [H⁺].

- Removing H⁺, adding bicarbonate or lowering

PCO_2 all cause the [H⁺] to fall.

- Primary problems with CO_2 excretion are reflected in PCO_2; these are called 'respiratory' acid–base disorders.

- Primary problems with H⁺ production or excretion are reflected in the [HCO_3^-], and these are called 'metabolic' acid–base disorders.

- The body has physiological mechanisms that try to restore [H⁺] to normal. These processes are called 'compensation'.

- The observed [H⁺] in any acid–base disorder reflects the balance between the primary disturbance and the amount of compensation.

22 | Metabolic acid–base disorders

Metabolic acid–base disorders are caused by an increase in H+ production or a loss of H+, resulting in the loss or gain of HCO_3^-. Direct loss or gain of HCO_3^- also will cause metabolic acid–base disorders. Metabolic acid–base disorders are recognised by inspecting the bicarbonate concentration (Fig. 22.1). Respiratory compensation takes place quickly, so patients with metabolic acid–base disorders will usually show some change in blood PCO_2 because of hyperventilation or hypoventilation (Fig. 22.2).

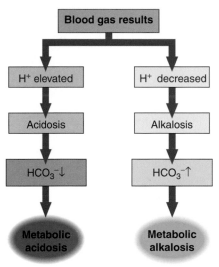

Fig. 22.1 Recognising primary metabolic acid–base disorders by inspecting the HCO_3^- concentration.

Metabolic acidosis

In metabolic acidosis the primary problem is a reduction in the bicarbonate concentration of the extracellular fluid. The main causes of metabolic acidosis are shown in Fig. 22.3. These are:
- increased production of hydrogen ions
- ingestion of hydrogen ions, drugs or other substances that are metabolised to acids
- impaired excretion of hydrogen ions by the kidneys
- loss of bicarbonate from the gastrointestinal tract or in the urine.

The anion gap

The cause of metabolic acidosis will often be apparent from the clinical history of the patient, but knowledge of the anion gap may be helpful. This can be assessed by looking at the serum electrolyte results and calculating the difference between the sum of the two main cations, sodium and potassium, and the sum of the two main anions, chloride and bicarbonate. There is no real gap, of course, as plasma proteins are negatively charged at normal [H+]. These negatively charged amino acid side chains on the proteins account for most of the apparent discrepancy when the measured electrolytes are compared. *The anion gap is thus a biochemical tool that is of help in assessing acid–base problems. It is not a physiological reality.*

In practice, because the potassium concentration is so small and will vary by so little, it is generally excluded when calculating the anion gap. Thus:

$$\text{Anion gap} = [Na^+] - [(Cl^-) + (HCO_3^-)]$$

In a healthy person, the anion gap has a value of between 8 and 16 mmol/L. When the bicarbonate concentration rises or falls, other ions must take its place to maintain electrochemical neutrality. If chloride substitutes for bicarbonate, the anion gap does not change. However, the anion gap value will increase in metabolic conditions in which acids (*unmeasured anions*), such as sulphuric, lactic or acetoacetic, are produced, or when salicylate is present.

Causes of metabolic acidosis

Metabolic acidosis with an elevated anion gap occurs in:
- *Renal disease.* Hydrogen ions are retained along with anions such as sulphate and phosphate.
- *Diabetic ketoacidosis.* Altered metabolism of fatty acids, as a consequence of the lack of insulin, causes endogenous production of acetoacetic and β-hydroxybutyric acids.
- *Lactic acidosis.* This results from a number of causes, particularly tissue anoxia. *In acute hypoxic states such as respiratory failure or cardiac arrest, lactic acidosis develops within minutes and is life-threatening.* Lactic acidosis also may be caused by liver disease. The presence of lactic acidosis can be confirmed, if necessary, by the measurement of plasma lactate concentration.
- *Certain cases of overdosage or poisoning.* The mechanism common to all of these is the production of acid metabolites. Examples include salicylate overdose where build-up of lactate occurs, methanol poisoning when formate accumulates or ethylene glycol poisoning where oxalate is formed.

Metabolic acidosis with a normal anion gap is sometimes referred to as 'hyperchloraemic acidosis' because a reduced HCO_3^- concentration is balanced by increased Cl- concentration. It is seen in:
- *Chronic diarrhoea or intestinal fistula.* Fluids containing bicarbonate are lost from the body.
- *Renal tubular acidosis.* Renal tubular cells are unable to excrete hydrogen ions efficiently, and bicarbonate is lost in the urine.

Clinical effects of acidosis

The compensatory response to metabolic acidosis is hyperventilation, since the

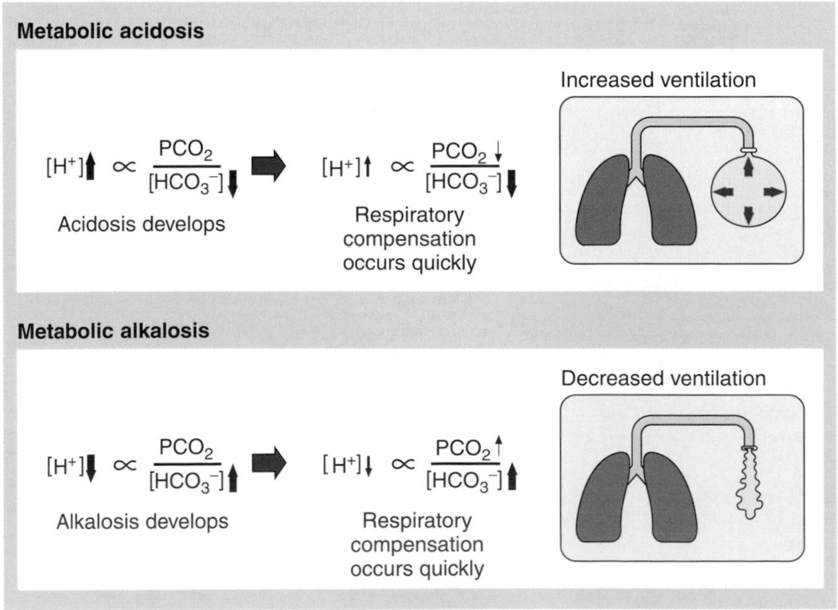

Metabolic acidosis

$[H^+]\uparrow \propto \dfrac{PCO_2}{[HCO_3^-]\downarrow}$ Acidosis develops

$\blacktriangleright$ $[H^+]\uparrow \propto \dfrac{PCO_2\downarrow}{[HCO_3^-]\downarrow}$ Respiratory compensation occurs quickly

Increased ventilation

Metabolic alkalosis

$[H^+]\downarrow \propto \dfrac{PCO_2}{[HCO_3^-]\uparrow}$ Alkalosis develops

$\blacktriangleright$ $[H^+]\downarrow \propto \dfrac{PCO_2\uparrow}{[HCO_3^-]\uparrow}$ Respiratory compensation occurs quickly

Decreased ventilation

Fig. 22.2 Compensation in primary metabolic disorders.

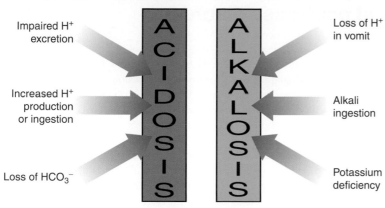

Fig. 22.3 Reasons for metabolic acidosis and alkalosis.

increased [H⁺] acts as a powerful stimulant of the respiratory centre. The deep, rapid and gasping respiratory pattern is known variously as acidotic or Kussmaul breathing or 'air hunger'. Hyperventilation is the appropriate physiological response to acidosis, and it occurs rapidly.

A raised [H⁺] leads to increased neuromuscular irritability. There is a hazard of arrhythmias progressing to cardiac arrest, and this is made more likely by the presence of hyperkalaemia, which will accompany the acidosis. Depression of consciousness can progress to coma and death.

Metabolic alkalosis

The causes of metabolic alkalosis are shown in Fig. 22.3. The condition may be due to:

- *Loss of hydrogen ions in gastric fluid during vomiting.* This is especially seen when there is pyloric stenosis preventing parallel loss of bicarbonate-rich secretions from the duodenum. Prolonged nasogastric suction following surgery may have a similar effect due to the aspiration of mostly gastric fluid.
- *Potassium deficiency.* In severe potassium depletion, often a consequence of diuretic therapy, hydrogen ions are retained inside cells to replace the missing potassium ions. In the renal tubule more hydrogen ions, rather than potassium, are exchanged for reabsorbed sodium. So, despite the presence of alkalosis, the patient passes acidic urine. This is often referred to as 'paradoxical' acidic urine, because in other causes of metabolic alkalosis, urinary [H⁺] usually falls.
- *Ingestion of an absorbable alkali such as sodium bicarbonate.* Very large doses are required to cause metabolic alkalosis unless there is renal impairment.

Clinical effects of alkalosis

The clinical effects of alkalosis include hypoventilation, confusion and eventually coma. Decrease in ionised calcium (as more of it is bound to the increased negative charge of albumin in alkalosis) may result in muscle cramps, paraesthesiae and even full-blown tetany.

Clinical note

As a diagnostic tool, the anion gap is most useful when it is normal, since the differential diagnosis is narrow. By contrast, most causes of metabolic acidosis are associated with a high anion gap.

Metabolic acid–base disorders

- In metabolic acidosis, the blood [H⁺] may be high or normal, but the [HCO₃⁻] is always low. In compensated conditions, PCO₂ is lowered.
- The commonest causes of metabolic acidosis are renal disease, diabetic ketoacidosis and lactic acidosis.
- Consideration of the anion gap sometimes may be helpful in establishing the cause of metabolic acidosis.
- In metabolic alkalosis, the [H⁺] is low and the [HCO₃⁻] is always raised. Respiratory compensation results in an elevated PCO₂.
- The commonest causes of metabolic alkalosis are hypokalaemia and prolonged vomiting.

Case history 14

A 28-year-old man is admitted to hospital with a week-long history of severe vomiting. He confessed to self-medication of his chronic dyspepsia. He was clinically severely dehydrated and had shallow respiration. Initial biochemical results were:

Arterial blood gases

H⁺	PCO₂	HCO₃⁻	PO₂
nmol/L	kPa	mmol/L	kPa
28	7.2	43	15

Na⁺	K⁺	Cl⁻	HCO	Urea	Creatinine
		mmol/L			μmol/L
146	2.8	83	41	31	126

Serum:

A random urine sample was obtained and had the following biochemical results: osmolality 630 mmol/kg, Na⁺ <20 mmol/L, K⁺ 35 mmol/L, pH 5.

- What is the acid–base disorder and how has it arisen?
- How might the urine results help in the diagnosis?
  Comment in Case history comments.

23 | Respiratory and mixed acid–base disorders

In respiratory acid–base disorders the primary disturbance is caused by changes in arterial blood PCO_2 (Fig. 23.1). Respiratory disorders are related to changes either in the amount of air moving in or moving out of the lungs (ventilation) or in the ability of gases to diffuse across the alveolar membrane (gas exchange). In both cases, PCO_2 changes and the carbonic acid concentration rises or falls.

It may appear confusing that carbonic acid can cause acidosis, since for each hydrogen ion produced, a bicarbonate molecule is also generated. However, the effect of adding one hydrogen ion to a concentration of 40 nmol/L is much greater than that of adding one bicarbonate molecule to a concentration of 25 mmol/L (25,000,000 nmol/L; almost a 'drop in the ocean').

Respiratory acidosis

Respiratory acidosis may be acute or chronic. Acute conditions occur within minutes or hours. They are uncompensated. Renal compensation has no time to develop as the mechanisms that adjust hydrogen ion secretion and bicarbonate reabsorption take 48 to 72 hours to become fully effective. The primary problem in acute respiratory acidosis is alveolar hypoventilation. If airflow is completely or partially reduced, the PCO_2 in the blood will rise immediately and the $[H^+]$ will rise quickly (Fig. 23.2). The resulting low PO_2 and high PCO_2 causes coma. If this is not relieved rapidly, death results.

Examples of acute, and hence uncompensated, respiratory acidosis are:
- choking
- rapid onset of severe bronchopneumonia
- acute exacerbation of asthma/chronic obstructive pulmonary disease (COPD)
- sedative overdose.

Chronic respiratory acidosis usually results from COPD and is usually a long-standing condition, accompanied by maximal renal compensation. In chronic respiratory acidosis the primary problem again is usually impaired alveolar ventilation, but renal compensation contributes markedly to the acid–base picture. Compensation may be partial or complete. The kidney increases hydrogen ion excretion, and extracellular fluid bicarbonate levels rise, by the regeneration mechanism outlined in Chapter 21. Blood $[H^+]$ tends back towards normal (Fig. 23.3).

It takes some time for the kidneys to respond to a high PCO_2 and a high $[H^+]$, and therefore compensation will be maximal only some days after the onset of the clinical problem. In many patients with chronic respiratory conditions, extensive renal compensation will keep the blood $[H^+]$ near normal, despite grossly impaired ventilation. In stable chronic bronchitis the $[H^+]$ may be within the reference interval despite a very high PCO_2. This is achieved only by maintaining a very high plasma bicarbonate concentration, sometimes twice that of normal. The PO_2 is usually depressed and becomes more so as lung damage increases with time. Examples of chronic respiratory disorders are:
- chronic bronchitis
- emphysema.

The causes of respiratory acidosis are summarised in Fig. 23.4.

Respiratory alkalosis

Respiratory alkalosis is much less common than acidosis but can occur when respiration is stimulated or is no longer subject to feedback control (see Fig. 23.4). Usually these are acute conditions, and there is no renal compensation. The treatment is to inhibit or remove the cause of the hyperventilation, and the acid–base balance should return to normal. Examples are:
- hysterical overbreathing
- mechanical over-ventilation in an intensive care patient
- direct stimulation of the respiratory centre. This can be caused by, e.g. raised intracranial pressure, hypoxia, salicylate overdose, hyperammonaemia

---

$$[H^+] = \frac{K\,PCO_2}{[HCO_3^-]} \qquad PCO_2 = kPa \qquad [HCO_3^-] = mmol/L$$
$$[H^+] = nmol/L \qquad K = 178$$

Normal control

$$[H^+] = 178 \times \frac{PCO_2\,(5.3)}{[HCO_3^-]\,(25)} = 38\ nmol/L$$

Hypoventilating patient: PCO_2 rises by 2 kPa

$$[H^+] = 178 \times \frac{PCO_2\,(7.3)}{[HCO_3^-]\,(25)} = 52\ nmol/L$$

Fig. 23.2 Why an increased PCO_2 causes acidosis.

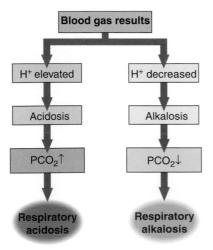

Fig. 23.1 Primary respiratory disorders are recognised by inspecting the PCO_2.

Respiratory acidosis

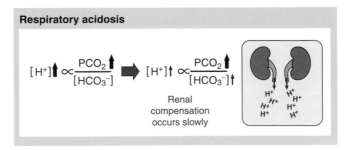

Fig. 23.3 Renal compensation in primary respiratory acidosis.

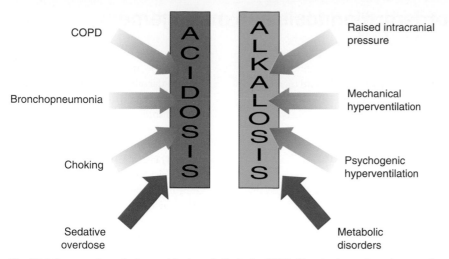

Fig. 23.4 Causes of respiratory acidosis and alkalosis. *COPD*, Chronic obstructive pulmonary disease

Mixed acid–base disorders

Patients sometimes have more than one acid–base disturbance at the same time. Patients in cardiorespiratory arrest have severe respiratory acidosis because they are not breathing and severe metabolic (lactic) acidosis because of reduced perfusion resulting from circulatory arrest. Each is a primary acid–base abnormality. The resulting acidosis (acidaemia) is so severe that it may help explain why patients in cardiac arrest often do not survive. A less extreme example of combined respiratory and metabolic acidosis is a patient with chronic bronchitis who develops renal impairment. In both of these examples, the PCO_2 will be increased and the bicarbonate concentration will be low.

When the two primary disorders are acidosis and alkalosis, they will tend to cancel each other out in terms of the impact on [H+], and so one of them may appear to be compensating for the other. Examples of mixed acid–base disorders commonly encountered are:
- hyperventilation causing respiratory alkalosis, with prolonged nasogastric suction that causes metabolic alkalosis
- a patient with respiratory acidosis due to COPD and diuretic-induced potassium depletion causing metabolic alkalosis
- salicylate poisoning in which respiratory alkalosis occurs due to stimulation of the respiratory centre, together with metabolic acidosis due to the effects of the drug on metabolism.

In these situations the history is all-important in teasing out what is going on – *knowledge of the clinical picture is essential.*

Interpretation of blood gas results is discussed further in the next chapter.

Clinical note

When interpreting acid–base results, the patient's clinical history is the most important factor in determining the nature of the disorder, or indeed in deciding if more than one disorder might be present. Biochemical measurements are the only means of quantifying the severity of the disorder(s) and the degree of compensation.

Respiratory and mixed acid–base disorders

- In respiratory acidosis, the PCO_2 is always high. The presence of compensation is signified by a high HCO_3. The H+ is usually high, but may be within the reference interval if the acidosis is fully compensated.
- Acute respiratory acidosis is a medical emergency and needs to be dealt with by removing the source of the respiratory problem.
- In contrast to respiratory compensation in metabolic disorders, the renal compensating mechanisms are much slower to take effect.
- In chronic respiratory disorders the [H+] often settles at a new steady state, which may be within the reference interval if compensation is complete.
- Respiratory alkalosis is uncommon and can result from mechanical over-ventilation or hysterical overbreathing.
- The interpretation of mixed acid–base disorders may be confusing if one of the disorders mimics the expected compensation. Knowledge of the clinical picture is important if the correct interpretation is to be placed on the results.

Case history 15

A 26-year-old woman was admitted to hospital with a crushed chest. On admission her arterial blood gases were:

H+	HCO_3^-	PCO_2	PO_2
nmol / L	mmol / L	kPa	kPa
63	29	10.1	6.4

- What do these results indicate?
  Comment in Case history comments.

24 | Acid–base disorders: diagnosis and management

Specimens for blood gas analysis

$[H^+]$ and PCO_2 are measured directly in an *arterial* blood sample. This is usually taken from the brachial or radial arteries (less commonly femoral) into a syringe that contains a small volume of heparin as anticoagulant. When the sample has been taken, any air bubbles in the sample should be expelled before analysis, which is almost always done at the point of care on dedicated blood gas analysers. If it has to be sent elsewhere for analysis, the syringe should be capped, and the sample placed on ice during transit. Otherwise, continued cellular metabolism may produce artefactual results, e.g. reduction in PO_2 and elevation in PCO_2, especially if there is a significant delay in transit.

Acid–base problems are considered with reference to the three components of the bicarbonate buffer system. In practice, blood gas analysers measure the $[H^+]$ of the sample and its PCO_2. There is no need to measure the third variable, the bicarbonate. By the law of mass action:

$$[H^+] \alpha \frac{PCO_2}{[HCO_3^-]}$$

If the $[H^+]$ and the PCO_2 are known, the bicarbonate can be calculated. Indeed blood gas analysers (Fig. 24.1) all provide this as the 'standard bicarbonate', i.e. bicarbonate calculated under standard conditions. Other parameters usually included are the PO_2 and the base excess, another way of assessing the metabolic component.

Bicarbonate may be measured, usually on a *venous* blood sample. This 'total CO_2' includes small amounts of dissolved carbon dioxide, carbonic acid and other carbamino compounds but should not differ from the calculated arterial standard bicarbonate by more than 3 mmol/L. A low bicarbonate in an electrolyte profile in venous plasma indicates a metabolic acidosis.

Interpreting results

The most important information available to interpret blood gases is provided by the patient's clinical history. The predicted compensatory responses in $[HCO_3^-]$ or PCO_2 when $[H^+]$ changes as a result of primary acid–base disorders are shown in Table 24.1.

A practical approach to the interpretation of blood gas results is shown in Fig. 24.2. The steps in classifying the acid–base disorder are:

- Look first at the $[H^+]$. Decide if an acidosis or an alkalosis is present.
- If the $[H^+]$ is elevated, decide what is the primary cause of the acidosis. Look at the PCO_2. If this is elevated, there is respiratory acidosis. Look at the bicarbonate. If this is decreased, there is metabolic acidosis.
- If the $[H^+]$ is decreased, determine the primary cause of the alkalosis. Look at the PCO_2. If low, then there is respiratory alkalosis. Look at the bicarbonate. If this is high, there is metabolic alkalosis.
- Having decided on the primary acid–base disorder, look to see if there is

Table 24.1 Primary acid–base disorders and compensatory responses

Primary Disorder	Compensatory Response
↑PCO_2 (Respiratory acidosis)	↑HCO_3^-
↓PCO_2 (Respiratory alkalosis)	↓HCO_3^-
↓HCO_3^- (Metabolic acidosis)	↓PCO_2
↑HCO_3^- (Metabolic alkalosis)	↑PCO_2

compensation. If there is, there will be a change in the other component (the one which was not used to determine the primary disorder), in the *same* direction as the primary abnormality, 'compensating' for the primary disorder, i.e. returning the ratio, and hence the $[H^+]$, towards normal. If there is not, the acid–base disorder may be uncompensated. If the change is in the opposite direction, a second acid–base disorder may be present. Even if it looks as if there is compensation, a second acid–base problem that mimics the compensatory response is possible (see Chapter 23).

- If there is compensation, decide if the disorder is fully compensated ($[H^+]$ within reference limits) or partially compensated ($[H^+]$ not within reference limits).

Clinical cases

The previous practical advice is best illustrated by some case examples.

- A patient who has had an acute asthmatic attack. Blood gas results are: $[H^+]$ = 24 nmol/L (*alkalosis*); PCO_2 = 2.5 kPa (*respiratory alkalosis*); $[HCO_3^-]$ = 20 mmol/L (not low, hence *uncompensated*). Therefore: *uncompensated respiratory alkalosis*.
- A patient with chronic bronchitis. Blood gas results are: $[H^+]$ = 44 nmol/L (normal, so either there is no acid–base disturbance, or a fully compensated one); PCO_2 = 9.5 kPa (*respiratory acidosis*); $[HCO_3^-]$ = 39 mmol/L (*metabolic alkalosis*). In view of the history, it will most likely be a *fully compensated respiratory acidosis*. The other possibility is a fully compensated metabolic alkalosis. This is unlikely for two reasons: (1) the degree of hypoventilation signified by the PCO_2 of 9.5 kPa is greater than what would be seen in compensatory hypoventilation – the associated hypoxia would override the acid–base signal to the respiratory centre; (2) the H^+ is high-normal – it would be unlikely for a compensatory mechanism to (almost) over-compensate.
- A young man with a history of dyspepsia and excessive alcohol intake who gives a history of vomiting. Blood gas results are $[H^+]$ = 28 nmol/L (*alkalosis*); $[HCO_3^-]$ = 48 mmol/L (*metabolic alkalosis* due to loss of H^+ from gut); PCO_2 = 7.2 kPa (*respiratory acidosis*, signifying *compensation*). Therefore the diagnosis is *partially compensated metabolic alkalosis*.

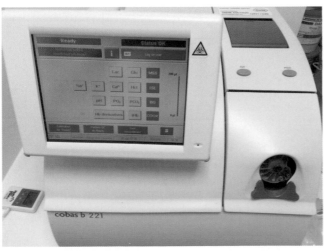

Fig. 24.1 Blood gas analyser.

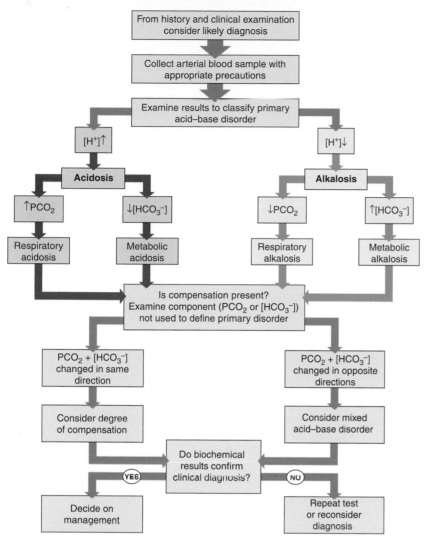

Fig. 24.2 Acid–base disorders: diagnosis and management.

Acid–base disorders: diagnosis and management

- Care should be taken to exclude air from the arterial blood sample taken for blood gas analysis, and speedy transportation to the laboratory should be arranged if the specimen cannot be analysed at the point of care.

- Blood gas analysers measure [H$^+$] and PCO$_2$ directly, and calculate [HCO$_3^-$]. This calculated bicarbonate is similar but not identical to the measured bicarbonate concentration obtained from the electrolyte profile in a serum venous sample.

- Acid–base disorders can be classified as acidosis or alkalosis, compensated or uncompensated and fully or partially compensated.

- The clinical status of the patient and the blood gas results should always agree.

- Management of acid–base disorders should be directed towards the correction of the underlying illness.

It could not be an over-compensated respiratory acidosis, because over-compensation does not occur.

Management of acid–base disorders

Many acid–base disorders are secondary to some other disorder. In most cases the management of an acid–base disorder is to treat the underlying illness. This may involve:

- fluid therapy and insulin in diabetic ketoacidosis
- artificial ventilation by intermittent positive pressure ventilation (IPPV) in acute status asthmaticus
- improvement of glomerular filtration rate by restoring blood volume in a patient with acute blood loss.

In cases of life-threatening acidosis (e.g. [H$^+$] >100 nmol/L), the infusion of sodium bicarbonate may be considered but only under the supervision of an experienced clinician, usually in the intensive care unit. Careful monitoring of the patient by repeatedly measuring the blood gases may be necessary. It should be noted, however, that once sodium bicarbonate has been administered, arterial blood gas results are very difficult to interpret.

Case history 16

A 56-year-old woman was admitted seriously ill and confused. The patient had systemic oedema and was being treated with furosemide (frusemide). On admission the following biochemical results were obtained:

Na$^+$	K$^+$	CL$^-$	HCO$_3^-$	Urea	H$^+$	PCO$_2$	PO$_2$
		mmol/L			nmol/L	KPa	KPa
135	2.6	59	53	6.8	33	9.3	12

- What is the evidence that this patient has a mixed acid–base disorder? Identify the components.
- Explain the aetiology of the present blood gas and electrolyte results.
- How should the patient be treated?
  Comment in Case history comments.

Want to know more?

http://maryland.ccproject.com/wp-content/uploads/sites/3/2013/12/Michael-Chansky-Acid-Base-Made-Easy-handout.pdf

There are lots of online acid–base teaching aids. This is one of the better ones. Good points include the provision of illustrative cases. Unfortunately, pH is used throughout rather than [H$^+$].

25 | Proteins and enzymes

Enzymes

Plasma enzymes in disease

Many students are introduced to biochemistry in the form of metabolic fuel pathways, where enzymes play critical roles related to their specific catalytic function. However, in routine clinical biochemistry, the focus, in terms of measurement of enzyme activity, is mostly not on what specific enzymes *do*, but rather on how they may be used as markers of tissue or organ damage. The basis for this lies in the fact that (1) enzymes that are predominantly intracellular are, along with other intracellular contents, released into the bloodstream when cells are damaged or die, and (2) some enzymes are located predominantly in one or a small number of tissues or organs. Thus, for example, alanine aminotransferase (ALT) is found predominantly in liver and is widely used as a marker of liver damage.

Enzymes that are used in this way are:

- *Alanine aminotransferase (ALT)*. An indicator of hepatocellular damage.
- *Amylase* and *lipase*. Indicators of pancreatic cell damage in acute pancreatitis.
- *Creatine kinase (CK)*. A marker of damage to muscle, including heart muscle (myocardium). Historically it was used as a marker of acute myocardial infarction but is now used almost exclusively to indicate damage to skeletal muscle.

- *Alkaline phosphatase (ALP)*. Increases in cholestatic liver disease and is also a marker of osteoblastic activity in bone disease.
- *Gamma-glutamyl transpeptidase (GGT)*. A sensitive but nonspecific marker of liver disease.
- *Aspartate aminotransferase (AST)*. An indicator of hepatocellular damage, muscle damage or red cell damage (haemolysis).
- *Lactate dehydrogenase (LDH)*. This enzyme is found in muscle, liver, kidney, brain and red blood cells. Its wide distribution means that its value as a marker of specific tissue damage is limited. However, it is still part of many so-called 'haemolytic screens' – groups of tests done to confirm suspected haemolysis.

Fig. 25.1 illustrates some of the main enzymes used to flag up damage or dysfunction of specific tissues or organs.

There are several points to note. First, increases in serum enzyme activity give only a rough idea of the extent of tissue damage or dysfunction. Second, some of the enzymes listed earlier, e.g. GGT and ALP, may increase as a result of alteration in the function of the cells in which they are located, rather than because of release from damaged or dying cells. Third, as pointed out earlier, some of these enzymes, e.g. ALP, AST, LDH, are found in several tissues or organs, limiting their value as specific markers. Fourth, other modalities

of investigation may complement – or surpass – the information provided by these markers. The resolution now provided by diagnostic imaging in particular has been revolutionised by technology.

Plasma proteins

More generically, biochemistry laboratories routinely measure 'total protein' and 'albumin' in plasma or serum; the 'globulin' fraction is the difference between these.

Total protein

Changes in total protein concentration are common. An elevated total protein concentration may indicate the presence of a paraprotein. A decreased total protein usually means that the albumin concentration is low.

Albumin

Albumin is the major plasma protein and is synthesised and secreted by the liver. It has a biological half-life in plasma of about 20 days and accounts for approximately 50% of the total hepatic protein production. Albumin makes the biggest contribution to the plasma oncotic pressure. A low plasma albumin concentration may result in oedema (Fig. 25.2) and can result from:

- *Abnormal distribution*. Albumin moves into the interstitial space as a result of increased capillary permeability in the acute phase response.

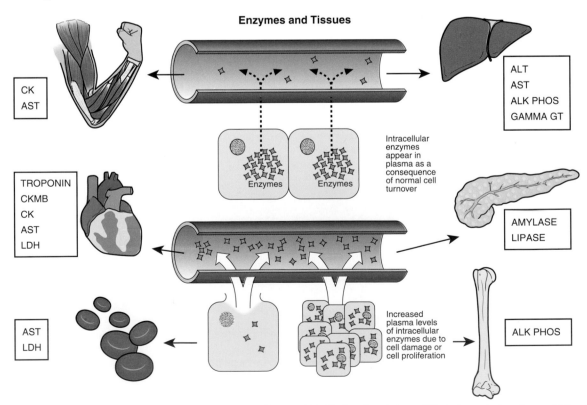

Fig. 25.1 Plasma levels of intracellular enzymes in diagnosis of disease. *ALP*, Alkaline phosphatase; *ALT*, alanine aminotransferase; *AST*, aspartate aminotransferase; *CK*, creatine kinase; *CKMB*, creatine kinase-MB; *LDH*, lactate dehydrogenase; *GGT*, gamma-glutamyl transpeptidase.

- *Decreased synthesis*. Due to advanced chronic liver disease, malabsorption and malnutrition.
- *Dilution*. Hypoalbuminaemia can be induced by overhydration.
- *Abnormal excretion or degradation*. The causes include nephrotic syndrome, protein-losing enteropathies, burns, haemorrhage and catabolic states.

Serum albumin measurements should not be used to monitor a patient's response to long-term nutritional support; they are unreliable and insensitive for this purpose.

Specific proteins

Table 25.1 outlines a number of specific proteins that give useful information in the diagnosis and management of disease. Characteristic changes in the concentration of certain plasma proteins are seen following surgery or trauma or during infection or tumour growth. The proteins involved are called *acute phase reactants* (see Chapter 55). These acute phase proteins may be used to monitor progress of the condition or its treatment.

Isoenzyme determination

Some enzymes are present in the plasma in two or more molecular forms, known as *isoenzymes*; despite different structures, they perform the same catalytic function. Different isoenzymes may be specific to different tissues. In principle this means that, for example, ALP isoenzymes may be used to distinguish between bone and liver involvement, e.g. in cancer patients in whom metastases of bone and/or liver are suspected. In practice, their ability definitively to establish the source is limited, and other investigations, e.g. isotope bone scans, are used to provide complementary information.

Cholinesterase

Cholinesterase, normally involved in the process of neuromuscular conduction, incidentally hydrolyses suxamethonium (succinylcholine), a muscle-relaxing drug used in anaesthesia. Patients with low cholinesterase fail to hydrolyse the drug normally and as a result suffer prolonged paralysis after anaesthesia. This is called scoline apnoea. In a completely different context, cholinesterase measurements are also useful in the diagnosis of poisoning with organophosphate pesticides that are cholinesterase inhibitors.

Proteins and enzymes

- Increased enzyme activities in serum indicate cell damage, altered cell function or increased cell proliferation.
- An increase in serum total protein usually reflects increased globulins and may indicate the presence of a paraprotein.
- A decreased total protein concentration is usually due to hypoalbuminaemia.
- Albumin is the main determinant of plasma oncotic pressure. Low albumin may be associated with oedema.
- Isoenzymes are forms of an enzyme that are structurally different but have similar catalytic properties.

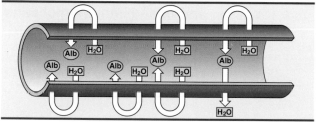

Normal

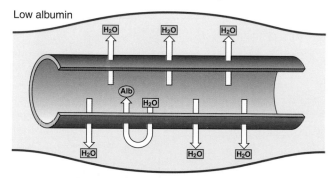

Low albumin

Fig. 25.2 Pathogenesis of oedema in hypoalbuminaemia.

Table 25.1 **Specific proteins that are measured in serum**

Protein Name	Function	Reason for Assay
α_1-antitrypsin	Protease inhibitor	Reduced in α_1-antitrypsin deficiency
β_2-microglobulin	Subunit of human leucocyte antigen on all cell membranes	Raised in renal tubular dysfunction
Caeruloplasmin	Copper transport	Reduced in Wilson's disease
C-reactive protein	Involved in immune response	Increased in acute illness, especially infection
Ferritin	Binds iron in tissues	Gives an indication of body iron stores
Haptoglobin	Binds haemoglobin	Reduced in haemolytic conditions
Thyroid-binding globulin	Thyroid hormone binding	Investigation of thyroid disease
Sex hormone-binding globulin	Binds testosterone and oestradiol	Investigation of androgen excess and/or insulin resistance
Transferrin	Iron transport	Assessment of iron status and/or response to nutritional support

26 | Immunoglobulins

Immunoglobulins, or antibodies, are proteins produced by the plasma cells of the bone marrow as part of the immune response. Plasma cells are B lymphocytes transformed after exposure to a foreign (or occasionally an endogenous) antigen. They are recognisable under a microscope because their nucleus is eccentric (at the edge of the cell) (Fig. 26.1).

Structure

All immunoglobulins consist of two identical light and two identical heavy polypeptide chains, held together by disulphide bridges (Fig. 26.2). These are conventionally known by the names of Greek letters. The light chains may be either kappa or lambda; the heavy chains may be alpha, gamma, delta, epsilon or mu. The immunoglobulins are named after their heavy chain type, as IgA, IgG, IgD, IgE and IgM.

Each immunoglobulin molecule has two functional areas:
- The *Fab* (fragment antigen-binding), or *variable* end, is the area that recognises and binds to the antigen.
- The *Fc* (fragment crystallisable) end is responsible for interaction with other components of the immune system, e.g. complement and T-helper cells.

The various classes of immunoglobulins have different tertiary structure and functions (Table 26.1). The major antibodies in the plasma are IgG, IgA and IgM.

Electrophoresis of serum proteins

Electrophoresis separates proteins on the basis of their charge/mass ratio and is widely used to study protein abnormalities. The normal pattern is shown in Fig. 26.3A. Each protein class may be quantitated by scanning the electrophoresis strip (Fig. 26.4). Immunoglobulins are seen primarily in the gamma-globulin area. Electrophoresis can show gross deficiency or excess of these and the presence of discrete bands (paraproteins) (see Fig. 26.3B). If an abnormality is detected, the particular type of immunoglobulin, or indeed of light or heavy chains where these are produced alone, may be confirmed by immunofixation or quantitatively by other means. Serum should be used for electrophoresis, as the fibrinogen of plasma (consumed during clotting) gives a discrete band that can easily be mistaken for a paraprotein.

Increased immunoglobulins

Immunoglobulins may be increased nonspecifically in many infections and also in autoimmune disease. This increased synthesis comes from a number of cell

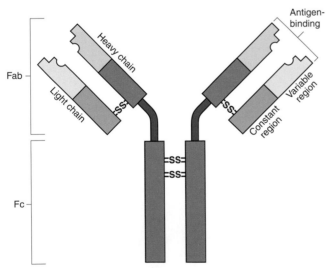

Fig. 26.1 Plasma cells are easily distinguished by their eccentric nucleus. Some of these nuclei are indicated by *arrows*.

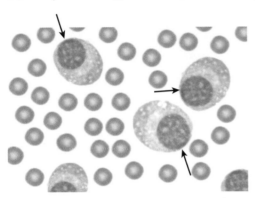

Fig. 26.2 Structure of an immunoglobulin. *Fab*, Antigen-binding fragment; *Fc*, crystallisable fragment.

Table 26.1 Classes of immunoglobulin

Immunoglobulin	Structure	Location	Function
IgG	Monomer	ECF	Neutralises toxins, activates complement
IgA	Dimer	ECF + secretions	Antimicrobial
IgM	Pentamer	Mainly intravascular	First to be made in immune response
IgD	Monomer	ECF + cell membrane	Cell surface antigen receptors
IgE	Monomer	ECF	Antiallergic, antiparasitic

ECF, Extracellular fluid.

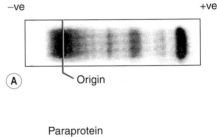

-ve   +ve

(A) Origin

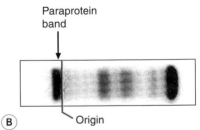

Paraprotein band

(B) Origin

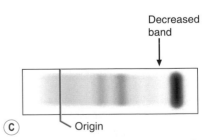

Decreased band

(C) Origin

Fig. 26.3 Electrophoresis of serum proteins. **(A)** Normal pattern; **(B)** paraprotein band; **(C)** α_1-antitrypsin deficiency.

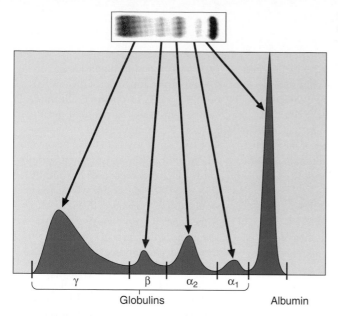

Fig. 26.4 Scan of an electrophoresis strip.

γ β α₂ α₁

Globulins   Albumin

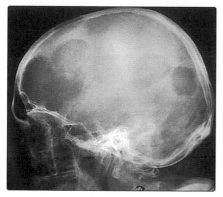

Fig. 26.5 Skull X-ray film showing osteolytic lesions of myeloma.

Table 26.2 **Causes of hypogammaglobulinaemia**	
Type	**Specific Causes**
Physiological	Levels of IgA and IgM are low at birth
Genetic	Bruton's X-linked agammaglobulinaemia
	Severe combined immunodeficiency (SCID)
Acquired	Malnutrition
	Malignancy
	Infections, e.g. HIV, measles
	Immunosuppressant drugs, e.g. azathioprine, ciclosporin

Deficiencies or absence of immunoglobulins

Deficiencies or absence of immunoglobulins can occur as a result of infection, genetic abnormalities or the effects of therapy (Table 26.2). Where this is irreversible, replacement therapy has been used, either by adding immunoglobulin-rich plasma or by transplanting bone marrow that contains competent (normal) plasma cells.

Clinical note

The diagnosis of myeloma requires that two of the following are present:

- a paraprotein in serum or urine
- plasma cell infiltration in bone marrow
- myeloma-related end-organ damage, including skeletal lesions (see Fig. 26.5).

Immunoglobulins

- Electrophoresis of serum may confirm the presence of a paraprotein in a specimen from a patient with a raised globulin fraction.
- Some myelomas produce immunological light chains only. These are best demonstrated by urine electrophoresis.
- Immunoglobulin measurements can give information on immune deficiency and response to infection.
- Serial study of immunoglobulin levels can be of help in following the progression of disease or monitoring of treatment.

Case history 18

A 45-year-old man presented with severe back pain and malaise. He had lost 3 kg weight in 3 months. His blood film showed many primitive red blood cells (RBCs) and white blood cells (WBCs). His bone marrow biopsy showed an excess of plasma cells. He did not have a paraprotein band on serum electrophoresis. Analysis of concentrated urine revealed an excess of free monoclonal light chains.

- What is the diagnosis?
  Comment in Case history comments.

Want to know more?

http://emedicine.medscape.com/article/780258-overview

This is quite a nice introduction to hyperviscosity syndrome. Waldenström's macroglobulinaemia accounts for most cases.

lines, each producing its own specific immunoglobulin. The response is therefore said to be *polyclonal* and results in a diffuse increase in proteins throughout the gamma-globulin region on electrophoresis. This is because the immunoglobulins produced by individual cell lines are each slightly different in terms of size and charge and so do not migrate to exactly the same place on electrophoresis. In contrast, cells from a single clone all make *identical* antibodies which do migrate to exactly the same place and therefore appear on electrophoresis as a single discrete *monoclonal* band. This is called a *paraprotein*. It may be an intact immunoglobulin or a fragment.

Paraproteins

Paraproteins may arise from any immunoglobulin class. Waldenström's macroglobulinaemia is multiple myeloma in which the antibody produced by the malignant clone is an IgM. This is a very large molecule because it is a pentamer (i.e. made up of five subunits), so gross over-production changes the physical properties of blood, resulting in hyperviscosity. Monoclonal light chains are produced in excess of heavy chains in 50% of cases of

myeloma, and in 15% of cases only light chains are found. These light chains are small enough to spill into the urine, where they are known as *Bence-Jones protein*.

Myeloma is characterised by osteolytic lesions (Fig. 26.5), and bone pain is often the presenting symptom. In the face of increasing synthesis of abnormal immunoglobulins, there is reduced bone marrow production of white cell and platelets, resulting in anaemia and increased susceptibility to infection. In addition, there is decreased production of normal immunoglobulins; on electrophoresis this feature – known as *immunoparesis* – is diagnostic of multiple myeloma when seen with a paraprotein band. The increased serum paraprotein may cause renal damage, leading to renal failure. Hypercalcaemia is also a feature of myeloma. Treatment of myeloma involves the use of bone marrow suppressant drugs.

Paraproteins are quite often found in elderly patients in the absence of associated pathology. This is called *benign paraproteinaemia* or *monoclonal gammopathy of uncertain significance* (MGUS). Regular and careful follow-up of such patients is required.

27 | Myocardial infarction

Infarction is defined as the process by which *necrosis* (cell or tissue death) results from *ischaemia* (loss of blood supply). Infarction of cardiac muscle (myocardial infarction (MI)) is one of the commonest causes of morbidity and mortality in adults living in industrialised societies.

Pathology

The underlying pathology in MI is atherosclerosis, an inflammatory process located within the arterial wall in the form of atheromatous plaques (Fig. 27.1). These develop over many years, causing progressive narrowing of the arterial lumen, resulting in reduced coronary perfusion,

the clinical manifestation of which is chest pain (angina pectoris). If an unstable plaque ruptures, the released contents precipitate the formation of a clot. This process, known as *thrombosis*, may result in sudden complete occlusion of the affected artery and infarction (death) of the area of myocardium it supplies.

Cardiac biomarkers

When myocardial cells die, they break up and release their contents. This is the basis for the role of cardiac biomarkers in MI diagnosis. Troponin I and T are cardiospecific, so increased levels in blood indicate myocardial necrosis. These are

part of the troponin complex found on the contractile apparatus of myocardial cells (Fig. 27.2). (Troponin C, the third component, is also present in skeletal muscle, so it cannot be used to diagnose MI in the same way as T and I.) Before the advent of troponin measurement, various 'cardiac enzymes' were used historically (Fig. 27.3). The ideal cardiac biomarker would allow clinicians to diagnose MI without delay. Troponins rise within a few hours of the onset of symptoms, and the current generation of highly sensitive troponin assays in principle permit diagnosis within as little as 3 hours. In addition, troponins remain elevated for over a week. This property enables late as well as early diagnosis.

Crucially, any elevation of troponin, i.e. detectable levels in the blood, especially with the newer highly sensitive assays, implies a greater risk of morbidity and mortality from a cardiac event over the next 30 to 60 days. Thus its application has extended beyond diagnosis of MI to risk stratification and other uses (Table 27.1). In addition, although troponins are considered very specific cardiac biomarkers, they also can increase in other cardiovascular pathologies such as myocarditis, pulmonary embolism and stroke, and noncardiac conditions such as severe sepsis.

Diagnosis

The essential components of diagnosis of MI are the history, the characteristic electrocardiographic (ECG) changes and the detection in blood of biochemical markers of myocardial injury. Patients experiencing MI classically complain of severe crushing central chest pain. However, such a characteristic history is not always obtained, and a minority of patients may even have a 'silent' MI. When present, the characteristic ECG changes (Fig. 27.4) are specific to MI, but they are equivocal or absent in up to 30% of patients. It is in this group of patients that cardiac markers are most useful.

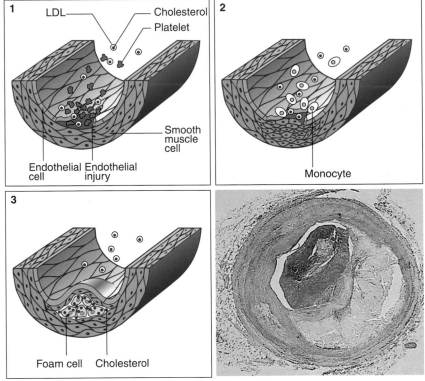

Fig. 27.1 Development of atheroma in coronary arteries, with histopathological section (bottom right). *LDL*, Low-density lipoprotein.

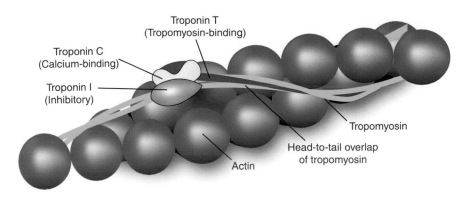

Fig. 27.2 Components of the contractile apparatus in muscle (sarcomere) including the troponin subunits.

Table 27.1 **Potential roles for troponin measurement**
• Diagnosis of acute myocardial infarction (MI)
• Prognosis in acute coronary syndrome
• Diagnosis of perioperative MI (where there is coexistent skeletal muscle damage)
• Monitoring thrombolytic therapy
• Identification of patients who will respond to interventions, e.g. low-molecular-weight heparins, platelet glycoprotein IIb/IIIa antagonists or angioplasty

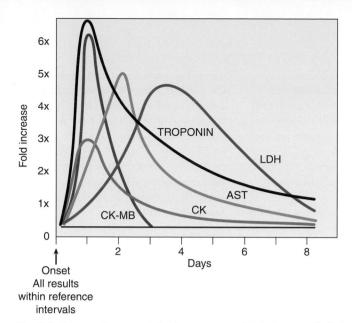

Fig. 27.3 Enzymes in serum following an uncomplicated myocardial infarction (MI).
AST, Aspartate aminotransferase; *CK*, creatine kinase; *CKMB*, creatine kinase-MB; *LDH*, lactate dehydrogenase.

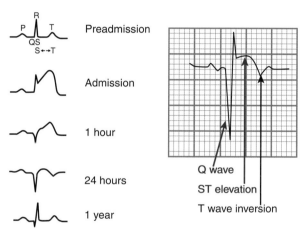

Fig. 27.4 ECG changes throughout an evolving myocardial infarction (MI), from preadmission through to 1 year later.

Clinical note

The classic feature of a myocardial infarction (MI) is crushing chest pain radiating down the left arm. Not all patients with an MI experience this. In addition to the many variants of angina-like pain, it is recognised that a proportion of MIs are 'silent' and are subsequently detected only by ECG and/or cardiac markers. In one European heart study, 2% of middle-aged men showed definite ECG evidence of a previously unrecognised MI.

Myocardial infarction

- Cardiac troponins I and T are among the most sensitive and specific tests routinely used in clinical biochemistry. Their use has led to a 'step-change' in the accuracy of diagnosis of myocardial infarction (MI).

- Despite this, troponins also can increase in other cardiovascular pathologies, as well as noncardiac conditions such as severe sepsis.

- Grossly elevated serum creatine kinase (>10,000 U/L) is not consistent with acute MI and points to rhabdomyolysis (skeletal muscle breakdown).

- Early diagnosis of MI is important – complications such as arrhythmias and heart failure are potentially fatal – and treatable.

Case history 19

A 52-year-old man presented at the accident and emergency department with severe chest pain which had been present for the past hour. He had previously attended the chest pain clinic and had a 2-year history of angina of effort.

- What specific tests would you request from the biochemistry laboratory? *Comment in Case history comments.*

Want to know more?

http://study.com/academy/lesson/tropomy-osin-definition-structure-function.html

This video clip outlines very nicely the background physiology of troponins, i.e. what they actually do. (In order to access the this link – and one or two other 'Want to know more?' links in this book – registration is required. It is worth the effort – overall this is a very useful resource. All content is available free of charge.)

Definitions

Acute coronary syndrome

The term *acute coronary syndrome* (ACS) applies to patients in whom myocardial ischaemia is suspected. It encompasses (1) ST segment elevation myocardial infarction (STEMI), (2) non–ST segment elevation myocardial infarction (NSTEMI) and (3) unstable angina. The first two of these are associated with a typical rise/ fall in cardiac markers. The ST segment is shown in Fig. 27.4. Pathologically, ACS is almost always associated with rupture of an atherosclerotic plaque and partial or complete thrombosis of a coronary artery. In some instances it may occur from increased demands on the heart, e.g. with severe blood loss, anaemia, tachycardia or severe infections.

Myocardial infarction

Acute MI is defined as a clinical event resulting from myocardial necrosis caused by ischaemia, as opposed to other pathologies such as myocarditis or trauma. In practical terms, this means a rise and fall in cardiac markers (usually troponin) associated with symptoms of ischaemia, such as chest pain, and/or fresh ECG changes (Q waves, ST changes, T wave inversion, left bundle branch block). (Q waves signify that the area of myocardial necrosis extends through the full thickness of the ventricular wall; their presence thus indicates a transmural MI.)

28 | Liver function tests

Introduction

The liver plays a major role in the metabolism of proteins, carbohydrates and lipids (Fig. 28.1). Glycolysis, the Krebs cycle, amino acid synthesis, amino acid degradation and oxidative phosphorylation are all carried out in hepatocytes, which are well-endowed with mitochondria that provide the required energy. The liver also contains an extensive reticuloendothelial system for synthesis and breakdown of blood cells. Liver cells metabolise, detoxify and excrete both endogenous and exogenous compounds. Excretion of water-soluble end products from the metabolism of both nutrients and toxins, and of digestive aids such as bile acids, occurs into the biliary tree.

Liver function tests

The term 'liver function tests' (LFTs) is a misnomer. LFTs merely flag up the existence, extent and, to a degree, type of liver damage. They do not assess quantitatively the capacity of the liver to carry out the functions described previously. Most LFT profiles include alanine aminotransferase (ALT), bilirubin, alkaline phosphatase (ALP) and albumin. These biochemical investigations can assist in differentiating the following:

- acute hepatocellular damage
- obstruction to the biliary tract
- chronic liver disease.

Bilirubin concentration and ALP activity indicate cholestasis, a blockage of bile flow. ALT activity is a measure of the integrity of liver cells, or parenchymal liver disease. In severe liver damage the distinction between cholestatic and parenchymal markers is less reliable, i.e. serum activities of all enzymes are likely to increase. The serum albumin concentration is a crude measure of the liver's synthetic capacity; prothrombin time is superior (see later).

The aminotransferases (ALT and AST)

The activity of ALT is widely used as a sensitive, albeit nonspecific, marker of acute damage to hepatocytes, irrespective of its aetiology. Causes of liver damage include hepatitis, regardless of the cause, and toxic injury due to any one of many "insults" to the liver, including drug overdose. Acute liver damage due to shock, severe hypoxia and acute cardiac failure also occur. Aspartate aminotransferase (AST), another aminotransferase found in liver cells, is less widely used in the assessment of liver disease because it is found in other tissues (see Chapter 25) and so provides less specific information.

Alkaline phosphatase

Increased ALP activity in liver disease reflects increased synthesis by cells lining the bile canaliculi, usually in response to cholestasis, which may be either intrahepatic or extrahepatic. Cholestasis, even of short duration, results in an increase in enzyme activity to at least twice the upper end of the reference interval. High ALP activity also may occur in infiltrative diseases of the liver, when space-occupying lesions (e.g. tumours) are present. It also occurs in cirrhosis.

ALP is also present in other organs: bone, small intestine, placenta and kidney. Normally, blood ALP activity is derived mainly from bone and liver, with small amounts from the intestine. Placental ALP appears in the maternal blood in the third trimester of pregnancy. Occasionally, the cause of a raised ALP is not immediately apparent. Although liver and bone isoenzymes can be separated by electrophoresis, in practice the finding of elevated gamma-glutamyl transpeptidase (GGT) (see later) is taken to indicate a hepatic source of the increased ALP.

Bilirubin

Bilirubin is derived from haem, an iron-containing protoporphyrin mainly found in haemoglobin (Fig. 28.2). An adult normally produces about 450 µmol of bilirubin daily from lysis of red blood cells. Unconjugated bilirubin is insoluble in water and is transported in plasma bound to albumin. It is taken up by liver cells and conjugated to form monoglucuronides and diglucuronides, which are much more soluble in water than unconjugated bilirubin. Conjugated bilirubin is then excreted into the bile. Normal bile contains bilirubin monoglucuronide as 25% and the diglucuronide as 75% of the total, accompanied by traces of unconjugated bilirubin. The main functional constituents of the bile are bile salts, which are involved in fat digestion and absorption from the small intestine. Serum bile acid concentrations are more sensitive indices

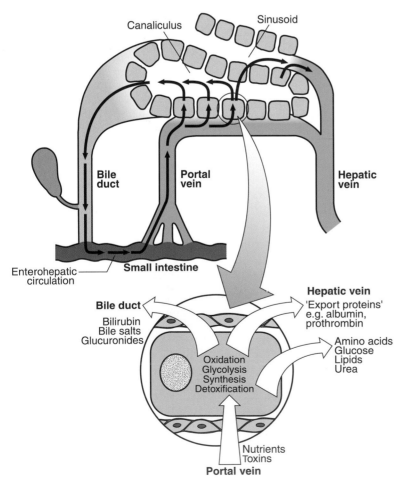

Fig. 28.1 Liver functions.

Haem

M − Methyl   P − Propionate
V − Vinyl   G − Glucuronide

Fig. 28.2 Structure of bilirubin and conjugated bilirubin. *UDP*, Uridine diphosphate.

of hepatic transport function than are total bilirubin measurements. (In pregnancy, the finding of raised maternal bile acids signifies increased fetal risk, for unrelated reasons.)

Bile reaches the gut through the ampulla of Vater at the end of the common bile duct. In the terminal ileum and colon, the bilirubin conjugates are degraded by bacteria to form a group of compounds known collectively as *stercobilinogen*, most of which are excreted in faeces. Some are absorbed and eventually reexcreted from the body by way of bile (the enterohepatic circulation). Small amounts of these tetrapyrroles are found in urine, in which they are known as *urobilinogen*.

When the biliary tract becomes blocked, bilirubin is not excreted and serum concentrations rise. The patient becomes jaundiced. The approach to the jaundiced patient is described in Chapter 29.

Gamma-glutamyl transpeptidase

GGT is a microsomal enzyme that is widely distributed; tissues include liver and renal tubules. Its activity is raised in cholestasis, and it is a very sensitive marker of liver pathology. Separately, alcohol and drugs such as phenytoin induce microsomal enzyme activity, and GGT is often used as a marker of this enzyme induction – it is increased by ingestion of alcohol, even in the absence of recognisable liver disease. In acute hepatic damage, changes in its activity parallel those of ALT.

Plasma proteins

Albumin is the major protein product of the liver. It has a long biological half-life in plasma (~20 days), so significant falls in albumin are slow to occur if synthesis is suddenly reduced. Hypoalbuminaemia is, however, a feature of advanced chronic liver disease. It also can occur in severe acute liver damage.

The total serum globulin concentration is sometimes used as a crude measure of the severity of liver disease.

Alpha-fetoprotein (AFP) is synthesised by the fetal liver and persists into the early neonatal period, after which it declines rapidly. In normal adults it is present in low concentrations (<3 kU/L). Its measurement is of value in suspected hepatocellular carcinoma, in which serum concentrations are increased in 80% to 90% of cases. AFP is also used as a marker for germ cell tumours (see Chapter 72).

Other proteins, such as α_1-antitrypsin and caeruloplasmin, are measured in the diagnosis of specific diseases affecting the liver (see Chapter 25).

Prothrombin time

The prothrombin time is a measure of the activities of certain coagulation factors made by the liver and is sometimes used as an indicator of hepatic synthetic function. Prothrombin has a very short half-life, and an increased prothrombin time may be the earliest indicator of reduced hepatic synthesis.

Clinical note

Diagnostic imaging techniques are at least as important as biochemical tests in the investigation of liver disease. The *arrow* in Fig. 28.3 highlights an area of defective isotope uptake, indicating the presence of a liver metastasis in a patient with disseminated malignant disease.

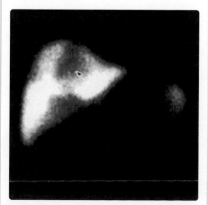

Fig. 28.3 Scintiscan of liver. *Arrow*, Area of defective isotope uptake.

Liver function tests

- Liver function test (LFT) profiles usually include bilirubin, alanine aminotransferase (ALT), alkaline phosphatase (ALP) and albumin.
- Raised ALT activity indicates hepatocellular damage.
- Increased bilirubin concentration indicates the presence of cholestasis, a blockage in bile flow.
- ALP and gamma-glutamyl transpeptidase (GGT) activities are a reflection of pathology of the biliary tree or its involvement by other pathology affecting the liver.
- Increased GGT activity may alternatively indicate hepatocellular enzyme induction due to drugs or alcohol.

Case history 20

A 60-year-old woman with a history of breast carcinoma treated by mastectomy 3 years previously is now complaining of general malaise and bone pain. Biochemistry showed that fluid and electrolytes, total protein, albumin and calcium values were all normal. LFTs were as follows:

Bilirubin µmol/L	AST	ALT	ALP	GGT
			U/L	
7	33	38	890	32

Liver function

- Evaluate these results and suggest a likely diagnosis.
  Comment in Case history comments.

Want to know more?

https://www.ncbi.nlm.nih.gov/pubmed/?term=liver+enzyme+alteration+a+guide+for+clinicians

This widely cited Canadian review from 2005 takes a detailed and critical look at the individual LFTs from a practical clinical perspective.

29 | Jaundice

Jaundice is a yellow discoloration of the skin or sclera (Fig. 29.1). It is due to the presence of excessive bilirubin in the blood and is not usually detectable until the concentration exceeds 50 μmol/L. Normally the bilirubin concentration is less than 21 μmol/L. Bilirubin is derived from the tetrapyrrole prosthetic group found in haemoglobin and the cytochromes. It is normally conjugated with glucuronic acid to make it more soluble, and excreted in the bile (Fig. 29.2). There are three main reasons why bilirubin levels in the blood may rise (Fig. 29.3):

- *Haemolysis.* Increased haemoglobin breakdown produces bilirubin, which overwhelms a normally functioning conjugating mechanism.
- *Failure of the conjugating mechanism within the hepatocyte.*
- *Obstruction in the biliary system.*

Both conjugated bilirubin and unconjugated bilirubin may be present in plasma. Conjugated bilirubin is water-soluble. Unconjugated bilirubin is water-insoluble and binds to albumin, from which it may be transferred to other proteins such as those in cell membranes. It can cross the blood-brain barrier and is neurotoxic; permanent brain damage can occur if levels are too high in neonates.

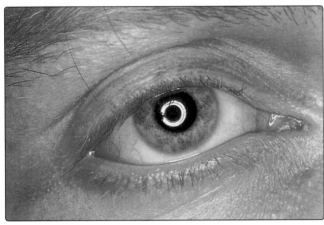

Fig. 29.1 Jaundice in the sclera of an eye.

Biochemical tests

Once conjugated, bilirubin is conveyed through the biliary tree into the gut via the common bile duct. Bilirubin in the gut is metabolised by bacteria to produce stercobilinogen, which gives faeces their brown colour. If it does not reach the gut, stools are pale. Stercobilinogen is partly reabsorbed and reexcreted in the urine as urobilinogen and may be detected by simple biochemical tests. When high levels of conjugated bilirubin are being excreted, urine may be a deep orange colour, particularly if allowed to stand.

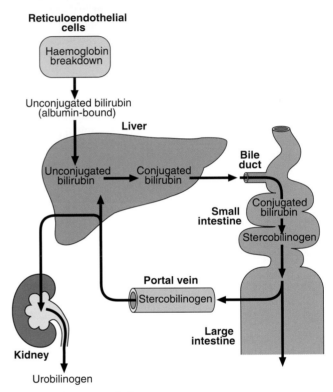

Fig. 29.2 Bilirubin metabolism.

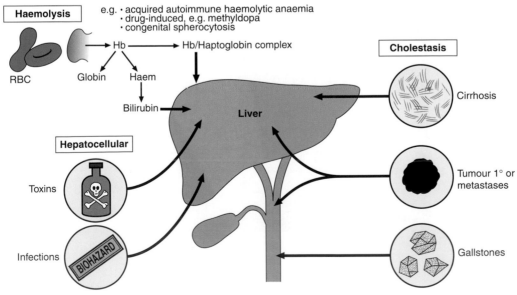

Fig. 29.3 Causes of jaundice. *RBC*, Red blood cell.

Table 29.1	**Laboratory differential diagnosis of jaundice**		
	Haemolytic	**Cholestatic**	**Hepatocellular**
Features	Bilirubin concentration variable	Bilirubin may be ↑↑↑ Bilirubin in urine	AST + ALT ↑↑ Bilirubin ↑ later
	No bilirubin in urine Reticulocytosis Haemoglobin ↓	ALP ↑, usually >3× upper limit of reference range	Bilirubin in urine ALP ↑ later
	Haptoglobin ↓ LDH, AST ↑	AST, ALT + LDH usually modestly ↑	

ALP, Alkaline phosphatase; *ALT*, alanine aminotransferase; *AST*, aspartate aminotransferase; *LDH*, lactate dehydrogenase.

The combination of pale stools and dark urine is characteristic of extrahepatic obstruction of the biliary tract.

Differential diagnosis

Jaundice may be a consequence of haemolysis, cholestasis or hepatocellular damage (see Fig. 29.3 and Table 29.1). There are also inherited disorders of bilirubin metabolism, of which Gilbert's disease is the commonest. This causes mild unconjugated hyperbilirubinaemia because of defective hepatic uptake. It has a normal life expectancy.

Haemolysis

Haemolysis increases bilirubin production and gives a mostly unconjugated hyperbilirubinaemia. This, and immature liver function, are common in newborn babies. Neonatal jaundice should be carefully monitored; unconjugated bilirubin is lipid-soluble and so may cross the blood-brain barrier. Within the brain it may get deposited in the basal ganglia (*kernicterus*), causing brain damage. If the concentration approaches 200 µmol/L, phototherapy should be used to break down the molecule in the skin and reduce the level. If the concentration rises above 300 µmol/L, exchange transfusion may be necessary.

Extrahepatic biliary obstruction

Gallstones, pancreatic cancer, and lymph nodes can block the bile duct (extrahepatic obstruction). Complete blockage is associated with a rise in both bilirubin and alkaline phosphatase (ALP), with little or no urobilinogen in urine, and pale stools. When the obstruction is removed, the stools regain their colour and urine again becomes positive for urobilinogen. Bilirubin may be normal in partial blockage, although ALP is usually high. This is classically seen with an isolated secondary neoplasm in the liver, partly disturbing the biliary tree. Unaffected liver tissue can still process and excrete bilirubin; the ALP mirrors the degree of obstruction. Intrahepatic biliary obstruction is much more difficult to diagnose than extrahepatic obstruction. The bile canaliculi can become blocked due to cirrhosis, liver cancer or infection. This leads to an increased concentration of conjugated bilirubin in serum.

Hepatocellular damage

Obstruction may be secondary to damage to the hepatocytes by infection or toxins, rather than damage to the biliary tract. The most common causes of acute jaundice seen in adults are viral hepatitis and paracetamol poisoning. In these cases, not only are the bilirubin and ALP levels raised but alanine aminotransferase (ALT) is elevated, indicating hepatocellular damage.

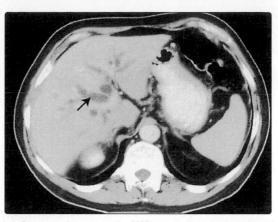

Fig. 29.4 Computed tomography (CT) scan of liver and gallbladder. *Arrow*, Dilated bile ducts.

Clinical note

Diagnostic imaging is invaluable in the investigation of the jaundiced patient. The dilated bile ducts (*arrow* in Fig. 29.4) are clearly visible in a computed tomography (CT) scan of a patient with extrahepatic obstructive jaundice due to carcinoma of the head of the pancreas.

Jaundice

- Jaundice indicates an elevated concentration of bilirubin in blood.

- In neonatal jaundice, it is important to know how much bilirubin is unconjugated since this can cause kernicterus and associated brain damage and is treatable.

- Complete extrahepatic obstruction produces a characteristic clinical picture of pale stools (due to absence of stercobilinogen from the gut) and dark urine (resulting from excess conjugated bilirubinuria).

Case history 21

A 65-year-old man came to his general practitioner's surgery with visible jaundice that he had noticed to be deepening in colour. He had no pain but had noticed some weight loss and that his stools were pale. He was a moderate drinker and was not on any drug therapy. His liver function tests (LFTs) were:

Bilirubin	AST	ALT		ALP
µmol/L			U/L	
250	87	92		850

- What is the differential diagnosis?
- What other investigations would be helpful in making a diagnosis? *Comment in Case history comments.*

Want to know more?

Rother RP, Bell L, Hillmen P, Gladwin MT. The clinical sequelae of intravascular hemolysis and extracellular plasma hemoglobin: a novel mechanism of human disease. *JAMA.* 2005;293(13):1653–1662 [Review].

Haemolysis is a key cause of unconjugated hyperbilirubinaemia. This interesting article asks a more profound question: why does the body scavenge haemoglobin? It suggests that free haemoglobin affects nitric oxide and endothelial function.

30 | Liver disease

Acute liver disease

Acute liver damage most commonly occurs for one of three reasons:
- poisoning
- infection
- inadequate perfusion.

Investigation

The transaminases such as alanine aminotransferase (ALT) will be raised, indicating hepatocyte damage. Elevated serum bilirubin and alkaline phosphatase (ALP) levels reflect the presence of associated cholestasis. Disease progression or recovery can be monitored by serial measurements of liver function tests (LFTs).

Poisoning

In practice, paracetamol overdose is the commonest scenario in which poisoning is encountered. In small amounts, paracetamol is metabolised uneventfully by the intact liver cell, but when present at high concentrations its toxic metabolites overwhelm the hepatocyte's natural antioxidant glutathione, leading to hepatocyte destruction and massive release of enzymes. The capacity of the liver to withstand an insult is reduced if there is underlying liver damage due to alcohol, malnutrition or other chronic disease.

Less commonly, some plant and fungal toxins, e.g. from mushrooms, cause catastrophic liver damage, resulting in fulminant liver failure within 48 hours (Fig. 30.1).

A third group of toxins are drugs that give rise to acute hepatocellular failure only in certain susceptible individuals. Important examples include sodium valproate, an anticonvulsant drug that causes toxicity in some children, and halothane, an anaesthetic agent.

Liver infection

Bacteria and viruses can give rise to infective hepatitis, which causes many deaths worldwide. Hepatitis A, hepatitis B and hepatitis C are the most common.

Inadequate perfusion

Inadequate perfusion of the liver usually occurs in the context of a wider perfusion problem, e.g. blood loss. In this situation, all organs and tissues are affected and the damage to the liver is predictable and therefore not a diagnostic dilemma. Treatment involves restoring perfusion as soon as possible.

'Shock liver' is a less well-defined entity. In patients who have undergone surgery, e.g. an abdominal operation, a significant unexplained rise in ALT is occasionally seen postoperatively. This is sometimes attributed to an intraoperative hypotensive episode; the presumption is that liver perfusion has been compromised resulting in liver damage.

Outcome

Acute liver damage can progress in three ways:
- It may resolve (the majority of cases).
- It may progress to acute hepatic failure.
- It may lead to chronic hepatic damage.

Acute hepatic failure

Acute hepatic failure is a medical emergency; failure of its complex metabolic functions cannot be compensated for by any other organ. In severe cases, there is extensive biochemical disruption. Electrolyte imbalance occurs, and sodium and calcium concentrations may both fall. There may be severe metabolic acid–base disturbances and hypoglycaemia.

Hepatic failure may give rise to renal failure due to exposure of the glomeruli to toxins usually metabolised by the liver. There may be an increase in blood ammonia as a result of the failure to detoxify this to urea. The pattern of abnormalities found in hepatic failure is shown in Fig. 30.2.

In acute hepatocellular damage, albumin synthesis is reduced or ceases, eventually leading to hypoalbuminaemia and the development of oedema and ascites. Failure to synthesise clotting factors leads to an increased haemorrhagic tendency or, in severe cases, to disseminated intravascular coagulation.

Recovery from acute hepatocellular damage may take weeks, during which monitoring of LFTs is helpful in detecting relapse and assisting prognosis.

Chronic liver disease

Examples of chronic liver damage are:
- alcoholic liver disease
- chronic active hepatitis
- primary biliary cirrhosis.
- nonalcoholic fatty liver disease.

All of these conditions may progress to cirrhosis, which is another name for liver fibrosis. Fibrosis is the formation of scar tissue, resulting in the disorganisation and shrinkage of liver architecture (Fig. 30.3). It also increases the pressure in the portal circulation (portal hypertension).

Aetiology of cirrhosis

Cirrhosis is the final stage of chronic liver damage and only occasionally follows an acute course. The most common causes of cirrhosis are:
- chronic excess alcohol ingestion
- viral hepatitis
- autoimmune diseases.

Cirrhosis is irreversible, although where alcohol is implicated, the preceding stage, that of chronic fatty liver, does respond to abstention from alcohol. For reasons that are not clear, only about 30% of patients with alcoholic liver disease progress to cirrhosis.

Clinical features

There are no good biochemical indicators of cirrhosis in the early and stable period,

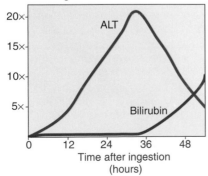

Fold increase above upper limit of reference range

Fig. 30.1 Pattern of liver function tests following ingestion of *Amanita phalloides* (a highly poisonous species of mushroom). *ALT*, Alanine aminotransferase.

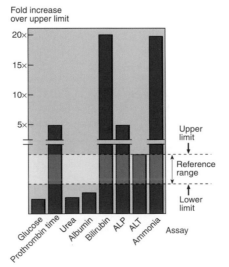

Fold increase over upper limit

Fig. 30.2 Laboratory findings in hepatic failure. *ALP*, alkaline phosphatase; *ALT*, alanine aminotransferase.

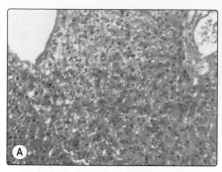
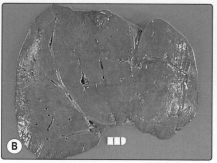
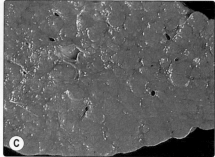

Fig. 30.3 Appearance of normal and diseased liver. (A) Normal liver histology. **(B)** Fatty liver. **(C)** Cirrhotic liver.

which may last for many years. In the later stages the features include jaundice, encephalopathy (due to toxins that are not removed), ascites (see Chapter 64), a bleeding tendency and, finally, terminal liver failure.

Patients with cirrhosis may be unable to cope with food, especially fatty meals, and have a reduced capacity to metabolise drugs. Some patients with cirrhosis suffer badly from itch, due to the failure to excrete bile acids, which accumulate in the skin. The immunological response of patients with cirrhosis may well be reduced, leading to increased susceptibility to infection. However, the cirrhotic liver has a reserve of function despite its macroscopic and microscopic appearance, and length of the clinical course may be difficult to predict.

Unusual causes of cirrhosis

Cirrhosis can develop in children as a result of α_1-antitrypsin deficiency or Wilson's disease and in adults due to haemochromatosis. α_1-antitrypsin deficiency can be detected in newborn infants in whom there may be a prolonged period of jaundice for several weeks. In some cases this progresses to juvenile cirrhosis. Haemochromatosis is a disorder of iron absorption, associated with deposition of iron in the hepatocytes and other tissues, which can lead to liver failure. The diagnosis is by measurement of serum iron, transferrin and ferritin (Chapter 58). Wilson's disease is an inherited disorder of copper metabolism that leads to failure to excrete copper, and its accumulation. It is biochemically characterised by low concentrations of its binding protein (caeruloplasmin) and deposition of copper in the liver and other tissues (Chapter 59). Cirrhosis also may occur following chronic ingestion of pyrrolizidine alkaloids, such as are found in some herbal teas.

Other liver problems

The liver is a common site of metastases from a wide variety of primary tumours, and jaundice may be the first indication of the presence of cancer in some patients. The primary malignancy of liver (hepatoma) is associated with conditions such as cirrhosis or hepatitis, as well as with carcinogens. Aflatoxins generated by specific fungi, infecting foodstuffs, have been identified. Alpha-fetoprotein is a useful marker of primary hepatic tumours (Chapter 72).

Clinical note

Liver biopsy is the definitive way of making a specific diagnosis. Before attempting a needle biopsy, it is essential that the patient's blood coagulation status is confirmed to be satisfactory.

Liver disease

- Acute liver damage may be caused by shock, toxins or infection.

- Biochemical monitoring of liver disease is by sequential measurements of alanine aminotransferase (ALT), bilirubin and alkaline phosphatase (ALP).

- In acute liver damage there is usually intrahepatic obstruction as well as hepatocellular damage.

- Severe cases of acute liver damage may progress to hepatocellular failure.

- Cirrhosis is the end-point of both acute and chronic liver damage, as well as being caused by a number of metabolic and autoimmune diseases.

- Biochemical tests are more useful in monitoring than in diagnosis. A liver biopsy is potentially definitive, whilst imaging may also provide diagnostic information.

Case history 22

A 49-year-old woman attended her general practitioner with an 8-day history of anorexia, nausea and flulike symptoms. She had noticed that her urine had been dark in colour over the past 2 days. Physical examination revealed tenderness in the right upper quadrant of the abdomen. LFTs were as follows:

Bilirubin µmol / L	AST	ALT U/L	ALP	GGT	Total protein g/L	Albumin
63	936	2700	410	312	68	42

- Comment on these results.
- What is the differential diagnosis?
  Comment in Case history comments.

Want to know more?

Tomasi TBR. Structure and function of alpha-fetoprotein. *Ann Rev Med.* 1977;28:453-465. http://www.annualreviews.org/doi/pdf/10.1146/annurev.me.28.020177.002321

Virtually all of the focus on alpha-fetoprotein is on its potential role in the detection of fetal malformations and as a tumour marker. For the curious, this elderly review article focuses on its biological role.

31 | Glucose metabolism and diabetes mellitus

Dietary carbohydrate is digested in the gastrointestinal tract to simple monosaccharides, which are then absorbed. Starch provides glucose directly, while fructose (from dietary sucrose) and galactose (from dietary lactose) are absorbed and also converted into glucose in the liver. Thus glucose is the common carbohydrate currency of the body. Fig. 31.1 shows the different metabolic processes that affect the blood glucose concentration. As always, this concentration reflects a balance between input and output, synthesis and catabolism.

Insulin

Insulin is the principal hormone affecting blood glucose concentrations, and an understanding of its actions is an important prerequisite to the study of diabetes mellitus. Insulin is a peptide hormone synthesised in the beta cells of the islets of Langerhans of the pancreas. It acts through membrane receptors, and its main target tissues are liver, muscle and adipose tissue. Insulin and glucose exist in a classic feedback loop; high concentrations of insulin lower glucose, while high glucose concentrations stimulate insulin secretion (Fig. 31.2).

Insulin signals the fed state, switching on pathways and processes involved in cellular uptake and storage of metabolic fuels, and switching off pathways involved in fuel breakdown (Fig. 31.3). Glucose cannot enter cells in the absence of insulin.

Insulin actions are opposed by, for example, glucagon, adrenaline, glucocorticoids and growth hormone. These are sometimes called stress (or 'anti-insulin') hormones; this explains why acutely ill (and therefore physiologically stressed) patients often have raised blood glucose.

Diabetes mellitus

Diabetes mellitus is the commonest endocrine disorder in clinical practice. It is characterised by hyperglycaemia due to insulin resistance and/or an absolute or relative lack of insulin.

Primary diabetes mellitus is generally subclassified into type 1 or type 2. These clinical entities differ in epidemiology, clinical features and pathophysiology. The contrasting features of types 1 and 2 diabetes mellitus are shown in Table 31.1.

Secondary diabetes mellitus may result from pancreatic disease, endocrine disease such as Cushing's syndrome, drug therapy and, rarely, insulin receptor abnormalities.

Type 1 diabetes mellitus

Type 1 diabetes accounts for approximately 10% of all diabetes. It is commonest in the young (peak incidence between 9 and 14 years of age). The absolute lack of insulin results from the autoimmune destruction of insulin-producing beta cells, and the presence of islet cell antibodies in serum predicts future development of diabetes. There may be an environmental precipitating factor such as a viral infection.

Type 2 diabetes mellitus

Type 2 diabetes accounts for approximately 90% of all diabetes and can occur at any age. It used to be known as maturity-onset diabetes, but is increasingly seen in younger patients, including children, as well. In this condition there is resistance of peripheral tissues to the actions of insulin, so the insulin level may be normal or even high. Family history and obesity are the most commonly associated clinical features.

Late complications of diabetes mellitus

Diabetes mellitus is not only characterised by the presence of hyperglycaemia but also by the occurrence of late complications:

- *Microangiopathy* is characterised by abnormalities in the walls of small blood vessels, especially thickening of the basement membrane. It is associated with poor glycaemic control.
- *Retinopathy* may lead to blindness because of vitreous haemorrhage from proliferating retinal vessels and maculopathy as a result of exudates from vessels or oedema affecting the macula (Fig. 31.4).
- *Nephropathy* leads ultimately to renal failure. In the early stage there is kidney hyperfunction, associated with an increased glomerular filtration

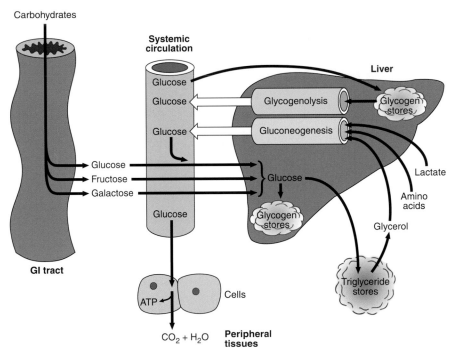

Fig. 31.1 Glucose homeostasis. *ATP*, Adenosine triphosphate; *GI*, gastrointestinal.

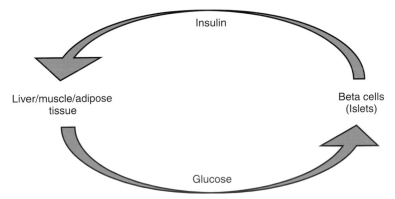

Fig. 31.2 Control of blood glucose.

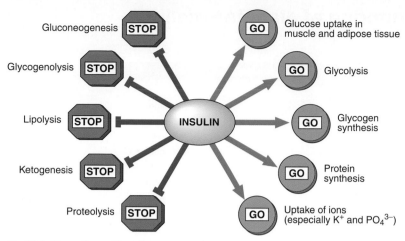

Fig. 31.3 The actions of insulin.

Table 31.1 **Type 1 versus type 2 diabetes mellitus**		
Main Features	**Type 1**	**Type 2**
Epidemiology		
Frequency in Northern Europe	0.7%–0.8%	6%–7%
Predominance	Northern European Caucasians	Worldwide
		Lowest in rural areas of developing countries
Clinical Characteristics		
Age at diagnosis	<30 years (peak 9–14 years)	>40 years (but emerging in younger people)
Weight	Low/normal	Increased
Onset	Rapid	Slow
Ketosis	Common	Under stress
Endogenous insulin	Low/absent	Present but insufficient
HLA associations	Yes	No
Islet cell antibodies	Yes	No
Pathophysiology		
Aetiology	Autoimmune destruction of pancreatic islet cells	Insulin resistance that eventually overwhelms insulin secretory capacity
Genetic associations	Polygenic	Strong
Environmental factors	Viruses and toxins implicated	Obesity, physical inactivity

HLA, Human leukocyte antigen.

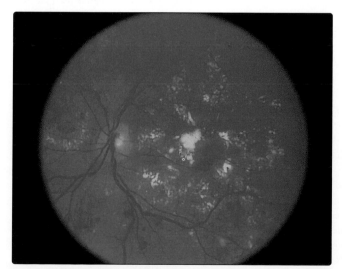

Fig. 31.4 Diabetic retinopathy.

rate, increased glomerular size and microalbuminuria (see Chapter 18, Albumin/creatinine ratio and 'microalbuminurria'). Later there is increasing proteinuria and a marked

decline in renal function, resulting in uraemia.

● *Neuropathy* may become evident as diarrhoea, postural hypotension, impotence, neurogenic bladder

and neuropathic foot ulcers, due to microangiopathy of nerve blood vessels and abnormal glucose metabolism in nerve cells.

● *Macroangiopathy (or accelerated atherosclerosis)* leads to premature coronary heart disease. The exact underlying mechanisms are unclear, although (compensatory) hyperinsulinaemia associated with insulin resistance and type 2 diabetes may play a key role. Certainly, the dyslipidaemia seen in these patients (increased triglycerides, decreased high-density lipoprotein (HDL) cholesterol, and a shift towards smaller, denser low-density lipoprotein (LDL)) is considered highly atherogenic.

Cardiovascular disease is the cause of death in 44% of fatalities in people with type 1 diabetes and 52% of fatalities in people with type 2 diabetes. Blindness is 25 times and chronic kidney disease 17 times more common in people with diabetes. There is increasing evidence that tight glycaemic control delays the onset of these sequelae.

Clinical note

Symptoms of hyperglycaemia include thirst, polyuria and polydipsia (also known as osmotic symptoms, since they result from increased osmolality due to hyperglycaemia), as well as lassitude, weight loss, pruritus vulvae and balanitis. However, some patients with undiagnosed type 2 diabetes may be completely asymptomatic.

Glucose metabolism and diabetes mellitus

● Glucose is the carbohydrate currency of the body. All other carbohydrates are converted to glucose after digestion and absorption.

● Insulin promotes the storage of metabolic fuels.

● Diabetes mellitus is characterised by hyperglycaemia and an absolute or relative lack of insulin.

● Type 1 diabetes mellitus is caused by a complete lack of insulin and is most common in the young.

● Type 2 diabetes mellitus accounts for 90% of all cases of diabetes and can occur at any age.

● Late complications of diabetes mellitus are a result of microangiopathies and macroangiopathies.

Want to know more?

Diabetes Statistics: https://www.diabetes.org.uk/professionals/position-statements-reports/statistics

This link provides various facts and figures which demonstrate the impact of diabetes.

32 | Diagnosis and monitoring of diabetes mellitus

The diagnosis of diabetes must be made with care, since it has far-reaching medical and social consequences. A number of biochemical tests are used in association with clinical assessment for both the initial diagnosis of this condition and long-term monitoring of patients.

Diagnosis of diabetes mellitus

Diabetes can be diagnosed using either venous plasma glucose or glycated haemoglobin (HbA1c). HbA1c is a modified form of haemoglobin, the concentration of which reflects the prevailing glucose concentration over a period of time. Unless accompanied by typical symptoms of diabetes (e.g. polyuria or thirst), a glucose or HbA1c result within the range consistent with diabetes should be confirmed by repeat sampling on a different day.

Plasma glucose

The current World Health Organisation (WHO) criteria for diagnosing diabetes mellitus on the basis of plasma glucose are shown in Table 32.1. The figures shown apply to the concentrations found in venous plasma; slightly different figures (not shown) apply to whole blood or capillary samples. Table 32.1 also shows the criteria for diagnosing diabetes on the basis of an oral glucose tolerance test (OGTT). This test is carried out if the patient has impaired fasting glycaemia (fasting plasma glucose of 6.1–6.9 mmol/L), as some patients will be found to have diabetes mellitus based on the glucose result 2 hours after consumption of a glucose load. As the name suggests, the patient consumes an oral glucose load, with plasma glucose measured (fasting) at the beginning of the test and 2 hours later. (It is important that the patient is sedentary following the consumption of the glucose load – otherwise the later glucose result may be uninterpretable). The 2-hour glucose result in an OGTT also can be used to diagnose impaired glucose tolerance (IGT), an intermediate category of glycaemia that falls short of the diagnosis of diabetes, but which defines an increased risk of developing diabetes. Typical plasma glucose concentrations after ingestion of an oral glucose load by people with and without diabetes are shown in Fig. 32.1.

Glucose is routinely measured in blood specimens that have been collected into tubes containing fluoride oxalate, an inhibitor of glycolysis. Although point-of-care blood glucose meters are central to self-monitoring of diabetes (see later), they should not be used to make a diagnosis of diabetes.

Glycated haemoglobin

Hyperglycaemia leads to the nonenzymatic attachment of glucose to a variety of proteins (glycation), which is virtually irreversible under physiological conditions, and the concentration of glycated protein is therefore a reflection of mean blood glucose concentration during the life of that protein. HbA1c reflects mean glycaemia over 2 months prior to its measurement, reflecting the half-life of haemoglobin. The HbA1c concentration is expressed as millimoles of glycated haemoglobin per mole of total haemoglobin (mmol/mol). Spurious results may sometimes be obtained in patients with inherited structurally abnormal haemoglobins (haemoglobinopathies). An HbA1c of 48 mmol/mol or greater is now accepted by the WHO as being diagnostic of diabetes; if not accompanied by typical symptoms, the result should be confirmed by repeat testing or by another diagnostic test on a different day. HbA1c should not be used for diagnosis if the patient has a condition that affects the lifespan of red blood cells, e.g. anaemia or haemolysis; it should not be used for diagnosis of diabetes in pregnancy and should not be used for diagnosis of suspected type 1 diabetes.

Monitoring of diabetes

HbA1c has a much more established role in monitoring the glycaemic control of diabetes. Targets for optimal control depend on the clinical situation but are generally around 48 to 53 mmol/mol.

Self-monitoring

Many people with diabetes monitor their blood glucose concentration using a point-of-care glucose meter (Fig. 32.2). This requires finger-prick whole blood capillary samples (a drop is usually adequate); the patient is usually advised to vary the time of self-testing in order to get an overall picture of their glycaemic control. Self-monitoring of blood glucose is generally recommended for people with type 1 diabetes, and for people with type 2 diabetes who are treated with insulin, suspected of having hypoglycaemic episodes, on oral medication that may increase their risk of hypoglycaemia, or are pregnant or planning to become pregnant. Many blood glucose meters can now have results downloaded to a computer for review in clinic.

Looking to the future, implantable insulin pumps that sense and respond in real time to the prevailing blood glucose are likely to become increasingly widely available, thus obviating the need for finger-prick testing. Continuous glucose monitoring systems (CGMSs) (see Clinical note and Fig. 32.3) are already in use.

Ketones in urine or blood

The term *ketone bodies* refers to acetone and the ketoacids acetoacetate and β-hydroxybutyrate. These are frequently found in uncontrolled diabetes (diabetic

---

Table 32.1 **Criteria for the diagnosis of diabetes mellitus**

Fasting Plasma Glucose

Nondiabetic	Impaired Fasting Glycaemia	Diabetes
≤6.0	6.1–6.9	≥7.0

Random Plasma Glucose

		Diabetes
		≥11.1

Oral Glucose Tolerance Test

	Fasting	2-hour
Impaired glucose tolerance	<7.0	7.8–11.0
Diabetes	≥7.0	≥11.1

All figures refer to glucose concentrations (mmol/L) in venous plasma.

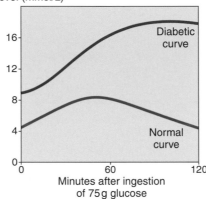

Fig. 32.1 **Plasma glucose concentrations following an oral glucose load in people with and without diabetes.**

ketoacidosis (DKA) – see Chapter 33). They are also found in normal subjects as a result of starvation or fasting and sometimes in alcohol-dependent patients with poor dietary intake (alcoholic ketoacidosis). People with type 1 diabetes are often advised to monitor ketones (in blood or urine) if they are unwell or hyperglycaemic, in order to detect DKA, an emergency situation requiring immediate treatment in hospital.

Clinical note

Despite optimal self-monitoring of blood glucose, some people with type 1 diabetes have problems with severe hypoglycaemia with no obvious precipitating cause, or may lose symptomatic awareness of hypoglycaemia. Some of these patients may benefit from use of a continuous glucose monitoring system – see Fig. 32.3 for an example of data that may be obtained.

Diagnosis and monitoring of diabetes mellitus

• The diagnosis of diabetes mellitus is made on the basis of plasma glucose concentrations or glycated haemoglobin (HbA1c).

• Fasting plasma glucose or HbA1c are the most commonly used first-line diagnostic tests for diabetes.

• HbA1c is widely used to monitor glycaemic control.

Case history 23

A 52-year-old man attends his general practice for a blood test as part of cardiovascular risk assessment. He has been asked to attend fasting. Blood glucose is found to be 7.1 mmol/L.

• What would you do next?
Comment in Case history comments.

Want to know more?

Use of Glycated Haemoglobin (HbA1c) in the Diagnosis of Diabetes Mellitus – https://www.who.int/publications/i/item/use-of-glycated-haemoglobin-(-hba1c)-in-diagnosis-of-diabetes-mellitus.

The use of HbA1c in the diagnosis, as opposed to monitoring, of diabetes mellitus is comparatively recent. This report summarises a WHO consultation on the role for HbA1c in the diagnosis of diabetes.

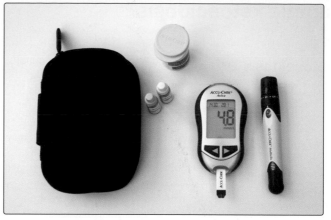

Fig. 32.2 Blood glucose testing device.

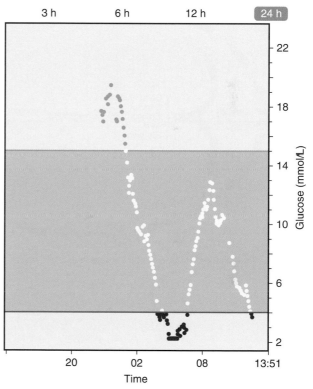

Fig. 32.3 Sample output from a continuous glucose monitoring system (CGMS). Note the episode of nocturnal hypoglycaemia. This record was from a 4-year-old child with a recent diagnosis of type 1 diabetes. She was asleep at the time, but the CGMS sent an alert to her mother's mobile phone, thus allowing the episode of hypoglycaemia to be treated.

33 | Diabetic ketoacidosis

How diabetic ketoacidosis develops

Diabetic ketoacidosis (DKA) is a medical emergency. All metabolic disturbances seen in DKA are the indirect or direct consequences of the lack of insulin (Fig. 33.1). Decreased glucose transport into tissues leads to hyperglycaemia, which gives rise to glycosuria. Increased lipolysis causes overproduction of fatty acids, some of which are converted into ketones, giving ketonaemia, metabolic acidosis and ketonuria. Glycosuria causes an osmotic diuresis, which leads to the loss of water and electrolytes – sodium, potassium, calcium, magnesium, phosphate and chloride. Dehydration, if severe, produces prerenal uraemia and may lead to hypovolaemic shock. The severe metabolic acidosis is partially compensated by an increased ventilation rate (acidotic or Kussmaul breathing). Frequent vomiting is also usually present and accentuates the loss of water and electrolytes. Thus the development of DKA is a series of interlocking vicious circles, all of which must be broken to aid the restoration of normal carbohydrate and lipid metabolism.

The most common precipitating factors in the development of DKA are omission of insulin, infection, myocardial infarction or trauma.

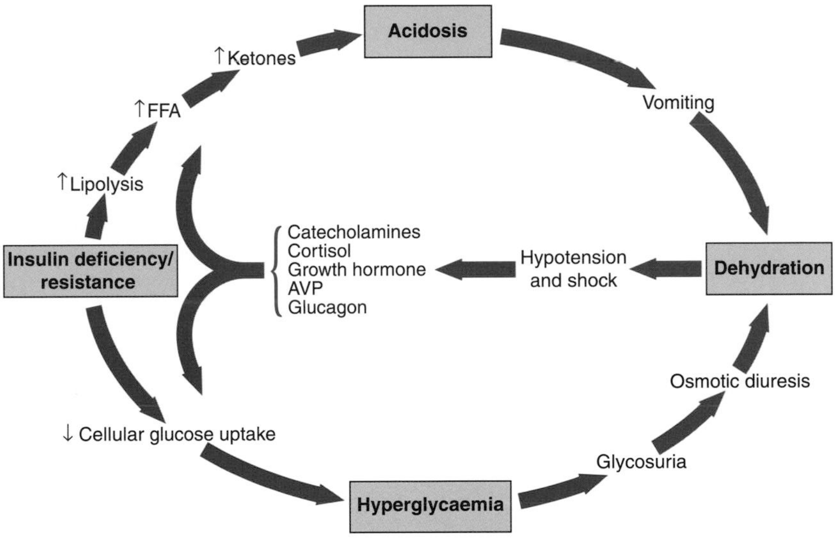

Treatment

The management of DKA requires the administration of three agents:

- *Insulin.* As the root cause in DKA is lack of insulin, prompt commencement of intravenous insulin therapy is required.
- *Fluids.* Patients with DKA are usually severely fluid depleted, and it is essential to expand their extracellular fluid volume with saline to restore their circulation.
- *Potassium.* Despite apparently normal or initially increased serum potassium levels, all patients with DKA have whole body potassium depletion that may be severe. Potassium should be included in intravenous fluids unless serum potassium is above the reference interval or the patient is anuric.

The detailed management of DKA is shown in Fig. 33.2. The importance of good fluid balance charts, as in any serious fluid and electrolyte disorder, cannot be overemphasised. The initial high input of physiological (0.9%) saline is cut back as the patient's fluid and electrolyte deficit improves. Intravenous insulin is given by continuous

Fig. 33.1 The development of diabetic ketoacidosis. *AVP*, Arginine vasopressin; *FFA*, free fatty acids.

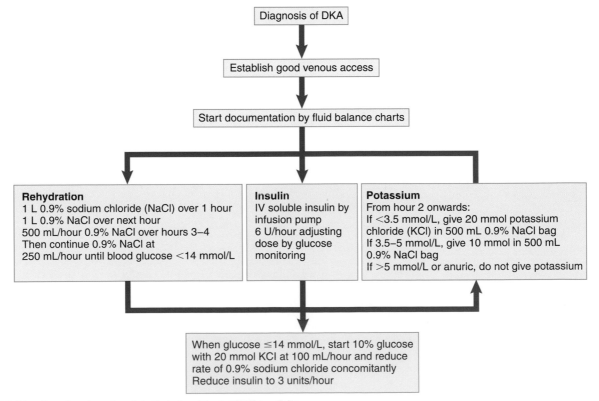

Fig. 33.2 A treatment regimen for diabetic ketoacidosis (DKA) in adults.

infusion using an automated pump, and potassium supplements are included in the fluid regimen. The hallmark of good management of a patient with DKA is close clinical and biochemical monitoring.

Laboratory investigations

Initially, urine (if available) or blood should be tested for glucose and ketones. Venous blood should be sent to the laboratory for plasma glucose and serum sodium, potassium, bicarbonate, urea and creatinine values. A venous blood sample also should be sent for measurement of blood gases.

It is important to highlight a clinically important consequence of laboratory methodology here. The presence of ketone bodies in serum interferes with creatinine measurement in some older assays; therefore serum creatinine can be falsely elevated in the acute stage. In this case, reliable creatinine values are obtained only after ketonaemia subsides.

For reasons that are not entirely clear, amylase activity in serum is also increased in DKA. Pancreatitis should be considered as a precipitating factor only if there is persistent abdominal pain; note, however, that abdominal pain also may be observed in DKA.

Blood glucose should be monitored hourly at the bedside until less than 14 mmol/L. Thereafter, checks may continue every 2 hours. The plasma glucose should be confirmed in the laboratory every 2 to 4 hours. Urea and electrolytes and bicarbonate should be checked at 2 and 4 hours, then every 4 hours for the first 24 hours (Fig. 33.3).

Hyperosmolar hyperglycaemic state (HHS)

This severe metabolic decompensation may occur in people with type 2 diabetes. Table 33.1 shows the principal features of this condition in comparison with DKA.

Diagnosis

HHS occurs mostly in elderly people with type 2 diabetes and develops relatively slowly over days or weeks. The level of insulin is sufficient to prevent significant ketosis but does not prevent hyperglycaemia and osmotic diuresis. Precipitating factors include severe illness, dehydration, glucocorticoids, diuretics, parenteral nutrition, dialysis and surgery. Extremely high blood glucose levels (>35 mmol/L, and sometimes >50 mmol/L) accompany severe dehydration, resulting in impaired consciousness.

Treatment

Treatment is similar to that of DKA, with the following modifications: rehydration should be slower to avoid neurological damage due to rapid osmotic shifts; dilute (0.45%) sodium chloride can be used where the serum osmolality is not declining despite adequate positive fluid balance. However, recent data indicate that in most cases the use of physiological (0.9%) sodium chloride is sufficient. In addition, the insulin dose requirements are usually lower than in DKA. There is also an increased risk of thromboembolism, and prophylactic low-molecular-weight heparin is recommended.

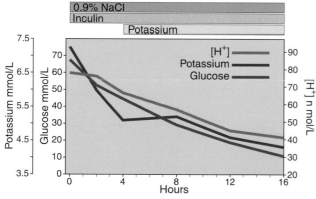

Fig. 33.3 Effective treatment of a severe case of diabetic ketoacidosis.

Table 33.1 **Principal features of diabetic ketoacidosis and hyperosmolar hyperglycaemic state**

Features	Diabetic Ketoacidosis	Hyperosmolar Hyperglycaemic State
Type of diabetes	Type 1	Type 2
Plasma glucose	High	Very high
Ketones	Present	Usually absent
Acidosis	Moderate/Severe	None
Dehydration	Prominent	Prominent
Hyperventilation	Present	None

Case history 24

A 22-year-old patient with diabetes comes to the emergency department. She gives a 2-day history of vomiting and abdominal pain. She is drowsy and her breathing is deep and rapid. There is a distinctive smell from her breath.

- What is the most likely diagnosis?
- Which bedside tests could you do to help you to confirm this diagnosis?
- Which laboratory tests would you request?
  Comment in Case history comments.

Clinical note

Always screen for infection in the patient with diabetes who presents with DKA, since this is a common precipitating factor. Blood, urine, sputum and any wound fluids should be sent for microbiological analysis at the earliest opportunity and certainly before antibiotics are introduced.

Diabetic ketoacidosis

- Diabetic ketoacidosis (DKA) arises from a number of metabolic derangements caused by insulin lack.
- Treatment is by intravenous fluids, insulin and potassium.
- Close clinical and biochemical monitoring are required to tailor the management protocol to the individual patient.
- Hyperosmolar hyperglycaemic state (HHS) is a less common, severe metabolic disturbance of type 2 diabetes.

Want to know more?

https://www.nhsggc.org.uk/media/260549/dkap1_revised4-sl2.pdf

Diabetic ketoacidosis care pathway 1. An example of a care pathway for DKA, it shows how the principles of treatment outlined earlier are applied in practice.

https://www.nhsggc.org.uk/media/260378/hhs-pathways-final-240420.pdf

A clinical guideline outlining the emergency management of hyperosmolar hyperglycaemic state.

These are examples of protocols that demonstrate how the principles of insulin, fluid and potassium replacement are applied in practice.

34 | Hypoglycaemia

Hypoglycaemia is defined as a low blood glucose concentration. In general, children and adults are not usually symptomatic unless the glucose falls below 2.2 mmol/L. Assessment of hypoglycaemia depends critically on the age of the patient, on whether it occurs in the fasting or postprandial state and on whether the patient has diabetes. A detailed drug history is important and should include over-the-counter and alternative preparations, as well as prescribed medications.

Clinical effects

Hypoglycaemia normally leads to suppression of insulin secretion, an increase in catecholamine secretion and stimulation of glucagon, cortisol and growth hormone. The catecholamine surge accounts for the signs and symptoms most commonly seen in hypoglycaemia, i.e. sweating, shaking, tachycardia and feeling weak, jittery and nauseated. Hypoglycaemia decreases the glucose fuel supply to the brain, and symptoms of cognitive impairment must always be sought since they reflect *neuroglycopenia*. They include confusion, poor concentration, detachment and, in more severe instances, convulsions and coma. The clinical effects of hypoglycaemia are summarised in Fig. 34.1.

Assessment

The diagnosis of hypoglycaemia is established when three criteria ('*Whipple's triad*') are satisfied:
- There must be symptoms consistent with hypoglycaemia.
- There must be laboratory confirmation of hypoglycaemia.
- Symptoms must be relieved by the administration of glucose.
  As a preliminary step to formal assessment, patients may be supplied with a blood glucose meter and asked, if they can, to take finger-prick blood samples

during symptomatic episodes. It may be necessary to try to precipitate symptoms, e.g. by prolonged fasting. If a blood sample is being collected for glucose analysis during a symptomatic episode, *an additional sample should be collected simultaneously for insulin*. This need not be analysed at the time, or indeed at all unless hypoglycaemia is confirmed, but the insulin level critically alters the differential diagnosis of causes of hypoglycaemia (Figs 34.2 and 34.3).

Specific causes of hypoglycaemia

Causes of hypoglycaemia may be divided into two groups: those which usually produce hypoglycaemia in the *fasting* patient and those in whom the low glucose is a response to a stimulus (*reactive* hypoglycaemia).

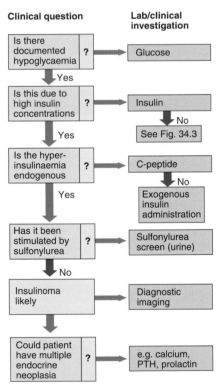

Fig. 34.2 The differential diagnosis of causes of hypoglycaemia in the presence of high insulin levels. *PTH*, Parathyroid hormone.

Fasting hypoglycaemia

Causes of fasting hypoglycaemia include:
- *Insulinoma.* These insulin-producing β-cell tumours of the pancreas may be isolated or part of the wider multiple endocrine neoplasia (MEN) syndrome (see Chapter 73). Insulin-induced weight gain is a characteristic feature. Localisation of the tumour may be difficult.
- *Malignancy.* Hypoglycaemia may be found with any advanced malignancy. Some tumours, e.g. retroperitoneal sarcomas, cause hypoglycaemia by producing insulin-like growth factors.
- *Hepatic and renal disease.* Both the liver and kidneys are capable of gluconeogenesis. Hypoglycaemia is occasionally a feature of advanced hepatic or renal impairment, but this is not usually a diagnostic dilemma.
- *Addison's disease.* Given the fact that glucocorticoids antagonise the actions of insulin, it should not be surprising that hypoglycaemia is occasionally a feature of adrenal insufficiency.
- *Sepsis.* Overwhelming sepsis may be associated with hypoglycaemia; the mechanism is unclear.

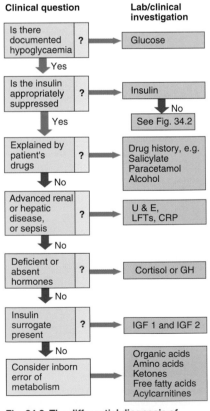

Fig. 34.3 The differential diagnosis of causes of hypoglycaemia in the absence of high insulin levels. *CRP*, C-reactive protein; *GH*, growth hormone; *IGF*, insulin-like growth factor; *LFTs*, liver function tests; *U&E*, urea and electrolytes.

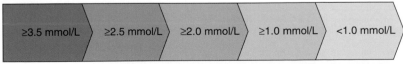
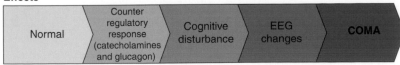

Fig. 34.1 The clinical effects of hypoglycaemia. *EEG*, Electroencephalogram.

Reactive hypoglycaemia

Causes of reactive hypoglycaemia include:

- *Insulin-induced.* Inappropriate or excessive insulin predictably produces hypoglycaemia. Occasionally it is important to distinguish between exogenous insulin (administered by the patient or someone else) and endogenous insulin. Standard assays for insulin cannot distinguish between the two kinds. However, insulin and its associated connecting peptide (or C-peptide) are secreted by the islet cells in equimolar amounts, and thus measurement of C-peptide along with insulin can differentiate between hypoglycaemia due to, for example, an insulinoma (high C-peptide) and that due to exogenous insulin (low C-peptide) (Fig. 34.4).

- *Drug-induced.* Oral hypoglycaemics, e.g. sulfonylureas, can produce hypoglycaemia. Urinary screens for sulfonylureas exist. Other drugs that occasionally give rise to hypoglycaemia less predictably include salicylate, paracetamol and β-blockers. More importantly, the last also may mask the patient's awareness of hypoglycaemia by blunting the β-receptor–mediated effect of adrenaline and reducing or eliminating the warning symptoms, e.g. palpitation or tremor.

- *Alcohol.* Hypoglycaemia is not uncommon in people who consume excess alcohol. Mechanisms include inhibition of gluconeogenesis, malnutrition and liver disease.

- *'Dumping syndrome'.* Accelerated gastric emptying following gastric resection (e.g. gastric bypass for weight loss) may result in the rapid absorption of large amounts of glucose with a resultant surge of insulin release. Smaller, more frequent meals and avoidance of large amounts of sugars may help to minimise this phenomenon.

Diabetes

In patients with diabetes, hypoglycaemia is rarely a diagnostic dilemma. Precipitating factors include:

- insufficient carbohydrate intake
- excess of insulin or sulfonylurea
- strenuous exercise
- excessive alcohol intake.

Neonatal hypoglycaemia

Certain groups of neonates are especially vulnerable to hypoglycaemia:

- *Small-for-gestational-age infants.* Depleted glycogen stores and impaired gluconeogenesis contribute.

- *Babies of diabetic mothers.* A fetus that is exposed to maternal hyperglycaemia will develop hyperplasia of the islet cells and associated hyperinsulinaemia. After delivery, the neonate is unable to suppress its high insulin levels that are now inappropriate, and hypoglycaemia results.

- *Nesidioblastosis.* Hyperplasia of the islet cells may develop even when the mother does not have diabetes; the reasons are unclear.

- *Inborn errors of metabolism.* Many inborn errors are associated with hypoglycaemia. Fatty acid oxidation defects, glycogen storage diseases and galactosaemia are important examples.

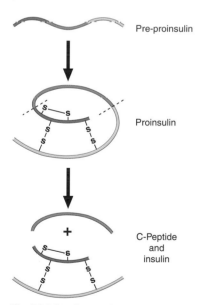

Fig. 34.4 Insulin and C-peptide.

Pre-proinsulin

Proinsulin

+

C-Peptide and insulin

Hypoglycaemia

- Hypoglycaemia is not a diagnosis but is a biochemical sign associated with a diverse group of diseases.

- Management is by glucose therapy and/or glucagon, irrespective of the underlying cause.

- Excess insulin, excess alcohol or low calorie intake in a patient with diabetes are the most common causes of hypoglycaemia.

- Insulinoma is characterised by hypoglycaemia in the face of inappropriately high plasma insulin.

- Hypoglycaemia in the neonate may result in brain damage.

Case history 25

A 25-year-old woman with type 1 diabetes mellitus complained of repeated episodes of sleep disturbances, night sweats and vivid, unpleasant dreams.

- What is the most likely cause of this woman's symptoms and how might the diagnosis be confirmed? *Comment in Case history comments.*

Want to know more?

https://metbio.net/wp-content/uploads/MetBio-Guideline-FUJA773994-19-11-2018.pdf

This guideline gives details of how to investigate hypoglycaemia in infants and children. There is a focus on inherited metabolic diseases which may present with hypoglycaemia.

35 | Calcium regulation and hypocalcaemia

Calcium homeostasis

The amount of calcium present in the extracellular fluid (ECF) is very small compared to what is stored in bone. Even in the adult, calcium in bone is not static; some bone is resorbed each day and the calcium returned to the ECF. To maintain calcium balance, an equal amount of bone formation must take place. Fig. 35.1 shows how much calcium is exchanged between one compartment and another daily.

Calcium homeostasis is modulated by hormones (Fig. 35.2). Parathyroid hormone (PTH) is secreted from the parathyroid glands in response to a low unbound plasma calcium. PTH causes bone resorption and promotes calcium reabsorption in the renal tubules, preventing loss in the urine. 1,25-dihydroxycholecalciferol (1,25 DHCC) maintains intestinal calcium absorption. This sterol hormone is formed from vitamin D (cholecalciferol), following hydroxylation in the liver and kidney. However, hydroxylation in the kidney is PTH-dependent, and so even the absorption of calcium from the gut relies (albeit indirectly) on PTH.

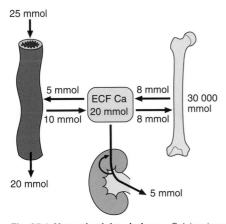

Fig. 35.1 **Normal calcium balance.** Calcium is exchanged each day, in the amounts shown, between the extracellular fluid *(ECF)* and the gut, bone and kidney.

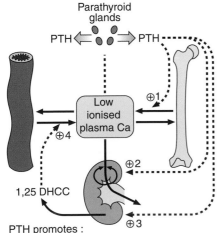

PTH promotes :
1 Bone resorption
2 Renal tubular reabsorption
3 1,25 DHCC synthesis
4 Calcium absorption from gut

Fig. 35.2 **The effects of parathyroid hormone *(PTH)* in restoring a low plasma calcium to normal.** PTH also promotes renal tubular excretion of phosphate. *1,25 DHCC*, 1,25-dihydroxycholecalciferol.

Plasma calcium

A healthy person has a total serum calcium of around 2.4 mmol/L. About half is bound to protein, mostly to albumin. Binding is H^+-dependent and is decreased in acidosis, because the amino acid side chains on albumin become more positively charged. Conversely, binding is increased if alkalosis is present. Hence, the percentage of unbound calcium increases in acidosis and decreases if there is an alkalosis.

Unbound or 'free' calcium exists in the ionised state and is sometimes referred to as ionised calcium. This is the biologically active fraction of the total calcium in plasma, and tight control is required for nerve function, membrane permeability, muscle contraction and glandular secretion. PTH acts to keep the unbound/ionised calcium concentration constant.

Laboratories routinely measure total calcium (bound plus unbound) in serum. However, changes in serum albumin concentration cause changes in total calcium concentration, and this may create problems with interpretation. If albumin falls, total serum calcium is low because the bound fraction is decreased. Remember that the homeostatic mechanisms for regulating plasma calcium respond to the unbound/ionised fraction, not to the total calcium. Patients with a low albumin have total serum calcium lower than the reference values, yet have normal unbound/ionised calcium. *These patients should not be thought of as hypocalcaemic.*

In order to circumvent this problem and ensure patients with a low albumin value are not mistakenly labelled as hypocalcaemic, clinical biochemists use the convention of the 'adjusted calcium' Laboratories measure total calcium and albumin and, if the albumin is abnormal (usually low), calculate what the total calcium would be if the albumin was normal. One such calculation is:

Adjusted calcium (mmol/L) = Total measured calcium + 0.02 (47 − Albumin)

Fig. 35.3 shows the relationship between blood calcium and PTH and helps in the differential diagnosis of common calcium-related disorders.

Hypocalcaemia

In health, serum calcium is tightly regulated between 2.2 and 2.6 mmol/L (in most laboratories).

The causes of hypocalcaemia include:

- *Vitamin D deficiency.* This may be due to malabsorption or an inadequate diet with little exposure to sunlight. If severe, it may lead to osteomalacia in adults and rickets in children (see Chapter 38).
- *Hypoparathyroidism.* This can be autoimmune, postsurgical or related to magnesium deficiency.
- *Magnesium deficiency.* This is a relatively common cause in hospital inpatients.
- *Renal disease.* The diseased kidneys fail to synthesise 1,25 DHCC (see Chapter 20). Increased PTH secretion in response to the resultant hypocalcaemia may lead to bone disease if untreated.
- *'Hungry bone' syndrome.* This classically occurs following parathyroidectomy for severe hyperparathyroidism. Rapid remineralisation of bone follows the sudden postoperative fall in PTH. There can be severe and potentially fatal hypocalcaemia with accompanying hypophosphataemia.

- *Pseudohypoparathyroidism.* PTH is secreted, but there is end-organ resistance – failure of target tissue receptors to respond to the hormone.
- *Rarer causes,* e.g. acute rhabdomyolysis, acute pancreatitis, ethylene glycol poisoning or bone marrow transplantation.

Clinical features

The clinical features of hypocalcaemia include neurological features such as tingling, tetany and mental changes; cardiovascular signs such as an abnormal electrocardiogram; and cataracts.

A strategy for the investigation and differential diagnosis of hypocalcaemia is shown in Fig. 35.4.

PTH

Low calcium and high PTH (Secondary hyperparathyroidism)	**High calcium and high PTH** (Primary hyperparathyroidism)
Renal impairment Vitamin D deficiency	Parathyroid adenoma(s) Parathyroid hyperplasia
Low calcium and low PTH (Hypoparathyroidism)	**High calcium and low PTH**
Idiopathic/autoimmune Surgical removal (neck surgery) Radiotherapy Magnesium deficiency	Malignancy Excess calcium intake Granulomatous disorders e.g. sarcoidosis, tuberculosis

Calcium

Fig. 35.3 Differential diagnosis of abnormal serum calcium. *PTH,* Parathyroid hormone.

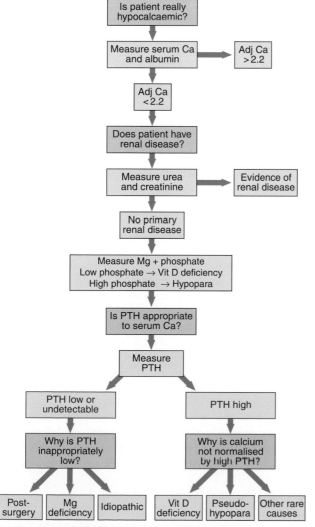

Fig. 35.4 The investigation of hypocalcaemia. *Adj ca,* Adjusted calcium; *PTH,* parathyroid hormone; *vit D,* vitamin D.

Treatment

The management calls for the treatment of the cause of the hypocalcaemia, if this is possible. Oral calcium supplements (often in combination with vitamin D) are commonly prescribed in mild disorders. Hypoparathyroidism or severe renal disease usually requires more potent forms of vitamin D – 1α-hydroxycholecalciferol, or calcitriol.

Clinical note

Trousseau's sign is the most reliable indication of latent tetany (Fig. 35.5). A sphygmomanometer cuff is inflated to above systolic pressure for at least 2 minutes while observing the hand. A positive response will be the appearance of typical carpal spasm, which relaxes soon after the cuff is released.

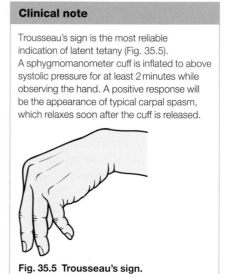

Fig. 35.5 Trousseau's sign.

Calcium regulation and hypocalcaemia

- 'Adjusted calcium' should be used to avoid the problems of interpreting the total calcium concentration in patients who have abnormal serum albumin concentrations.

- If a hypocalcaemic patient has low or undetectable parathyroid hormone (PTH) in serum, they are hypoparathyroid. This may be because of hypomagnesaemia.

- If PTH concentrations are appropriately elevated to the low calcium, the reason for the hypocalcaemia is most likely to be vitamin D deficiency.

- Patients with chronic renal failure often have hypocalcaemia due to the inability of renal cells to synthesise 1,25-dihydroxycholecalciferol. Secondary hyperparathyroidism and bone disease may result.

Case history 26

A 70-year-old woman attended her general practitioner complaining of generalised bone pain. Biochemistry results on a serum specimen taken at the surgery showed the following:

Calcium	Phosphate	Albumin	Ca (adj)
	mmol/L	g/L	mmol/L
1.80	1.1	39	1.96

- What further investigations would be appropriate? *Comment in Case history comments.*

Want to know more?

http://bestpractice.bmj.com/best-practice/monograph/517.html

This BMJ Best Practice monograph breaks down osteomalacia into bite-sized chunks of information.

36 | Hypercalcaemia

Calcium analysis is part of a 'bone profile' and is frequently requested along with other biochemical tests. Therefore unsuspected hypercalcaemia can be detected long before symptoms become apparent. Certainly, patients today are unlikely to present with gross bone disease or severe renal calculi as a consequence of untreated primary hyperparathyroidism, as used to happen in the past. A high serum calcium concentration may be an unexpected finding in a patient in any clinic or hospital ward, as the symptoms of hypercalcaemia are nonspecific. All such findings should be followed up.

Clinical features

Symptoms of hypercalcaemia include:

- neurological and psychiatric features, e.g. lethargy, confusion, irritability and depression
- gastrointestinal problems such as anorexia, abdominal pain, nausea, vomiting and constipation
- renal features such as thirst, polyuria and renal calculi
- cardiac arrhythmias.

Diagnosis

The commonest causes of hypercalcaemia are primary hyperparathyroidism and hypercalcaemia of malignancy.

A diagnostic decision chart is shown in Fig. 36.1. *Primary hyperparathyroidism* is most often due to a single parathyroid

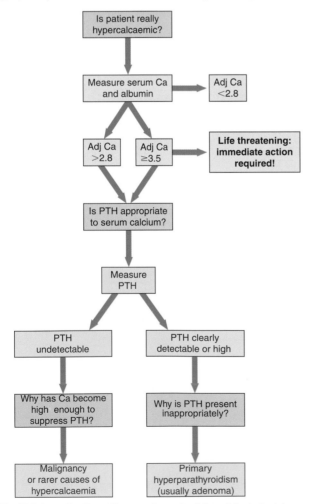

Fig. 36.1 Investigation of hypercalcaemia. *Adj ca,* Adjusted calcium; *PTH,* parathyroid hormone.

adenoma, which secretes parathyroid hormone (PTH) autonomously, i.e. not responding to feedback control by plasma calcium. *Hypercalcaemia associated with malignancy* is the commonest cause of high calcium in hospital inpatients and signifies a poor prognosis. Some tumours secrete a protein called parathyroid hormone-related peptide (PTHrP), which has PTH-like properties, causing hypercalcaemia, but is not detected in the assay for PTH.

Rarer causes of hypercalcaemia include:

- *Inappropriate dosage of vitamin D or metabolites,* e.g. in the treatment of hypoparathyroidism or renal disease or due to self-medication.
- *Granulomatous diseases* (e.g. sarcoidosis or tuberculosis) or certain tumours (e.g. lymphomas) synthesise 1,25-dihydroxycholecalciferol (1,25 DHCC).
- *Thyrotoxicosis* very occasionally leads to increased bone turnover and hypercalcaemia.
- *Thiazide therapy.* The hypercalcaemia is usually mild.
- *Immobilisation.* Especially in association with quadriplegia or paraplegia.
- *Renal disease.* PTH secretion may become independent of calcium feedback after a long-standing cause of secondary hyperparathyroidism is removed (classically described following renal transplantation). This is termed *tertiary hyperparathyroidism* and is biochemically indistinguishable from primary hyperparathyroidism. It is very rarely seen.
- *Calcium therapy.* Patients are routinely given calcium-containing solutions during cardiac surgery and may have transient hypercalcaemia afterwards.
- *Diuretic phase of acute renal failure or in the recovery from severe rhabdomyolysis.*
- *Milk alkali syndrome.* The combination of an increased calcium intake together with bicarbonate, as in a patient self-medicating with proprietary antacid, may cause hypercalcaemia, but the condition is rare.

Treatment

Treatment is *urgent* if the adjusted serum calcium is greater than 3.5 mmol/L; the priority is to reduce it to a safe level. Hypercalcaemia inhibits proximal tubular reabsorption of sodium; as a result patients are dehydrated due to loss of sodium and water. Intravenous saline is administered to replace these losses and in so doing to restore the glomerular filtration rate. Although steroids, mithramycin, calcitonin and intravenous phosphate have been used, parenteral bisphosphonates (zoledronic acid and pamidronate) and denosumab have been found to have the best calcium-lowering effects and are the treatment of choice in patients with hypercalcaemia of malignancy (Fig. 36.2). They act by inhibiting bone resorption. In the absence of renal failure or heart failure, routine use of loop diuretics (e.g. furosemide) to increase urinary calcium excretion is not recommended due to potential complications.

The cause of the hypercalcaemia should be treated if possible. Surgical removal of a parathyroid adenoma usually provides a complete cure for a patient with primary hyperparathyroidism. Immediately after successful surgery, transient hypocalcaemia ('hungry bone syndrome') may have to be treated with vitamin D metabolites, until the remaining parathyroid glands begin to operate normally.

Familial benign hypercalcaemia

Although a definitive differential diagnosis of hypercalcaemia often can be made, there is one rare condition in which an

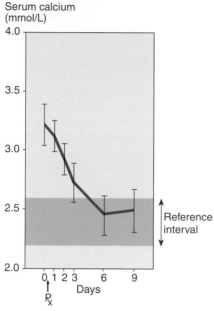

Fig. 36.2 Treatment of hypercalcaemia of malignancy with pamidronate. The graph shows the response of serum calcium in 12 patients treated with a single dose of the bisphosphonate pamidronate in 0.9% saline infused over 6 h, after initial rehydration.

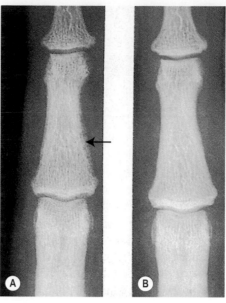

Fig. 36.3 Classic subperiosteal resorption in a patient with severe primary hyperparathyroidism. (A) Radiograph shows resorption in the phalanges. **(B)** Same finger 5 months after removal of parathyroid adenoma.

incorrect diagnosis can lead to unnecessary surgery. In *familial benign hypercalcaemia* (FBH) (also known as familial hypocalciuric hypercalcaemia), genetic mutations in the calcium-sensing receptor in the parathyroid glands result in reduced receptor sensitivity. As a result, suppression of PTH release by negative feedback occurs at a higher calcium concentration than normal. Because of this alteration in the 'set point' for calcium sensing, a high calcium is sensed by the parathyroid glands as normal. The patient therefore has normal or modestly elevated levels of PTH in association with hypercalcaemia, a combination of results which may lead to them being labelled incorrectly as hyperparathyroid. On neck exploration, no parathyroid adenoma is found and it may be discovered subsequently that family members also have asymptomatic

hypercalcaemia. Patients with the condition require no treatment; the hypercalcaemia is usually mild and asymptomatic.

Urine calcium excretion in this condition is lower than would be expected for the serum calcium and usually lower than in primary hyperparathyroidism, although the values in both conditions overlap. However, it may be difficult to distinguish the conditions biochemically. Other modalities of investigation, e.g. isotope (sestamibi) scans, may be helpful. FBH always must be considered when investigating the cause of asymptomatic hypercalcaemia in a relatively young patient.

Clinical note

If hypercalcaemia is not detected early, the high circulating parathyroid hormone (PTH) causes a characteristic pattern of bone resorption, known as *osteitis fibrosa cystica* (Fig. 36.3). As pointed out earlier, such severe bone abnormalities are seen much less frequently than in the past.

Hypercalcaemia

- Consideration of both serum calcium and albumin concentrations, as an 'adjusted' calcium, will give a correct assessment of the severity of the hypercalcaemia.

- Hypercalcaemia will most likely be due to the presence of a parathyroid adenoma or will be associated with a malignancy. In the former, serum parathyroid hormone (PTH) will be high or inappropriately detectable, whereas in hypercalcaemia of malignancy the high calcium suppresses parathyroid function and serum PTH is very low or undetectable.

- Serum calcium in excess of 3.5 mmol/L is a medical emergency.

- Parenteral bisphosphonates and denosumab have the ability to reduce serum calcium rapidly by inhibiting bone resorption.

Case history 27

A 48-year-old woman came to her general practitioner (GP) with a 12-month history of increasing tiredness and muscle fatigue. In recent weeks she had been increasingly thirsty and had polyuria. Her GP tested a urine sample for glucose, which he found to be negative, and then arranged that her urea and electrolytes be measured. He decided to request a calcium profile on the serum sample as well.

Biochemistry results in a serum specimen were:

Na⁺	K⁺	Cl⁻	HCO₃⁻	Urea	Creatinine
		mmol/L			*μmol/L*
149	3.5	109	20	7.5	160
Calcium	Phosphate		Albumin		Ca (adj)
mmol/L	*mmol/L*		*g/L*		*mmol/L*
3.30	0.51		35		3.54

- What are the most likely diagnoses in this patient?
- What other investigations would be appropriate?
  Comment in Case history comments.

Want to know more?

Minisola S, Pepe J, Piemonte S, Cipriani C. The diagnosis and management of hypercalcaemia. *BMJ.* 2015;350:27–30.

This article outlines an approach to the diagnosis and management of hypercalcaemia.

37 | Phosphate and magnesium

Phosphate

Phosphate is abundant in the body and is an important intracellular and extracellular anion. Much of the phosphate inside cells is covalently attached to lipids and proteins. Phosphorylation and dephosphorylation of enzymes are important mechanisms in the regulation of metabolic activity. Much of the body's phosphate is in bone (Fig. 37.1). Phosphate changes accompany calcium deposition or resorption of bone. Control of extracellular fluid (ECF) phosphate concentration is achieved by the kidney, where tubular reabsorption is reduced by parathyroid hormone (PTH). The phosphate that is not reabsorbed in the renal tubule acts as an important urinary buffer.

Inorganic phosphate

At physiological hydrogen ion concentrations, phosphate exists in the ECF both as monohydrogen phosphate and dihydrogen phosphate. Both forms together are termed 'phosphate', and the total is normally maintained within the limits of 0.80 to 1.50 mmol/L. Sometimes the term *inorganic phosphate* is used to distinguish these forms from organically bound phosphate such as in adenosine triphosphate (ATP). Approximately 20% of plasma phosphate is attached to protein, although in contrast to the binding of calcium, this is of little physiological significance.

Hyperphosphataemia

Persistent hyperphosphataemia may result in calcium phosphate deposition in soft tissues. It is classically seen in patients with end-stage renal disease undergoing dialysis. Keeping the calcium-phosphate product in the blood (obtained by multiplying the blood calcium and phosphate concentrations) as low as possible, reduces the risk of this happening.

Causes of a high serum phosphate concentration include:
- *Renal failure*. Phosphate excretion is impaired. This is the commonest cause of hyperphosphataemia.
- *Hypoparathyroidism*. Low circulating PTH decreases phosphate excretion by the kidneys.
- *Redistribution*. Cell damage (lysis), e.g. haemolysis, chemotherapy and rhabdomyolysis, results in release of intracellular phosphate.
- *Acidosis*. Impairs glycolysis and therefore decreased intracellular utilisation of phosphate.
- *Pseudohypoparathyroidism*. There is tissue resistance to PTH.

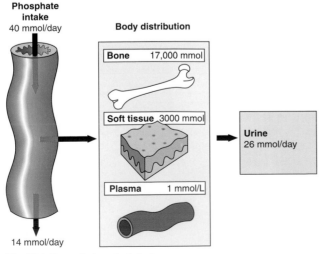

Fig. 37.1 Normal phosphate balance.

Hypophosphataemia

Severe hypophosphataemia (<0.3 mmol/L) is rare and causes muscle weakness, which may lead to respiratory impairment. This requires immediate intravenous infusion of phosphate. Modest hypophosphataemia is much more common. Alcoholic patients are especially prone to hypophosphataemia.

Causes of a low serum phosphate include:
- *Hyperparathyroidism*. This results in increased phosphate excretion by the kidneys.
- *Treatment of diabetic ketoacidosis*. The effect of insulin in causing the shift of glucose into cells causes similar shifts of phosphate.
- *Alkalosis*. Especially respiratory, increases glycolysis and results in movement of phosphate into cells.
- *Refeeding syndrome*. Hypophosphataemia is frequently encountered when malnourished patients are first fed, due to movement of phosphate into cells.
- *Oncogenic hypophosphataemia*. This is a rare cause of hypophosphataemia seen in some tumours and is due to renal phosphate wasting caused by over-expression of fibroblast growth factor 23.
- *'Hungry bone' syndrome*. See Chapter 35.
- *Ingestion of non-absorbable antacids, such as aluminium hydroxide*. These prevent phosphate absorption by binding to it in the gut.
- *Congenital defects of tubular phosphate reabsorption*. In these conditions phosphate is lost from the body in the urine.

Magnesium

Although the biological and biochemical importance of magnesium ions (Mg^{2+}) is well understood, the role of this cation in clinical medicine is sometimes overlooked. Magnesium is the second most abundant intracellular cation, after potassium. Some 300 enzyme systems are magnesium activated, and many aspects of intracellular biochemistry are magnesium-dependent, including glycolysis, oxidative metabolism and transmembrane transport of potassium and calcium.

As well as these intracellular functions, the electrical properties of cell membranes are affected by any reduction in the *extracellular* magnesium concentration. Any detailed consideration of magnesium biochemistry must take into account the interactions among Mg^{2+}, K^+ and Ca^{2+} ions.

Magnesium influences the secretion as well as the action of PTH. Severe hypomagnesaemia may lead to hypoparathyroidism and refractory hypocalcaemia, which is easily correctable by magnesium supplementation. This secondary cause of hypocalcaemia is often missed in clinical practice.

Magnesium homeostasis

Since magnesium is an integral part of chlorophyll, green vegetables are an important dietary source, as are cereals and animal meats. Average dietary intake is around 15 mmol/day, which generally meets the recommended dietary intake. Children and pregnant or lactating women have higher requirements. About 30% of the dietary magnesium is absorbed from the small intestine and widely distributed to all metabolically active tissue (Fig. 37.2).

Serum magnesium

Hypermagnesaemia is uncommon but is occasionally seen in renal failure or following administration of therapeutic magnesium. Hypomagnesaemia is usually associated with

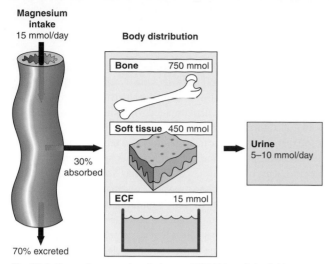

Fig. 37.2 Normal magnesium balance. *ECF*, Extracellular fluid.

magnesium deficiency. The symptoms of hypomagnesaemia are very similar to those of hypocalcaemia: impaired neuromuscular function such as tetany, hyperirritability, tremor, convulsions and muscle weakness.

Magnesium deficiency

Since magnesium is present in most common foodstuffs, low dietary intake of magnesium is associated with general nutritional insufficiency. Symptomatic magnesium deficiency can be expected as a result of:

- dietary insufficiency accompanied by intestinal malabsorption, severe vomiting, diarrhoea or other causes of intestinal loss
- osmotic diuresis such as occurs in diabetes mellitus
- prolonged use of diuretic therapy, especially when dietary intake has been marginal
- prolonged nasogastric suction
- cytotoxic drug therapy such as cisplatin, which impairs renal tubular reabsorption of magnesium
- other drugs: ciclosporin, proton pump inhibitors.

Laboratory diagnosis

The repeated demonstration of a magnesium concentration of less than 0.7 mmol/L in a serum specimen is evidence of intracellular depletion. However, intracellular magnesium depletion may exist where the serum magnesium concentration is within the reference interval. Research procedures have been used to investigate these marginal states. These include the use of nuclear magnetic resonance spectroscopy to detect 'free' Mg^{2+} inside cells, and direct determination of Mg^{2+} in peripheral white blood cells or in muscle biopsy samples.

Management

The provision of magnesium supplements orally is complicated by the fact that they often cause diarrhoea and may counter-productively increase magnesium losses. Indeed, oral magnesium salts are often given as laxatives for this reason. A variety of oral, intramuscular and intravenous regimens have been proposed.

Administration of magnesium salts, by whatever route, is relatively contraindicated when there is a significant degree of renal impairment. In these circumstances, any supplementation must be monitored carefully, and dose adjusted accordingly, to avoid toxic effects associated with hypermagnesaemia.

Clinical note

Intravenous magnesium is the treatment of choice in severe preeclampsia to prevent convulsions and lower the blood pressure.

Phosphate and magnesium

- Hyperphosphataemia is commonly a consequence of renal impairment.
- Hypophosphataemia may be due to the effects of a high circulating parathyroid hormone (PTH) concentration, or to redistribution into cells.
- Magnesium deficiency results from a combination of poor dietary intake and increased urinary or intestinal losses.
- Magnesium deficiency may occur as a complication of intestinal disease or surgery, renal damage by nephrotoxins, diuretics or in diabetes.
- The demonstration of a persistently low serum magnesium suggests severe deficiency, whereas marginal magnesium deficiency states may be present even when serum magnesium is within reference limits.

Case history 28

A 46-year-old woman, known to have radiation enteritis with chronic diarrhoea and associated malabsorption syndrome, presented to the outpatient department complaining of severe tingling of recent onset in her hands and feet. The patient had a past history of hypocalcaemic tetany 18 months previously, but serum calcium had since remained normal on therapy with 1α-hydroxycholecalciferol, 0.75 µg/day, plus oral calcium supplements.

Calcium	Phosphate	Albumin	Ca (adj)	ALP	Magnesium
	mmol/L	g/L	mmol/L	U/L	mmol/L
1.30	1.1	39	1.46	110	0.25

The patient did not respond to treatment with increased calcium supplements and continued 1α-hydroxycholecalciferol.

- What would you predict the patient's PTH status to be?
- What treatment is appropriate and why?
  Comment in Case history comments.

Want to know more?

https://www.researchgate.net/profile/Michael_Murphy11/publication/43147742_Reflex_and_reflective_testing_Efficiency_and_effectiveness_of_adding_on_laboratory_tests/links/55780b9c08aeacff20005d71.pdf

This article examines (among other things) how low serum potassium and/or calcium can point to low serum magnesium.

38 | Metabolic bone disease

Metabolic bone disease covers a broad spectrum of disorders of altered bone structure and/or function. In many of them, serum calcium (and phosphate) concentration may be normal; conversely, the finding of hypercalcaemia or hypocalcaemia does not imply that there will be marked bone changes. The main metabolic bone diseases are:

- osteoporosis
- osteomalacia and rickets
- Paget's disease.

Bone metabolism

Bone is constantly being broken down and re-formed in the process of bone remodelling; this is also referred to as *bone turnover* (Fig. 38.1). Bone disease is often associated with alterations in bone turnover. Theoretically at least, biochemical markers of bone turnover may be useful in assessing the extent of disease, as well as monitoring treatment. However, partly because of their biological and analytical variation, their analysis is restricted to specific conditions and usually requested by specialists.

Urinary hydroxyproline, from the breakdown of collagen, can be used to monitor bone resorption. However, urinary excretion of hydroxyproline is markedly influenced by dietary gelatin and therefore is not a clinically reliable marker. Another collagen degradation product, deoxypyridinoline, is not metabolised or influenced by diet. This fragment of collagen contains the pyridinium cross-links and is specific to bone.

Activity of the enzyme alkaline phosphatase has traditionally been used as an indicator of bone turnover. This enzyme is found in the osteoblasts that lay down the collagen framework and the mineral matrix of bone, and increased osteoblastic activity is indicated by elevated alkaline phosphatase activity. Indeed, children who have active bone growth compared with adults have higher 'normal' alkaline phosphatase activity in serum. However, alkaline phosphatase is not specific to bone – it is also produced by the cells lining the bile canaliculi and hence is a marker for cholestasis. The bone isoenzyme of alkaline phosphatase may be measured, but there is need for a more specific and more sensitive marker.

Osteocalcin meets some of these requirements. It is synthesised by osteoblasts and is an important noncollagenous constituent of bone. Not all of the osteocalcin that an osteoblast makes is incorporated into the bone matrix. Some is released into plasma and provides a sensitive indicator of osteoblast activity.

Common bone disorders

Osteoporosis

Osteoporosis is the commonest bone disorder and is discussed separately in Chapter 39.

Osteomalacia and rickets

Osteomalacia and rickets are the names given to defective or inadequate bone mineralisation in adults and children, respectively (Fig. 38.2). It is primarily due to vitamin D deficiency, and in certain countries, the addition of vitamin D to foodstuffs has reduced the prevalence of the condition. Groups at risk of vitamin D deficiency include the elderly or housebound and certain ethnic groups. Causative factors include inadequate dietary consumption of vitamin D and limited exposure to sunlight. Vitamin D status can be assessed by measurement of the main circulating metabolite, 25-hydroxycholecalciferol, in a serum specimen. The metabolism of vitamin D is shown in Fig. 38.3.

In severe osteomalacia due to vitamin D deficiency, serum calcium falls, resulting in an appropriate increase in parathyroid hormone (PTH) secretion (secondary hyperparathyroidism); PTH increases renal excretion of phosphate, and low serum phosphate may also be an important tell-tale biochemical finding. Elevated serum alkaline phosphatase activity reflects associated osteoblastic activity, trying to compensate for the resulting bone loss. Clinically, patients usually present with muscle aches and bone pain, which respond to high-dose vitamin D supplementation.

Paget's disease of bone

Paget's disease of bone is common in the elderly and characterised by increased osteoclastic activity, which leads to increased bone

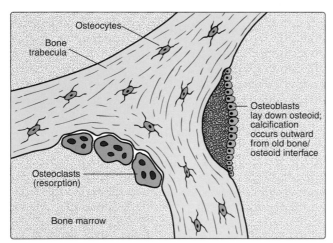

Fig. 38.1 Bone remodelling.

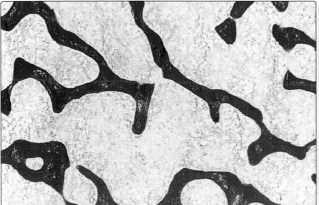
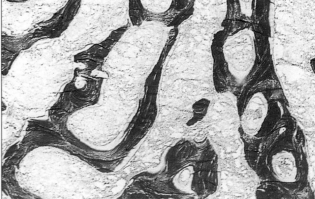

Fig. 38.2 Bone biopsy showing normal *(left)* and osteomalacic *(right)* bone.

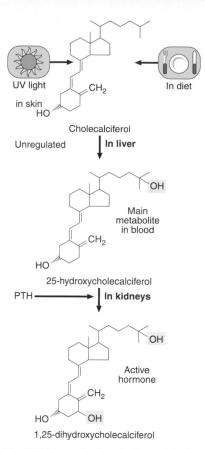

Fig. 38.3 The main steps in the metabolism of vitamin D. *PTH*, Parathyroid hormone.

resorption. Just as with osteomalacia, discussed previously, increased osteoblastic activity repairs resorbed bone, but the new bone is laid down in a disorganised way. Bone turnover is grossly increased, and the new bone formed is more 'plastic', i.e. malleable, than normal bone; as a result, clinical features include bone deformities in addition to bone pain. Serum alkaline phosphatase is very high, and urinary hydroxyproline excretion is elevated. These can be used to monitor the disease. The cause of Paget's disease has not been established definitively; viral and genetic aetiologies have been proposed, the latter probably predisposing individuals to developing the condition. Paget's disease is very common in the white population affecting about 3% of individuals over the age of 55 years, the vast majority of whom may remain asymptomatic and therefore undiagnosed.

Other bone diseases

Examples of other bone diseases include:
- *Vitamin D–dependent rickets*. These rare bone diseases result from genetic disorders leading to the inability to make the active vitamin D metabolite or from receptor defects that do not allow the hormone to act.
- *Tumoral calcinosis*. This is characterised by ectopic calcification around the joints.
- *Hypophosphatasia*. This deficiency of alkaline phosphatase is associated with a form of rickets-like bony deformities.
- *Hypophosphataemic rickets*. There are different hereditary forms of this, resulting in renal phosphate losses and resultant demineralisation of bone.
- *Osteopetrosis*. This rare condition is characterised by defective bone resorption leading to excessively dense bones (the opposite of osteoporosis).
- *Osteogenesis imperfecta (brittle bones)*. This inherited disorder is due to a genetic defect in collagen formation and results in babies and young adults developing multiple and recurrent fractures.

Table 38.1 Biochemical profiles in bone diseases	
Disease	**Profile**
Bone metastases	Calcium may be high, low or normal
	Phosphate may be high, low or normal
	Parathyroid hormone (PTH) is usually low
	Alkaline phosphatase (ALP) may be elevated or normal
Osteomalacia/rickets	Calcium will tend to be low or may be clearly decreased
	PTH will be elevated
	25-hydroxycholecalciferol will be decreased if the disease is due to vitamin D deficiency
Paget's disease	Calcium is normal
	ALP is significantly elevated
Osteoporosis	Biochemistry is unremarkable
Renal osteodystrophy	Calcium is decreased; phosphate is high
	PTH is very high
Primary hyperparathyroidism	Calcium is elevated
	Phosphate is low or normal
	PTH is increased, or clearly detectable and thus 'inappropriate' to the hypercalcaemia

Biochemistry testing in calcium disorders or bone disease

First-line tests include measurement of calcium, albumin, phosphate and alkaline phosphatase in a serum specimen. Follow-up tests that may be requested include:
- PTH
- magnesium
- 25-hydroxycholecalciferol
- urine calcium excretion
- specific markers of bone turnover.

Characteristic biochemistry profiles in some common bone diseases are shown in Table 38.1.

Bone disease

- Alkaline phosphatase is a marker for bone formation. Urinary hydroxyproline is a marker for bone resorption. Other markers for bone turnover are available in specialised laboratories but have limited utility.

- Osteomalacia due to vitamin D deficiency can be confirmed by finding a low 25-hydroxycholecalciferol concentration. Other characteristic biochemical features include hypocalcaemia, elevated parathyroid hormone (PTH) and elevated alkaline phosphatase.

- The characteristic biochemical marker of Paget's disease is a significantly increased alkaline phosphatase activity, as a consequence of increased bone turnover.

Case history 29

A 66-year-old man presented to the bone clinic with severe pains in his right leg and pelvis. Radiological examination revealed Pagetic lesions in his legs, pelvis and skull. Biochemical results in a serum sample were unremarkable except for alkaline phosphatase, which was grossly elevated at 2700 U/L. It was decided to treat him with zoledronic acid (a parenteral bisphosphonate).

- How would you monitor this patient's response?
  Comment in Case history comments.

Want to know more?

Shetty S, Kapoor N, Bondu JD, Thomas N, Paul TV. Bone turnover markers: emerging tool in the management of osteoporosis. *Indian J Endocrinol Metab*. 2016;20(6):846–852. https://www.ncbi.nlm.nih.gov/pmc/articles/PMC5105571/

This article discusses the role of bone turnover markers in the management of osteoporosis.

39 | Osteoporosis and fragility fractures

Osteoporosis is a major public health problem and a major cause of morbidity and mortality in the elderly, as it predisposes to major fractures, including those of the hip and spine.

Bone is in a constant state of turnover, kept in balance by opposing actions of osteoblasts (bone-forming cells) and osteoclasts (bone-resorbing cells). Osteoporosis results when this balance is disturbed in favour of resorption. It is characterised by low bone mineral density (BMD), deterioration of the microarchitecture of bone tissue and susceptibility to fracture (Fig. 39.1). It therefore encompasses a reduction in both the quality and quantity of bone tissue. The World Health Organization (WHO) has proposed a clinical definition based on BMD measurement: a patient is osteoporotic if BMD is 2.5 standard deviations or more below typical peak bone mass of young healthy white women (the so-called T score). A T score of –2.5 (and below) is defined as *osteoporosis*, and a T score of –1 to –2.4 is defined as *osteopenia*.

Risk factors

Age and menopause are the two main nonmodifiable risk factors for osteoporosis. Peak bone mass is reached at around 25 to 30 years (Fig. 39.2). Contributing factors include genetic factors, dietary intake of calcium and vitamin D, and physical exercise.

Other risk factors include history of previous fracture, family history of osteoporosis and hip fracture, sex hormone deficiency, smoking, alcohol, immobility and sedentary lifestyle. Osteoporosis also may be secondary to corticosteroid use (Fig. 39.3), and is seen in various endocrine disorders: Cushing's syndrome, primary hyperparathyroidism, hypovitaminosis D (classically associated with osteomalacia), hypogonadism, hyperthyroidism as well as systemic illnesses such as rheumatoid arthritis, chronic kidney and liver diseases and malignancies.

Diagnosis

A detailed clinical history helps to determine the presence of risk factors. Clinical examination is not always informative. Measurement of bone density by dual-energy X-ray absorptiometry (DEXA) scan is the mainstay of diagnosis. Biochemical markers of bone turnover have limited use in diagnosis of osteoporosis. They can help to select and monitor treatment.

Principles of treatment

Treatment is aimed at improving bone density and quality and preventing fractures. First-line drugs are oral bisphosphonates. These inhibit osteoclastic function, thereby slowing bone loss. However, in practice this does not always result in increased BMD on DEXA scans. Other agents also shift the balance between bone osteoblasts and osteoclasts in favour of the former so that there is net increase in bone formation. They include denosumab, teriparatide and most recently romosozumab.

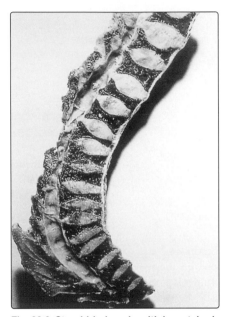

Fig. 39.3 Steroid-induced multiple vertebral fractures.

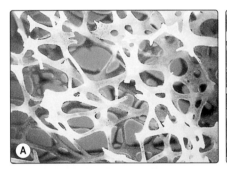
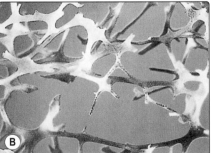

Fig. 39.1 Bone showing (A) normal trabeculae and (B) bone loss in osteoporosis.

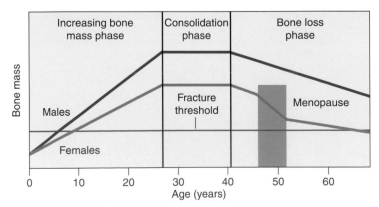

Fig. 39.2 Changes in bone mass with age.

Osteoporosis

- Osteoporosis is a major cause of morbidity and mortality in the elderly.

- It is characterised by a reduction in bone density.

- Although both sexes show a gradual bone loss throughout life, women lose bone rapidly in the postmenopausal years.

- Bone loss causing secondary osteoporosis may be accelerated by a number of factors, e.g. the use of corticosteroids, smoking and immobilisation.

Want to know more?

https://www.sign.ac.uk/media/1812/sign-142-osteoporosis-v3.pdf

This guideline takes an evidence-based approach to the management of osteoporosis.

3

Endocrinology

40 | Endocrine control

Biochemical regulators

Homeostasis, the tendency to maintain stability, is essential to survival. It is achieved by a system of control mechanisms. Endocrine control is achieved by biochemical regulators. Some of these are hormones, i.e. they are released from specialised glands into the blood to influence the activity of cells and tissues at distant sites. Others are paracrine factors, which are not released into the circulation, but which act on adjacent cells, e.g. in the regulation of the immune system. Finally, autocrine factors act on the very cells responsible for their synthesis. These different kinds of regulation are illustrated in Fig. 40.1.

Hormone structure

The diverse biological effects of different hormones are reflected in different molecular structures. Three broad classes are recognised:
- *Peptides or proteins*. Most hormones fall into this class, although they vary enormously in size. For example, the hypothalamic factor thyrotrophin-releasing hormone (TRH) has just three amino acids, whilst the pituitary gonadotrophins are large glycoproteins with subunits.
- *Amino acid derivatives*. Examples include the thyroid hormones and adrenaline (epinephrine).
- *Steroid hormones*. This large class of hormones includes glucocorticoids and sex steroid hormones, all of which are derived structurally from cholesterol.

Assessment of endocrine control

Many endocrine diseases arise from failure of control mechanisms (Table 40.1). Assessment of endocrine control presents particular difficulties:
- *Low concentrations*. Hormone concentrations in blood are sometimes so low that they are at or below the lower limit of

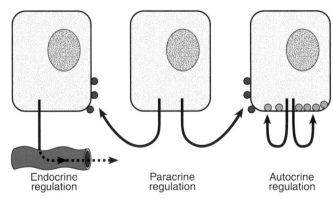

Fig. 40.1 Biochemical regulation of cell function.

Endocrine regulation   Paracrine regulation   Autocrine regulation

Table 40.1 Examples of endocrine disease

Oversecretion

Cushing's disease, in which a pituitary adenoma secretes ACTH

Undersecretion

Primary hypothyroidism, in which the thyroid gland is unable to make sufficient thyroid hormone despite continued stimulation by TSH

Failure of hormone responsiveness

Pseudohypoparathyroidism, in which patients become hypocalcaemic despite elevated plasma PTH concentrations because target organs lack a functioning receptor signalling mechanism

ACTH, Adrenocorticotrophic hormone; *PTH*, parathyroid hormone; *TSH*, thyroid-stimulating hormone.

analytical detection. In the past, it was often the biological response to hormones that formed the basis of relatively crude bioassays of hormone activity. The advent of immunoassays in the 1960s revolutionised endocrinology by permitting the measurement of hormones at very low concentrations. However, despite the refinement of immunoassay technology by, for example, the introduction of monoclonal antibodies, measurement of structurally related hormones continues to be a challenge for the clinical biochemistry laboratory, as is immunoassay interference (see Chapter 82). This problem has been overcome, to an extent, by the use of methods based on highly specific mass spectrometry, but these are not routinely available for all hormone analyses.
- *Variability*. Even where it is possible to measure the concentration of a hormone accurately, the result of a single measurement may be difficult to interpret. This is because the concentration may vary substantially for various reasons, some of which are illustrated in Fig. 40.2. For example, because growth hormone is released in a pulsatile fashion, an undetectable level is largely meaningless. The marked circadian rhythm of cortisol likewise makes interpretation of a random cortisol measurement on an untimed sample potentially challenging.
- *Hormone binding*. Steroid and thyroid hormones bind to specific hormone-binding glycoproteins in plasma. It is the unbound or 'free' fraction of the hormone that is biologically active. Failure to measure the binding protein may lead to misinterpretation of hormone results. For example, testosterone is significantly bound to sex hormone-binding globulin.

Types of endocrine control

Negative feedback

The basic operation of a negative feedback loop is shown in Fig. 40.3. It is perhaps easier to understand the features of such a loop with reference to a particular axis, e.g. the thyroid. Hormone A in this axis is TRH, hormone B is thyroid-stimulating hormone (TSH) and hormone C is thyroid hormone (T_4). Like a dial on a thermostat, the hypothalamus sets the point of optimal control for the system by secreting TRH at a certain level; this will correspond to a certain intended concentration of T_4. By means of negative feedback from T_4, the hypothalamus senses any difference between the actual concentration of T_4 and the intended concentration and readjusts the TRH level (set point) accordingly. This stimulates TSH release from the pituitary in a log-linear fashion, i.e. TSH rises exponentially with increasing TRH, thus permitting an extremely precise degree of control.

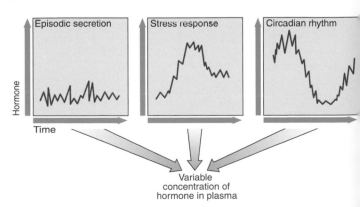

Episodic secretion   Stress response   Circadian rhythm

Hormone

Time

Variable concentration of hormone in plasma

Fig. 40.2 Reasons why a single blood hormone measurement may have little clinical value.

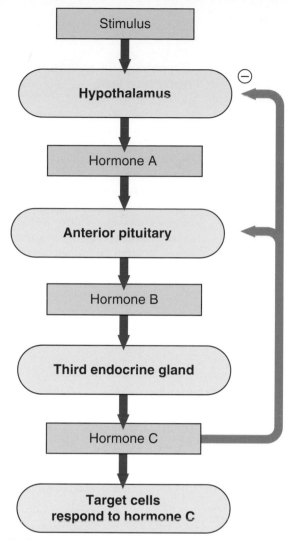

Fig. 40.3 Negative feedback in a hypothalamic pituitary endocrine gland system.

Positive feedback

Negative feedback control is ubiquitous in endocrinology, but there is one notable example of positive feedback. During the follicular phase of the menstrual cycle, the release by the hypothalamus of gonadotrophin-releasing hormone (GnRH) fluctuates. Both follicle-stimulating hormone (FSH) and luteinising hormone (LH) are released in response by the pituitary; FSH stimulates the developing follicles to produce increasing amounts of oestrogen. At a particular point in the cycle the feedback from oestrogen on LH production switches from being negative to being positive, and the resulting LH surge triggers ovulation. The reasons for this switch are not entirely clear (after all, the hypothalamic–pituitary–ovarian axis normally operates as a negative feedback loop), but positive feedback requires a threshold concentration of oestradiol (thought to be in the region of 700 pmol/L) to persist for at least 48 hours. The hormonal changes during a normal menstrual cycle are illustrated in Chapter 50.

Pitfalls in interpretation

- *Immunoassay interference.* Up to 40% of the population may have unsuspected antibodies that can interfere with immunoassays, by interacting either with the analyte being measured or with the antibody being used in the immunoassay reaction mixture. These antibodies can produce falsely lowered or falsely raised results, with potentially serious consequences. Crucially, these interferences are specific to the patient's serum, so *quality control will not detect the problem*. If there is a discrepancy between the clinical and biochemical pictures, or if a result is totally unexpected, this possibility should always be considered. This kind of problem is well recognised for some assays, e.g. thyroglobulin, prolactin. It is dealt with in more detail in Chapter 82.
- *Log-linear responses.* In response to alterations in TRH, TSH rises exponentially. This kind of relationship means the biological significance of a rise in TSH from 1 to 5 mU/L is the same as a rise from 10 to 50 mU/L. Moreover, this kind of relationship applies to all trophins released by the anterior pituitary, including growth hormone, the trophic hormone for insulin-like growth factors. Interestingly, the (skewed) distribution of serum prolactin behaves in a similar way, as if it too was a trophin, like TSH or adrenocorticotrophic hormone (ACTH), even though, as yet, no prolactin-controlled hormone has been identified.

Dynamic function tests

Where the results of clinical assessment and baseline biochemical investigations fail to rule in or rule out a serious endocrine diagnosis, dynamic function tests may be required. Indeed, these are routine in the investigation of some disorders, e.g. acromegaly. They are dealt with in detail in Chapter 41.

Clinical note

The overriding influence of stress on the endocrine system makes the diagnosis of endocrine disorders in the critically ill patient very difficult. Ill patients may have hyperglycaemia, high serum cortisol or abnormal thyroid hormone results. These could be misinterpreted as diabetes mellitus, Cushing's syndrome or thyroid disease, respectively.

Endocrine control

- Endocrinology is the study of hormones, a class of biochemical regulators secreted into blood to act at distant sites in the body.
- Hormone concentrations in plasma are very variable.
- For a clear demonstration of abnormalities of hormone secretion or regulation, dynamic tests are often necessary.

Want to know more?

Wilkin TJ. Endocrine feedback control in health and disease. In: Bittar N, Bittar EE, eds. *The Principles of Medical Biology.* Greenwich, CT: JAI Press; 1998.

This stimulating chapter explores theoretical aspects of endocrine control, noting similarities between natural negative feedback loops and servocontrol loops.

41 | Dynamic function tests

Much of clinical endocrinology is concerned with diseases that involve either a deficiency or an excess of hormones. It is not always possible to diagnose these diseases on the basis of clinical assessment and baseline laboratory investigations. Dynamic function tests (DFTs) involve either stimulating or suppressing a particular hormonal axis and observing the appropriate hormonal response. In general, if a deficiency is suspected, a stimulation test should be used; if excess is suspected, a suppression test is used. Often, the stimulus is an exogenous analogue of a trophic hormone; in other cases it is provided by biochemical or physiological stress, e.g. hypoglycaemia or exercise.

On subsequent pages, individual DFT procedures are discussed in the context of specific hormonal axes. Here, we describe the principles that underpin some of these DFTs and look at aspects of interpretation. The abbreviations used for the various hormones and the tests are listed in Tables 41.1 and 41.2, respectively.

Insulin stress test

This test is carried out when hypopituitarism is suspected. It is also known as the insulin tolerance test. Enough insulin is administered to produce hypoglycaemic stress (blood glucose <2.2 mmol/L). This tests the ability of the anterior pituitary to produce adrenocorticotrophic hormone (ACTH) and growth hormone (GH) in response. Cortisol is measured instead of ACTH (which is unstable); this assumes that the adrenals can respond normally to ACTH. A peak GH in excess of 6 µg/L is regarded as evidence of adequate reserve. For cortisol there is less consensus about what should be regarded as an adequate response, mainly due to different analytical methods; an acceptable response may vary from 420 to 550 nmol/L. An example of the results of an insulin stress test (IST) is shown in Fig. 41.1.

Thyrotrophin-releasing hormone test

Thyrotrophin-releasing hormone (TRH) is given as an intravenous bolus; blood sampling is at 0, 20 and 60 minutes (Fig. 41.2). In normal subjects, TRH elicits a brisk release of both thyroid-stimulating hormone (TSH) and prolactin. This test may be used to assess the adequacy of anterior pituitary reserve or to evaluate suspected hypothalamic disease, in which the TSH response to TRH is characteristically delayed (TSH higher at 60 minutes than at 20 minutes).

Table 41.1 Abbreviations for some hormones

Adrenocorticotrophic hormone	ACTH
Arginine vasopressin	AVP
Corticotrophin-releasing hormone	CRH
Follicle-stimulating hormone	FSH
Gonadotrophin-releasing hormone	GnRH
Growth hormone	GH (or HGH)
Growth hormone-releasing hormone	GHRH
Luteinising hormone	LH
Parathyroid hormone	PTH
Thyroid-stimulating hormone	TSH
Thyrotrophin-releasing hormone	TRH
Thyroxine	T_4
Triiodothyronine	T_3

Table 41.2 Commonly used abbreviations for various dynamic function tests

IST	Insulin stress test
OGTT	Oral glucose tolerance test
SST	Short Synacthen test
DST	Dexamethasone suppression test
CAPFT	Combined anterior pituitary function test

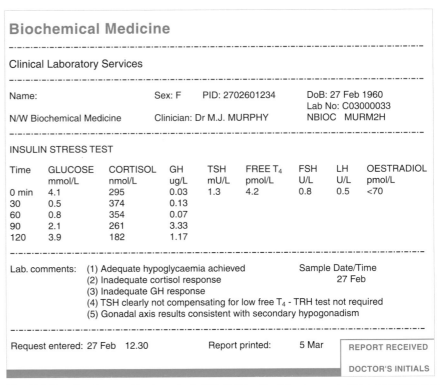

Biochemical Medicine

Clinical Laboratory Services

Name:	Sex: F	PID: 2702601234	DoB: 27 Feb 1960
			Lab No: C03000033
N/W Biochemical Medicine	Clinician: Dr M.J. MURPHY		NBIOC MURM2H

INSULIN STRESS TEST

Time	GLUCOSE mmol/L	CORTISOL nmol/L	GH ug/L	TSH mU/L	FREE T₄ pmol/L	FSH U/L	LH U/L	OESTRADIOL pmol/L
0 min	4.1	295	0.03	1.3	4.2	0.8	0.5	<70
30	0.5	374	0.13					
60	0.8	354	0.07					
90	2.1	261	3.33					
120	3.9	182	1.17					

Lab. comments:	(1) Adequate hypoglycaemia achieved	Sample Date/Time
	(2) Inadequate cortisol response	27 Feb
	(3) Inadequate GH response	
	(4) TSH clearly not compensating for low free T₄ - TRH test not required	
	(5) Gonadal axis results consistent with secondary hypogonadism	

Request entered: 27 Feb 12.30	Report printed:	5 Mar	REPORT RECEIVED
			DOCTOR'S INITIALS

Fig. 41.1 Results of an insulin stress test. *FSH*, Follicle-stimulating hormone; *GH*, growth hormone; *LH*, luteinising hormone; *T₄*, thyroxine; *TSH*, thyroid-stimulating hormone.

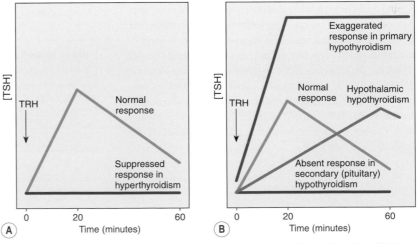

Fig. 41.2 Pituitary responses to TRH. (A) Used in the investigation of hyperthyroidism. **(B)** Used in the investigation of pituitary or hypothalamic hypothyroidism. *TRH*, Thyrotrophin-releasing hormone; *TSH*, thyroid-stimulating hormone.

It is sometimes done also in suspected hyperthyroidism, hypothyroidism or subclinical thyroid disease. Where there has been prolonged negative feedback due to hyperthyroidism, the pituitary response to TRH is flat (TSH rises by <2 mU/L); conversely, an exaggerated TSH response (>25 mU/L) is seen in hypothyroidism.

Gonadotrophin-releasing hormone test

In normal adults, gonadotrophin-releasing hormone (GnRH) produces a marked rise in luteinising hormone (LH) and a smaller rise in follicle-stimulating hormone (FSH); typical expected increments in adults are greater than 15 U/L for LH and greater than 2 U/L for FSH. In children the FSH response is greater than the LH response. This test is indicated where there is clinical or biochemical evidence of hypogonadism, particularly in the absence of the expected compensatory rises in LH and FSH. It may be performed alone or as part of a combined anterior pituitary function test. The latter simply consists of the three separate DFTs described previously (IST, TRH test and GnRH test) performed simultaneously. Collectively they provide a comprehensive assessment of anterior pituitary reserve.

Oral glucose tolerance test with GH measurement

Just as hypoglycaemia stimulates GH secretion, so hyperglycaemia suppresses it. This forms the basis for performing an oral glucose tolerance test (OGTT) with GH measurement. Normal adults suppress GH to less than 1 µg/L, but acromegalic patients do not; failure to suppress is therefore highly suggestive of acromegaly. Following treatment, patients who fail to suppress GH below 2 µg/L have a higher prevalence of diabetes, heart disease and hypertension.

Synacthen tests

Short Synacthen test

The short Synacthen test (SST) is one of the most commonly performed DFTs. The procedure is described in Chapter 48. Of the three criteria used to define a normal response (see Fig. 48.2), the final cortisol is the most important, and the increment the least important. As with the IST, there is lack of agreement on what constitutes an adequate cortisol response to Synacthen; cut-offs for the final level vary between 420 and 550 nmol/L.

Long Synacthen test

Where the response to an SST is inadequate or equivocal, it may not be clear whether the adrenal insufficiency is primary, or secondary to pituitary or hypothalamic disease. Secondary adrenal insufficiency is most frequently seen following the use of long-term steroid therapy, which causes central suppression of the axis. If the SST is repeated after the administration of a much larger dose of Synacthen (1 mg), a normal response may be observed, confirming the diagnosis.

Dexamethasone suppression tests

Dexamethasone is an exogenous steroid that mimics the negative feedback of endogenous glucocorticoids. Dexamethasone suppression tests (DSTs) are important in the investigation of suspected overactivity of the hypothalamic–pituitary–adrenal axis.

Low-dose DST

In its simplest form, the low-dose DST – usually performed on an outpatient basis – involves the patient taking 1 mg dexamethasone orally at 23:00 and attending for a cortisol blood test the following morning at 08:00 or 09:00. If the cortisol has suppressed to less than 50 nmol/L, cortisol overproduction is unlikely and no further action is normally required.

High-dose DST

Failure to suppress in response to low-dose dexamethasone may occur because of autonomous ACTH production by the pituitary (Cushing's disease), ectopic ACTH production (usually malignant), or adrenal production of cortisol (see Chapter 49). The high-dose DST (8 mg) is used to distinguish the first two of these options. ACTH production in Cushing's disease does usually suppress in response to high-dose dexamethasone, whereas malignant production of ACTH usually does not.

Dynamic function tests – protocol variation

Protocols for individual DFTs vary from one centre to another. For example, an additional cortisol specimen is collected at 60 minutes in some SST protocols, although this rarely alters the interpretation of the SST. Likewise, the long Synacthen test (LST) may be performed as a day-long procedure, with 1 mg Synacthen administered in the morning and cortisol samples collected for up to 24 hours; others perform this test as outlined in Chapter 48. The reasons for the different protocols are often practical rather than evidence-based, but it is always wise to check with the local laboratory before proceeding with any DFT.

Clinical note

Insulin-induced hypoglycaemia is designed to induce stress. If a patient requires intravenous glucose therapy to correct severe hypoglycaemia, the test should not be abandoned. Obviously in such cases, adequate stress has been induced and useful information may still be obtained.

Dynamic function tests

- Dynamic function tests (DFTs) are often required for the diagnosis of endocrine disorders.
- These tests involve either stimulating or suppressing a particular hormonal axis.
- Many of these tests are complex and require careful attention to appropriate timing of samples for their results to be meaningful.

Want to know more?

http://www.bartsendocrinology.co.uk/resources/PITUITARY_Barts_protocol_$5Bfinal$5D.pdf

This collection of endocrine protocols provides practical advice about procedures and interpretation of quite a few dynamic function tests (DFTs). It would be even better if it explained the principle of each test.

42 | Pituitary function

The pituitary gland

Pituitary function is regulated by the hypothalamus, to which it is connected via the pituitary stalk, which comprises portal blood capillaries and nerve fibres. The anterior pituitary is influenced by a variety of stimulatory and inhibitory hormones through these capillaries. The posterior pituitary is a collection of specialised nerve endings that derive from the hypothalamus.

Anterior pituitary hormones

- *Thyroid-stimulating hormone (TSH)* acts on the thyroid gland to elicit secretion of thyroid hormones.
- *Adrenocorticotrophic hormone (ACTH)* acts on the adrenal cortex to elicit secretion of cortisol and other steroids.
- *Luteinising hormone (LH) and follicle-stimulating hormone (FSH)*, known jointly as the gonadotrophins, act cooperatively on the ovaries in women and the testes in men to stimulate sex hormone secretion and reproductive processes.
- *Growth hormone (GH)* acts on many tissues to modulate metabolism. Metabolic fuels (e.g. glucose, free fatty acids) in turn modify GH secretion.
- *Prolactin* acts directly on the mammary glands to control lactation. Gonadal function is impaired by elevated circulating prolactin concentrations.

Hyperprolactinaemia

Hyperprolactinaemia is common and can cause infertility in both sexes. An early indication in women is amenorrhoea and galactorrhoea, whereas in men there may be no early signs and the first indication of the presence of a prolactinoma may be when a large growing tumour begins to interfere with the optic nerves causing visual disturbance. Causes of hyperprolactinaemia include:

- stress (venepuncture is sufficient to raise plasma prolactin in some patients)
- drugs (e.g. oestrogens, some antipsychotic medications, metoclopramide, α-methyl dopa)
- seizures (acutely)
- primary hypothyroidism (prolactin is stimulated by the raised thyrotrophin-releasing hormone (TRH))
- other pituitary disease.

If these causes are excluded, the differential diagnosis is between:

- a prolactinoma (a prolactin-secreting pituitary tumour, commonly a microadenoma)
- idiopathic hypersecretion, which may be due to impaired secretion of dopamine, the hypothalamic factor that inhibits prolactin release.

Differentiating between these, after exclusion of stress, drugs and other disease, is done by detailed pituitary imaging together with dynamic tests of prolactin secretion. A rise in serum prolactin following administration of TRH or metoclopramide is observed in idiopathic hyperprolactinaemia but not in the presence of a pituitary tumour.

In some cases, a raised prolactin is due to the presence of *macroprolactin*, an immune complex. Prolactin combines with an immunoglobulin, and the resultant complex is too large (hence 'macro') to be excreted by the kidneys, resulting in high blood prolactin levels; this is a nonpathological condition but can result in unnecessary investigations and anxiety to the patient. The biochemistry laboratory can do a relatively simple screening test to look for the presence of macroprolactin.

Posterior pituitary hormones

Hypothalamic neurons synthesise arginine vasopressin (AVP) and oxytocin, which pass along axonal nerve fibres in the pituitary stalk to the posterior pituitary, where they are stored in granules in the terminal bulbs of nerves in close proximity to systemic veins.

Secretion of AVP, also known as antidiuretic hormone (ADH), is stimulated by:

- increased plasma osmolality via hypothalamic osmoreceptors
- blood volume depletion via cardiac baroreceptors
- stress and nausea.

The role of AVP in fluid and electrolyte regulation is discussed in Chapter 8. A pituitary tumour arising in the anterior gland may cause impaired secretion of this posterior pituitary hormone, with consequent diabetes insipidus.

Oxytocin is released in response to suckling of the breast and uterine contraction at the onset of labour.

Fig. 42.1 illustrates the various pituitary endocrine axes.

Pituitary tumours

Diagnosis

Pituitary tumours may be either functional (i.e. they secrete hormones) or nonfunctional (i.e. they do not). The incidence of different tumour types is shown in Fig. 42.2. Local effects include headaches, papilloedema and visual field defects. There may be specific signs of hormone excess, particularly in acromegaly, Cushing's syndrome and prolactinoma. There may be signs of hypopituitarism in skin, hair and musculature.

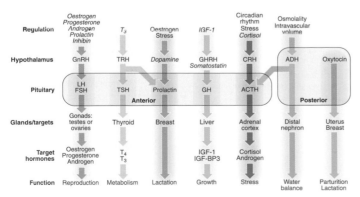

Fig. 42.1 Pituitary endocrine axes. *IGF-BP3*, Insulin-like growth factor-binding protein-3; T_3, triiodothyronine; T_4, thyroxine. (See text for remaining abbreviations.) *(From Innes JA, ed.* Davidson's Essentials of Medicine, *3rd ed. Elsevier; 2021.)*

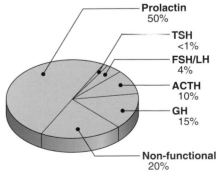

Fig. 42.2 Incidence of different types of pituitary tumours. *ACTH*, Adrenocorticotrophic hormone; *FSH*, follicle-stimulating hormone; *GH*, growth hormone; *LH*, luteinising hormone; *TSH*, thyroid-stimulating hormone.

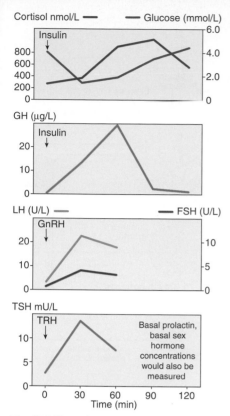

Fig. 42.3 Normal responses in a combined anterior pituitary function test. *FSH*, Follicle-stimulating hormone; *GH*, growth hormone; *GnRH*, gonadotrophin-releasing hormone; *LH*, luteinising hormone; *TSH*, thyroid-stimulating hormone; *TRH*, thyrotrophin-releasing hormone.

The impact of the tumour on pituitary function requires formal assessment by dynamic function tests. GH- and ACTH-secreting cells are most vulnerable, and an insulin stress test (see Chapter 41) may suffice. However, comprehensive assessment of anterior pituitary reserve requires a combined anterior pituitary function test (Fig. 42.3). TRH, gonadotrophin-releasing hormone (GnRH) and insulin are administered. All hormones are assessed at 0, 30 and 60 minutes and GH additionally at 90 and 120 minutes. It is usual also to assess basal thyroid (thyroxine) and gonadal (testosterone or oestradiol) function.

The administration of insulin is contraindicated if there is established coronary disease or epilepsy. A clinician must be on hand throughout the test, and intravenous dextrose and hydrocortisone (as well as good venous access) must be readily available in the event of severe or prolonged hypoglycaemia resulting in neuroglycopenia, e.g. loss of consciousness or fits.

Because of its associated dangers, insulin-induced hypoglycaemia is sometimes avoided by administration of growth hormone-releasing hormone (GHRH) and corticotrophin-releasing hormone (CRH) to investigate GH and cortisol secretion.

Another alternative is the *prolonged glucagon test*. Here, the initial glucagon-induced rise in glucose falls back to normal; this fall in glucose acts as a (much) milder – and safer – pituitary stressor.

Treatment

- *Medical.* Dopamine agonist drugs, e.g. bromocriptine and cabergoline, are widely used to treat hyperprolactinaemia, especially when due to microprolactinomas. They also may be used to shrink large suprasellar prolactinomas before surgery.
- *Surgery.* Transsphenoidal hypophysectomy is the standard procedure. Patients undergoing this are routinely given steroid cover (usually hydrocortisone), in case they cannot mount an adequate cortisol response to the stress of the operation. For the same reason, postoperative assessment of pituitary reserve should be deferred for several days.
- *Radiation.* The impact of radiation on pituitary function is cumulative, and irradiated patients require lifelong annual dynamic function testing of their anterior pituitary reserve thereafter.

Hypopituitarism

There are many causes of hypopituitarism, a relatively uncommon condition in which there is failure of one or more pituitary functions. These causes include tumour, infarction, trauma, congenital malformation, infection and hypothalamic disorder. Where several hormonal axes are affected by inadequate pituitary function, it is referred to as *panhypopituitarism*.

The clinical presentation of hypopituitarism depends on the age of the patient. In infancy, short stature or impaired development may point to the condition. In the reproductive years, women may present with amenorrhoea or infertility. Men may present with decreased libido or a lack of male secondary sex characteristics. Elderly patients may present with problems relating to ACTH or TSH deficiency such as hypoglycaemia or hypothermia.

Clinical note

Some antipsychotic drugs, e.g. phenothiazines, inhibit dopamine secretion by the hypothalamus, and thus predictably result in marked hyperprolactinaemia. This property is used by psychiatrists to assess patient compliance with these drugs.

Pituitary function

- Adenomas secreting each of the anterior pituitary hormones have been identified.
- Around 20% of pituitary tumours appear not to secrete hormone (i.e. are nonfunctioning).
- It is important to establish if a pituitary tumour, whether hormone-secreting or not, has interfered with the other hypothalamic–pituitary connections.
- Hyperprolactinaemia is common. Once stress, drugs or other disease have been eliminated as possible causes, dynamic tests and detailed radiology are used to differentiate between prolactinoma and idiopathic hypersecretion.
- Hypopituitarism is uncommon; the clinical presentation depends on the age of the patient.

Case history 30

A 36-year-old man complained of impaired vision while driving, particularly at night. After clinical and initial biochemical assessment, a combined anterior pituitary stimulation test was performed (intravenous insulin 0.1 U/kg, TRH 200 µg, GnRH 100 µg).

Time (min)	Glucose mmol/L	Cortisol nmol/L	GH µg/L	PRL mU/L	FSH —— U/L ——	LH	TSH mU/L	Free T₄ pmol/L	Testosterone nmol/L
0	3.6	320	0.5	17 000	<0.7	<1.0	<1.0	6	6.1
30	0.9	310	0.6	16 400	0.8	3.7	2.7		
60	1.8	380	0.5	18 000	1.2	3.7	4.1		
90	2.7	370	0.7						
120	3.3	230	0.4						

- A lower than normal dose of insulin was used. Why?
- What is the most likely diagnosis?
- What precautions should be taken before surgery?
  Comment in Case history comments.

Want to know more?

https://www.ncbi.nlm.nih.gov/pmc/articles/PMC2585697/pdf/259.pdf

This article describes aetiology, diagnosis and treatment of hypopituitarism in adults.

43 | Growth disorders and acromegaly

Normal growth

Growth in children can be divided into three stages (Fig. 43.1). Rapid growth occurs during the first 2 years of life; the rate is influenced by conditions *in utero*, as well as the adequacy of nutrition in the postnatal period. The next stage is relatively steady growth for around 9 years and is controlled mainly by growth hormone (GH). If the pituitary does not produce sufficient GH, the yearly growth rate during this period may be reduced and the child will be of short stature. The growth spurt at puberty is caused by the effect of the sex hormones in addition to continuing GH secretion. The regulation of GH secretion is outlined in Fig. 43.2.

GH is only one of many hormones involved in growth; others include insulin-like growth factors (IGF-1), thyroxine, cortisol, the sex steroids and insulin.

Growth hormone insufficiency

Any child whose height for age falls below the 3rd centile on a standard chart, or who exhibits a slow growth rate, requires further investigation. If GH deficiency is diagnosed and treatment is required, then the earlier it is given the better the chance that the child will eventually reach normal height.

GH insufficiency is a rare cause of impaired physical growth. It is important to differentiate between children whose slow growth or growth failure is due to illness or disease and those whose short stature is a normal variant of the population. Causes of short stature are:

- having parents who are both short
- inherited diseases such as achondroplasia
- poor nutrition
- systemic chronic illness, such as renal disease, gastrointestinal disorders or respiratory disease
- psychological factors such as emotional deprivation
- hormonal disorders.

Standard graphs relating age and height are available for the normal population. Accurate measurements of height should be made to establish whether a child is small for chronological age. These measurements are repeated after 6 and 12 months to assess the growth rate. The height of the parents also should be assessed. The bone age is the best predictor of final height in a child with short stature; this is determined by radiological examination of hand and wrist. In most growth disorders, bone age is delayed and by itself is of little diagnostic value, but taken together with height and chronological age, a prediction of final height may be obtained.

Tests of growth hormone insufficiency

GH deficiency may be present from birth or due to later pituitary failure. A variety of stimulation tests have been used to evaluate GH deficiency. Serum GH concentrations rise in response to exercise, and this may be used as a preliminary screening test. They also rise during sleep, and high concentrations in a nocturnal sample may exclude GH deficiency. The lack of GH response to the stress of exercise, or clonidine, a potent stimulant of GH secretion, is diagnostic. Some centres have now abandoned the use of insulin-induced hypoglycaemia as a diagnostic test in children because of its hazards and instead use the arginine stimulation test.

The GH response to stimulation requires the presence of sex steroids. Thus, prepubertal children

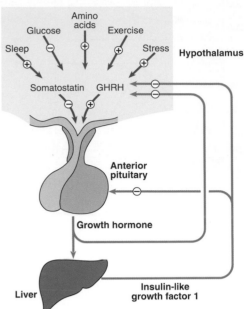

Fig. 43.2 The normal regulation of growth hormone (GH) secretion. *GHRH*, Growth hormone–releasing hormone.

> **Clinical note**
>
> In the investigation of normal-looking children with short stature, coeliac disease must be considered. The diagnosis is frequently overlooked, especially in the absence of obvious gastrointestinal symptoms.

and hypogonadal adults require *'priming'* by the administration of either testosterone or oestrogen before GH reserve is assessed.

Random serum IGF-1 analyses are also useful in assessing possible GH lack in children, though levels within reference limits do not exclude GH deficiency.

Treatment

Genetically engineered GH is available and is used in the treatment of children with proven GH deficiency.

Excessive growth

GH excess in children is characterised by extremely rapid linear growth (gigantism). The condition is uncommon and is most often due to a GH-secreting pituitary tumour. Other causes of tall stature in children are rare and include:

- *Hyperthyroidism*. An increased growth rate, with advanced bone age, is a feature of hyperthyroidism in children or hypothyroid children over-replaced with thyroxine.
- *Inherited disorders* such as Klinefelter's syndrome (a 47XXY karyotype). The relative deficiency of testosterone is

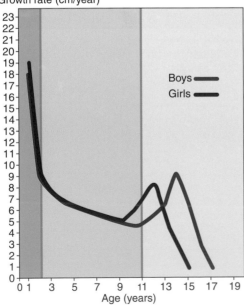

Fig. 43.1 Median height velocity curve for boys and girls showing the three growth stages.

associated with delayed epiphyseal closure.

- *Congenital adrenal hyperplasia.* This may cause rapid somatic growth in children but usually leads to suboptimal adult height due to premature epiphyseal closure, as a result of androgen excess.

Acromegaly

Increased GH secretion later in life, after fusion of bony epiphyses, causes acromegaly (Fig. 43.3). The most likely cause is a pituitary adenoma. Clinical features include:

- coarsening facial features
- soft tissue thickening, e.g. the lips
- characteristic 'spade-like' hands
- protruding jaw (prognathism)
- sweating
- impaired glucose tolerance or diabetes mellitus, hypertension, headaches, joint pains.

Diagnosis

Formal diagnosis of acromegaly requires an oral glucose tolerance test with GH measurement. Patients with acromegaly do not suppress fully in response to hyperglycaemia (Fig. 43.4), and indeed in some patients a paradoxical rise in GH may be observed.

IGF-1 is produced in response to GH and provides useful additional biochemical information. It is now routinely measured in the diagnosis and especially monitoring of treated acromegaly, with an elevated level suggestive of active disease. Other measurements, e.g. IGF binding protein-3, have not yet attained widespread clinical use.

Treatment

- *Surgery.* Transsphenoidal hypophysectomy is the first-line treatment for most acromegalic patients. Its success depends on the size of the tumour.
- *Radiation.* This is usually reserved for patients whose disease remains active despite surgery. It may take years after pituitary irradiation before safe levels of GH are achieved. Medical treatment is required in the interim.
- *Medical.* Dopamine agonists such as bromocriptine were widely used in the

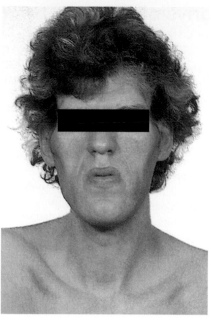

Fig. 43.3 Clinical picture of an acromegalic patient.

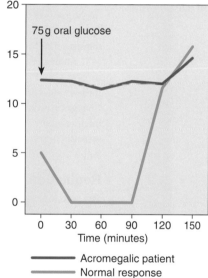

Serum GH (µg/L)

75 g oral glucose

Time (minutes)

— Acromegalic patient
— Normal response

Fig. 43.4 The response of growth hormone (GH) in a glucose tolerance test in a normal and acromegalic patient.

Growth disorders and acromegaly

- Growth hormone (GH) deficiency is a rare cause of short stature in children. Diagnosis of GH deficiency is made on the failure of serum GH to rise in response to stimuli.
- Gigantism in children is caused by increased GH secretion, usually from a pituitary tumour. Acromegaly is the consequence of increased GH secretion in adults.
- Lack of suppression of serum GH levels in response to a glucose tolerance test is the diagnostic test for acromegaly.
- Serum insulin-like growth factor (IGF-1) concentrations are of value in the diagnosis of acromegaly and the monitoring of treatment.

Case history 31

James is 5 years old and is much smaller than his classmates at school. His growth rate has been monitored and has clearly dropped off markedly in the past year. He is an active child and on examination has normal body proportions. His mother and father are of average height. His bone age is that of a 3-year-old child.

- What biochemical tests would be appropriate in the investigation of this boy?
  Comment in Case history comments.

Want to know more?

Ribeiro-Oliveira A, Barkan A. The changing face of acromegaly: advances in diagnosis and treatment. *Nat Rev Endocrinol.* 2012;8(10):605–611.

This paper discusses developments in diagnosis and treatment of acromegaly.

past, but response rates were low. The advent of long-acting synthetic analogues of somatostatin, such as octreotide, has transformed the medical management of acromegaly. Prior to treatment, patients may be screened for responsiveness by demonstrating reduction in serum GH levels after administering octreotide (octreotide suppression test).

44 | Thyroid pathophysiology

Thyroxine (T_4) and triiodothyronine (T_3) are together known as the 'thyroid hormones'. They are synthesised in the thyroid gland by the iodination and coupling of two tyrosine molecules whilst attached to a complex protein called thyroglobulin. T_4 has four iodine atoms, whereas T_3 has three (Fig. 44.1).

The thyroid gland secretes mostly T_4, the concentration of which in plasma is around 100 nmol/L. Peripheral tissues, especially liver and kidney, deiodinate T_4 to produce approximately two-thirds of the circulating T_3, present at a concentration of around 2 nmol/L. Most cells are capable of taking up and deiodinating T_4 to T_3. T_3 is more biologically active: it binds to receptors and triggers the end-organ effects of the thyroid hormones. T_4 can alternatively be metabolised to *reverse T_3* (rT_3), which is biologically inactive. Tissues can thus 'fine tune' their local thyroid status by modulating the relative production of T_3 and rT_3. Exactly how this is accomplished is not yet fully understood.

Goitre

A goitre is an enlarged thyroid gland (Fig. 44.2). This may be associated with hypothyroidism, hyperthyroidism or a euthyroid state. Globally, iodine deficiency is the commonest cause of goitre.

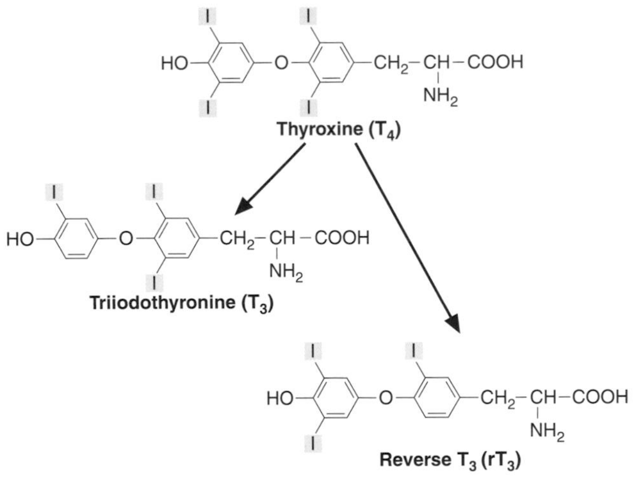

Fig. 44.1 The chemical structures of T_4, T_3 and rT_3.

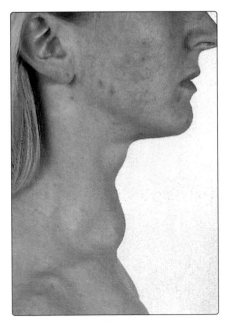

Fig. 44.2 A patient with a goitre.

The World Health Organization estimates that approximately 2 billion people have an inadequate iodine intake, making it the commonest preventable cause of neurodevelopmental problems. In many developed countries this problem has been overcome by the addition of iodine to staple foods, e.g. salt.

Thyroid hormone action

Thyroid hormones are essential for normal maturation and metabolism of all body tissues. Their effects on tissue maturation are most dramatically seen in congenital hypothyroidism, a condition which, unless treated within 3 months of birth, results in permanent brain damage. Hypothyroid children have delayed skeletal maturation, short stature and delayed puberty.

Thyroid hormone effects on metabolism are diverse. The rates of protein and carbohydrate synthesis and catabolism are influenced. For example, in hypothyroidism, down-regulation of low-density lipoprotein (LDL) receptors on hepatocytes results in reduced clearance of LDL cholesterol. This explains why hypothyroidism is associated with raised cholesterol and cardiovascular disease.

Binding in plasma

In plasma, over 99.95% of T_4 is transported bound to proteins. T_4-binding globulin carries 70% of T_4, albumin approximately 25% and transthyretin (formerly called prealbumin) around 5%. Over 99.5% of T_3 is transported by the same proteins. It is, however, the unbound, or 'free', T_4 and T_3 concentrations that exert the biological effects of the hormones, including feedback to the pituitary and hypothalamus. Changes in binding protein concentration complicate the interpretation of thyroid hormone results, e.g. in pregnancy (oestrogen increases the binding protein). For this reason, most laboratories now report free, rather than total, T_4 and T_3 concentrations.

Regulation of thyroid hormone secretion

The components of the hypothalamic–pituitary–thyroid axis are thyrotrophin-releasing hormone (TRH), thyroid-stimulating hormone (TSH) and thyroid hormones. TRH, a tripeptide, is secreted by the hypothalamus and in turn causes the synthesis of a large glycoprotein hormone, TSH, from the anterior pituitary. This drives the synthesis of thyroid hormones by the thyroid. Production of TSH is regulated by feedback from circulating unbound thyroid hormones (Fig. 44.3). A knowledge of these basics is essential for the correct interpretation of results in the investigation of primary thyroid disease. Remember:

- If the thyroid is producing too much thyroid hormone, this will suppress the circulating TSH.
- If the thyroid is not secreting enough thyroid hormone, TSH will be high – attempting to stimulate the gland to secrete more.

Thyroid function tests

Biochemical measurements in the diagnosis of thyroid disease are traditionally known as thyroid function tests. TSH and some estimate of T_4 status (either total T_4 or free T_4) are the first-line tests.

- *TSH*. Measurement of TSH is a good example of how better technology has helped diagnose and monitor disease. Early assays for TSH could not reliably distinguish pathologically low concentrations from the concentrations at the low end of the reference interval in healthy subjects – the detection limits overlapped significantly. Now, very sensitive TSH assays can detect much lower concentrations, and it is possible to tell with a greater degree of certainty whether TSH secretion really is lower than normal.

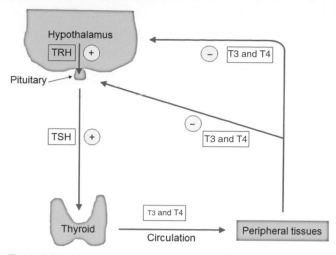

Fig. 44.3 The hypothalamic–pituitary–thyroid (HPT) axis showing release of the hormones thyrotrophin-releasing hormone (*TRH*), thyroid-stimulating hormone (*TSH*), triiodothyronine (*T₃*), and thyroxine (*T₄*) and their actions in feedback control of the axis.
(From Darbre P, ed. Endocrine Disruption and Human Health. *2nd edn. Elsevier; 2022.)*

- Because of its log-linear relationship with TRH, TSH is very sensitive to derangements in thyroid control, and many laboratories use TSH alone as the first-line thyroid function test. There is, however, one situation in which TSH cannot be used to diagnose thyroid disease, or to monitor replacement, i.e. hypopituitarism, where the feedback loop is broken. For example, TSH is undetectable post hypophysectomy and an estimate of T₄ status must be used instead to monitor the adequacy of T₄ replacement.
- *Total T₄ or free T₄.* Following the introduction of replacement T₄ or of antithyroid treatment, e.g. carbimazole, or indeed following any alteration in dosage, TSH may take many weeks to adjust to its new level. During this time, it is essential to have some estimate of T₄ status. This applies particularly to the monitoring of antithyroid treatment; patients can become profoundly hypothyroid quite quickly.
- *Total T₃ or free T₃.* Occasionally, it may be useful to have an estimate of T₃ status in addition to T₄. In hyperthyroidism, the rise in T₃ is almost always disproportionate to the rise in T₄; an estimate of T₃ status may in principle permit earlier identification of thyrotoxicosis. In some patients, only the T₃ rises – the T₄ remains within the reference interval (T₃ toxicosis).
- *Antibodies.* The titre of autoantibodies to thyroid tissue antigens may be helpful in the diagnosis and monitoring of autoimmune thyroid disease. Antithyroid peroxidase may be useful in hypothyroidism, and TSH receptor antibodies in thyrotoxicosis (specifically, Graves' disease).

Drugs and the thyroid

Various drugs affect thyroid function tests. The effects of some of these are summarised in Table 44.1.

Thyroid pathophysiology

- The thyroid gland synthesises, stores and secretes thyroxine (T₄) and triiodothyronine (T₃), which are important for normal development and metabolism.
- The secretion of thyroid hormones is controlled primarily by thyroid-stimulating hormone (TSH) from the anterior pituitary.
- Most T₄ and T₃ circulate in plasma bound to protein. Only a small proportion is not bound, yet it is this 'free' fraction that is biologically important.
- Knowledge of TSH, thyroid hormone and binding protein concentrations in serum may all be needed in the assessment of a patient's thyroid status.
- A patient may have severe thyroid disease, such as a large goitre or thyroid cancer, yet have normal concentrations of thyroid hormones in blood.

Case history 32

A 49-year-old woman was referred to the lipid clinic for evaluation of hypercholesterolaemia, after her general practitioner found her total cholesterol to be 9.0 mmol/L and low-density lipoprotein (LDL) cholesterol to be 5.5 mmol/L.

Thyroid function tests checked in clinic showed:

TSH (mU/L)	Free T₄ (pmol/L)
>100	<5

- What is the patient's thyroid status?
- Does this explain the patient's lipid profile results?
Comment in Case history comments.

Want to know more?

Thyroid disease: assessment and management. https://www.acb.org.uk/resource/ng145-thyroid-disease-assessment-and-management-pdf.html

This document summarises guidance from the National Institute for Health and Care Excellence (NICE) on appropriate use of thyroid function tests.

Table 44.1 Drugs affecting thyroid function tests

Drug	Mechanism	Major Effects
Amiodarone	Reduces peripheral deiodination. Amiodarone also can stimulate or inhibit release of thyroid hormones from thyroid.	↑T₄, ↓T₃, transient ↑ in TSH Hyperthyroidism Hypothyroidism
Lithium	Reduces thyroid uptake of iodine. Reduces release of thyroid hormone	Goitre Hypothyroidism
Anticonvulsants (phenytoin, carbamazepine, phenobarbital)	Displace T₄ and T₃ from binding proteins. Carbamazepine also may reduce free T₄ by increasing hepatic metabolism.	↑ Free T₄, ↑ free T₃ Possible ↓ free T4 with carbamazepine
Heparin	Releases lipoprotein lipase into plasma with resultant increase in free fatty acids. These displace T₄ and T₃ from binding proteins.	↑ Free T₄, ↑ free T₃
Aspirin	In high concentrations displaces T₄ from transthyretin.	↑ Free T₄

↑, Increase; ↓, decrease; TSH, thyroid-stimulating hormone; T₃, triiodothyronine; T₄, thyroxine.

45 | Hypothyroidism

Hypothyroidism usually develops slowly. It is therefore easily missed clinically, and clinical biochemistry has an important role to play in diagnosis.

Clinical features

The clinical features of hypothyroidism include:
- lethargy and tiredness
- cold intolerance
- weight gain
- dryness and coarsening of skin and hair
- hoarseness
- slow relaxation of muscles and tendon reflexes
- many other associated signs, including anaemia, dementia, constipation, bradycardia, muscle stiffness, carpal tunnel syndrome, subfertility and galactorrhoea.

Causes

Over 90% of cases of hypothyroidism occur as a consequence of:
- autoimmune destruction of the thyroid gland (Hashimoto's disease)
- radioiodine or surgical treatment of hyperthyroidism.
  Rarer causes include:
- transient hypothyroidism due to treatment with drugs such as lithium carbonate
- thyroid-stimulating hormone (TSH) deficiency, which may be a component of panhypopituitarism
- congenital defects such as blocks in the biosynthesis of thyroxine (T_4) and triiodothyronine (T_3) or end-organ resistance to their action
- severe iodine deficiency.

Diagnosis

Hypothyroidism is caused by a deficiency of thyroid hormones. Primary hypothyroidism is failure of the thyroid gland itself and is one of the most commonly encountered endocrine problems. The demonstration of an elevated TSH concentration is usually diagnostic. Secondary hypothyroidism, i.e. failure of the pituitary to secrete TSH, is much less common. Isolated pituitary deficiency of TSH is rare, but impairment of the hypothalamic–pituitary–thyroid axis may happen as a result of any pituitary disease or damage.

Clinical features other than those of hypothyroidism may indicate the need for investigation of pituitary function (see Chapter 42), and the thyrotrophin-releasing hormone (TRH) test will be included in such a protocol. A strategy for the biochemical investigation of clinically suspected hypothyroidism is shown in Fig. 45.1.

Treatment

Replacement therapy with T_4 is the treatment of choice since the hormone is readily available and is inexpensive. Monitoring TSH concentrations are helpful in assessing the adequacy of treatment. Once the dosage is established, the patient will be required to continue treatment for life (Fig. 45.2).

Fig. 45.3 shows the need for careful monitoring of treatment. This graph shows the changes in thyroid hormone results as a hyperthyroid female patient became hypothyroid after radioiodine treatment, and it subsequently proved difficult to stabilise her on a replacement dose of thyroxine.

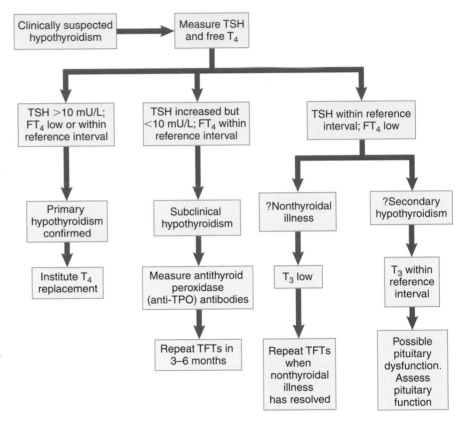

Fig. 45.1 Strategy for the biochemical investigation of suspected hypothyroidism. *FT₄*, Free thyroxine; *T₃*, triiodothyronine; *TFTs*, thyroid function tests; *TSH*, thyroid-stimulating hormone.

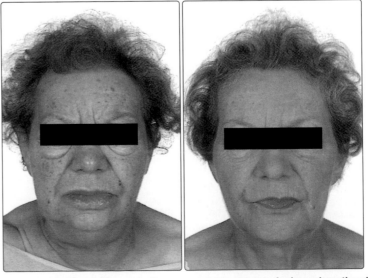

Fig. 45.2 A patient before and after successful treatment of primary hypothyroidism.

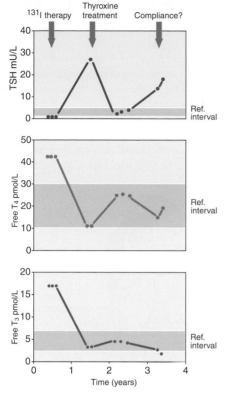

Fig. 45.3 Biochemical monitoring of a patient during treatment for thyroid disease. This 55-year-old woman was first diagnosed as having hyperthyroidism and received radioiodine therapy. She became profoundly hypothyroid and was treated with thyroxine (T_4). Her thyroid hormone results at first indicated good replacement, but subsequently they indicated under-replacement, suggesting that she was not taking her thyroxine tablets regularly. T_3, Triiodothyronine; *TSH*, thyroid-stimulating hormone.

Screening for neonatal hypothyroidism

Congenital hypothyroid disorders occur with a frequency of 1 in every 4000 live births. If these disorders are diagnosed at an early age, replacement thyroid hormone can be given and normal development can occur. Delays in treatment result in impaired brain development, learning difficulties and impaired physical growth (see Chapter 79). Elevated TSH, measured in blood spots, is diagnostic of disorders of the thyroid itself, i.e. primary neonatal hypothyroidism. However, the neonatal TSH screening test does not pick up pituitary dysfunction in the newborn.

Nonthyroidal illness

In health the major factor that regulates the serum concentration of TSH is the feedback of thyroid hormone activity on the pituitary and hypothalamus. Other factors also play a role. There is a diurnal rhythm, with the serum TSH reaching a peak between 2 and 4 a.m. and a nadir in the afternoon. In systemic illness the normal regulation of TSH, T_4 and T_3 secretion, and the subsequent metabolism of the thyroid hormones, is disturbed. Increased amounts of T_4 are converted to the biologically inactive reverse T_3, rather than to T_3. The resultant reduction in thyroid hormone activity does not result in an increased serum TSH concentration. TSH secretion is suppressed (hypothesised to be due to increased circulating levels of endogenous steroids, dopamine and prostaglandins); T_4 and T_3 concentrations are usually decreased.

The concentrations of the transport proteins also decrease. A low serum albumin and transthyretin (prealbumin) are classic features of the metabolic response to illness, and increased free fatty acid concentrations compete with T_4 and T_3 for their binding sites.

These changes result in sick patients having low serum free T_4, free T_3 and TSH, and if thyroid function tests are requested, the results may well be misinterpreted. A typical nonthyroidal illness pattern might be:

Free T_4	Free T_3	TSH
(11.5–22.7)	(3.3–6.1)	(0.4–4)
pmol/L	pmol/L	mU/L
6.0	0.6	0.1

These results were obtained in a man with acute pancreatitis. In developing hypothyroidism, the free T_3 would be maintained within the reference range (and the TSH would rise). A low free T_3 is almost invariably due to the presence of nonthyroidal illness.

Disturbances in the normal regulation of the hypothalamic–pituitary–thyroid axis in systemic illness are usually referred to as the *sick euthyroid syndrome*. As this term implies, the patients are euthyroid and there is no evidence to support treating them with either T_4 or T_3. Studies have shown that 90% of acutely ill patients in whom the TSH is less than 0.04 or greater than 20.0 U/L, i.e. clearly outside the reference interval, are not found to have thyroid dysfunction when they recover. In clinical practice, one should postpone measuring thyroid function tests until the patient has recovered from the acute illness, unless there is good clinical evidence that hypothyroidism or hyperthyroidism is a primary cause of their acute condition.

Clinical note

Patients with primary hypothyroidism who have, or are suspected of having, cardiac disease, should be initially treated with very small doses of thyroxine – 25 µg (i.e. 0.025 mg) daily. At higher doses, patients are at an increased risk of developing angina or suffering a myocardial infarction. The dose should be slowly increased over a number of months until the patient is euthyroid.

Hypothyroidism

- Hypothyroidism is common and is most often due to the destruction of the thyroid gland by autoimmune disease, surgery or radioiodine therapy.

- Primary hypothyroidism is confirmed by elevated thyroid-stimulating hormone (TSH) and low free thyroxine (FT₄) in a serum specimen.

- A thyrotrophin releasing hormone (TRH) test is used to investigate secondary hypothyroidism due to pituitary or hypothalamic causes.

- Hypothyroidism is managed by thyroxine replacement, and therapy is monitored by measuring the serum TSH concentration.

- Patients with severe nonthyroidal illness may show apparent abnormalities in thyroid hormone results, known as the 'sick euthyroid syndrome' or nonthyroidal illness pattern of results.

Case history 33

Investigation of a 63-year-old woman with effort angina revealed a serum thyroid-stimulating hormone (TSH) of 96 mU/L and a serum free thyroxine (FT₄) of 3.7 pmol/L. Electrocardiography showed some evidence of ischaemia but was not diagnostic of myocardial infarction. Further biochemical investigation revealed:

Cholesterol (mmol/L)	Creatine Kinase (U/L)	aAsparate aminotransferase
9.3	450	70

- How should these results be interpreted?
  Comment in Case history comments.

Want to know more?

Okosieme O, Gilbert J, Abraham P, et al. Management of primary hypothyroidism: statement by the British Thyroid Association Executive Committee. *Clin Endocrinol.* 2016;84(6):799–808. doi:0.1111/cen.12824. http://www.british-thyroid-association.org/sandbox/bta2016/bta_statement_on_the_management_of_primary_hypothyroidism.pdf

This statement from the British Thyroid Association addresses some frequently asked questions regarding management of primary hypothyroidism.

46 | Hyperthyroidism

Thyrotoxicosis occurs when tissues are exposed to high levels of the thyroid hormones. Used correctly, the term *hyperthyroidism* refers specifically to overactivity of the thyroid gland; *thyrotoxicosis* can also occur from ingestion of too much thyroxine (T_4) or, very rarely indeed, from increased pituitary stimulation of the thyroid.

Clinical features

The clinical features of hyperthyroidism may be dramatic and include (Fig. 46.1):
- weight loss despite normal or increased appetite
- sweating and heat intolerance
- fatigue
- palpitations – sinus tachycardia or atrial fibrillation
- agitation and tremor
- generalised muscle weakness; proximal myopathy
- angina and heart failure
- diarrhoea
- oligomenorrhoea and subfertility
- goitre
- eyelid retraction and lid lag.

Causes

Hyperthyroidism can result from:
- Graves' disease (diffuse toxic goitre)
- toxic multinodular goitre
- solitary toxic adenoma
- thyroiditis
- exogenously administered iodine and iodine-containing drugs, e.g. amiodarone
- excessive T_4 and/or triiodothyronine (T_3) ingestion.

Graves' disease is the most common cause of hyperthyroidism and is an autoimmune disease in which antibodies to the thyroid-stimulating hormone (TSH) receptor on the surface of thyroid cells mimic the action of the pituitary hormone. As a result, although pituitary secretion of TSH is completely inhibited by the high concentrations of thyroid hormones in the blood, the normal regulatory control of T_4 synthesis and secretion is lacking.

Although the eyelid retraction commonly seen in the patient with Graves' disease (Fig. 46.2) is partly due to the effects of high thyroid hormone concentration, not all of the eye signs are caused by this. The thyroid and orbital muscle may have a common antigen that is recognised by the circulating autoantibodies. The inflammatory process in the eye may lead to severe exophthalmos. This may occur independently of the thyroid disease, i.e. even when the patient is euthyroid.

Diagnosis

In most cases, primary hyperthyroidism is easily diagnosed on finding a suppressed TSH with an increased free T_4 concentration. Identification of the cause of hyperthyroidism may influence choice of treatment options; thus measurement of thyroid autoantibodies may be helpful. The presence of TSH-receptor antibodies is indicative of Graves' disease; antithyroid peroxidase antibodies, being a less specific indicator of autoimmune thyroid disease, are suggestive, but not diagnostic.

If a patient is found to have suppressed TSH with free T_4 concentration within the reference interval, free T_3 should be measured. This is because in some cases (especially early in the course of Graves' disease, and in some cases of toxic multinodular goitre) free T_3 is increased (and TSH suppressed) without an increase in free T_4 – this is known as T_3 toxicosis.

Subclinical hyperthyroidism is defined as having a low TSH concentration with free T_4 and free T_3 within the reference intervals. Some patients with subclinical hyperthyroidism are at increased risk of subsequently developing overt primary hyperthyroidism.

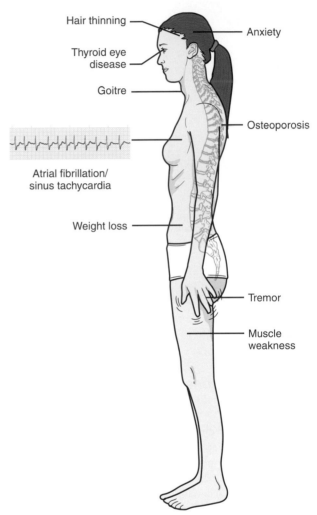

Hair thinning
Thyroid eye disease
Goitre
Atrial fibrillation/ sinus tachycardia
Weight loss
Anxiety
Osteoporosis
Tremor
Muscle weakness

Fig. 46.1 Clinical features of hyperthyroidism.

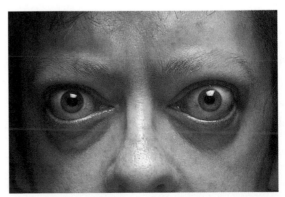

Fig. 46.2 Lid retraction and exophthalmos in a patient with Graves' disease. *(From Walker BR, Colledge NR, Ralston SH, Penman I, eds.* Davidson's Principles and Practice of Medicine. *22nd ed. Philadelphia: Elsevier; 2014.)*

On identifying a case of subclinical hyperthyroidism, nonthyroidal illness and drug causes should be excluded, and thyroid antibodies measured. Thereafter, thyroid function tests should be monitored at intervals as guided by the clinical situation – an interval of 3 to 6 months is likely to be appropriate in most cases.

Occasionally, results of thyroid function tests show an 'inappropriate' TSH level; this is the case when free T_4 and/or free T_3 are increased but TSH is not suppressed. Potential explanations for this pattern of results include analytical (antibody) interference or, very rarely, conditions such as a TSH-secreting pituitary tumour or thyroid hormone resistance. In the first instance, results fitting this pattern should be discussed with the laboratory. A strategy for the biochemical investigation of clinically suspected hyperthyroidism is shown in Fig. 46.3.

Treatment

There are three methods for the treatment of Graves' disease:
- *Antithyroid drugs* (such as carbimazole and propylthiouracil). These are of most use in patients with a higher likelihood of remission, e.g. those with mild disease or small goitres.
- *Radioiodine*. Therapy with ^{131}I is irreversible – patients will eventually require permanent replacement thyroxine. Thus thyroid function tests must be checked regularly to detect developing hypothyroidism.
- *Surgery*. Many patients who have a subtotal thyroidectomy may later require thyroxine replacement. Occasionally, the parathyroids may be damaged and the patient may become hypocalcaemic postoperatively due to lack of parathyroid hormone. Surgery is of use when there is a large goitre or symptoms of compression from a goitre, e.g. hoarseness (due to pressure on the recurrent laryngeal nerve) or stridor.

Thyroid function tests play a central role in the monitoring of all of these modalities of treatment. It takes a number of weeks before the tissue effects of thyroid hormones accurately reflect the concentration in the serum. In particular, TSH may take several months to adjust to its new level.

Thyroid eye disease

Clinically, thyroid eye disease can be a prominent feature of Graves' disease (Fig. 46.2). It may pursue a separate or similar course to the thyroid disease; typically it takes longer to resolve. It may be exacerbated by the administration of radioiodine, and temporary steroid treatment ('cover') may be required.

Clinical note

Elderly patients with thyrotoxicosis frequently do not exhibit many of the clinical features of hyperthyroidism. This is called 'apathetic hyperthyroidism'. Isolated idiopathic atrial fibrillation may be the only manifestation in some patients. Others may present with weight loss that may lead to anxiety and a futile search for malignant disease.

Hyperthyroidism

- Autoimmune disease is the commonest cause of hyperthyroidism.
- Diagnosis of hyperthyroidism is confirmed by suppressed thyroid-stimulating hormone (TSH) and elevated free thyroxine (T_4) in a serum specimen, although total or free triiodothyronine (T_3) concentration is needed if T_3 toxicosis is suspected.
- The management of hyperthyroidism is by antithyroid drugs, radioiodine therapy or thyroidectomy. TSH and free T_4 are used to monitor thyroid function after all of these treatments.

Case history 34

A 28-year-old woman with thyrotoxicosis has had two courses of carbimazole. Results from her recent visit to the thyroid clinic now show:

TSH	Free T_4
mU/L	pmol/L
<0.05	66

- What has happened?
- What treatment options are there?
  Comment in Case history comments.

Want to know more?

Ross DS, Burch HB, Cooper DS, et al. 2016 American Thyroid Association guidelines for diagnosis and management of hyperthyroidism and other causes of thyrotoxicosis. *Thyroid*. 2016;26(10):1343-1421. http://online.liebertpub.com/doi/full/10.1089/thy.2016.0229

American Thyroid Association guidance provides comprehensive details of the current approach to evaluation and treatment of hyperthyroidism, including details of the circumstances in which each potential treatment for hyperthyroidism might be the preferred option.

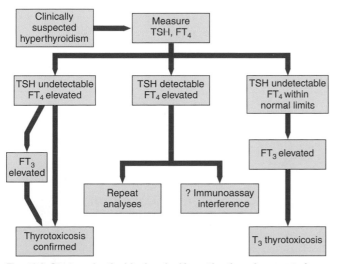

Fig. 46.3 Strategy for the biochemical investigation of suspected hyperthyroidism. *FT_3/FT_4:* Free triiodothyronine/free thyroxine; *TSH*, thyroid-stimulating hormone.

47 | Adrenocortical pathophysiology

There are two adrenal glands, one located on top of each kidney (hence also known as suprarenal glands). Each gland consists of a cortex and medulla. The cortex is further subdivided into three zones: zona glomerulosa, zona fasciculata, zona reticularis (Fig. 47.1). The hormones they make are essential for survival. Aldosterone and cortisol are two important steroid hormones made by the adrenal cortex. The adrenal medulla is part of the sympathetic nervous system and is embryologically and histologically distinct from the cortex. Medullary cells synthesise, store and secrete adrenaline, along with noradrenaline and dopamine. The adrenal medullary hormones are discussed further in Chapter 70.

Cortisol

Cortisol is produced in the zona fasciculata and zona reticularis of the adrenal cortex and is the end-product of a cascade of hormones that make up the hypothalamic–pituitary–adrenocortical (HPA) axis. *Corticotrophin-releasing hormone* (CRH) is secreted by the hypothalamus under the influence of cortical factors. *Adrenocorticotrophic hormone* (corticotrophin, or simply ACTH) is secreted by the anterior pituitary under the control of CRH to stimulate the secretion of cortisol from the adrenal cortex. Hypothalamic secretion of CRH and pituitary secretion of ACTH are modulated by cortisol in classic negative feedback loops (Fig. 47.2).

Adrenal cortex cells have low-density lipoprotein receptors, enabling them to take up cholesterol, from which the adrenal steroid hormones are synthesised (Fig. 47.3). The conversion of cholesterol to pregnenolone is the rate-limiting step in cortisol biosynthesis. It is stimulated by ACTH and involves the action of a specific reductase/isomerase and three separate hydroxylase enzymes. Inherited defects of all of these enzymes have been characterised.

Cortisol is a vital hormone with effects on many tissues. It plays a major role in metabolism by promoting protein breakdown in muscle and connective tissue and the release of glycerol and free fatty acids from adipose tissue. Thus, cortisol provides the substrates for gluconeogenesis, which it promotes in the liver. *Glucocorticoids* are natural synthetic steroids with cortisol-like effects, many of which are antiinflammatory or immunosuppressant. Synthetic glucocorticoids are used in a wide range of inflammatory conditions, e.g. asthma and connective tissue disorders.

Adrenal androgens

The adrenal androgens are androstenedione, dehydroepiandrosterone (DHEA) and DHEA sulphate. They are produced predominantly by the zona reticularis. These compounds probably owe their androgenic activity to peripheral conversion to testosterone. In females the adrenal cortex is an important source of androgens, but in adult males this source is insignificant compared with testosterone made by the testes.

Assessing the function of the HPA axis

Cortisol secretion fluctuates widely throughout the day (see Fig. 5.2B), and single serum measurements are of limited value in clinical practice. Dynamic tests of cortisol production involve stimulation of the adrenal cortex by synthetic ACTH, or alternatively stimulation or suppression of the whole HPA axis. They form an important part of investigation of adrenocortical hyperfunction or hypofunction and are discussed on the following pages.

Aldosterone

Aldosterone is produced exclusively by the zona glomerulosa and is primarily controlled by the renin–angiotensin system (Chapter 8). The synthesis of aldosterone utilises many of the same enzymes involved in cortisol biosynthesis. The zona glomerulosa lacks the 17-hydroxylase enzyme and has the additional 18-hydroxylase and 18-hydroxysteroid dehydrogenase enzymes necessary for aldosterone synthesis. Other factors, including ACTH, also are involved in regulation of aldosterone synthesis.

Aldosterone promotes sodium reabsorption and potassium excretion in the kidney; this is called *mineralocorticoid* activity. All of the 21-hydroxylated steroids have mineralocorticoid effects to varying degrees. As with glucocorticoid activity, there are many natural or synthetic steroids with mineralocorticoid activity.

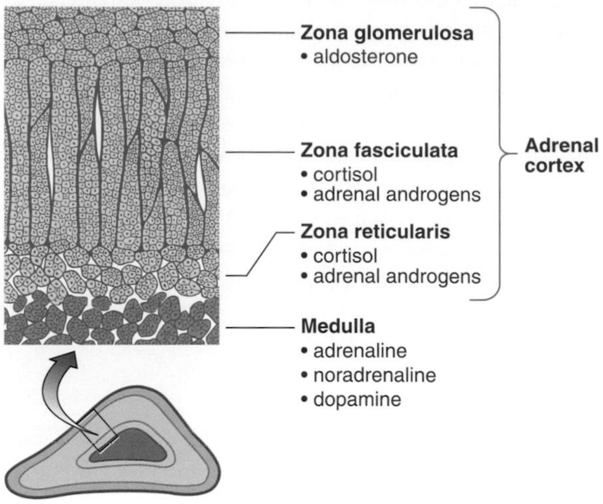

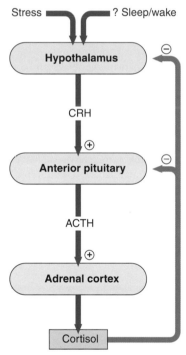

Fig. 47.1 The histology of an adrenal gland.

Fig. 47.2 The hypothalamic–pituitary–adrenocortical axis. *ACTH*, Adrenocorticotrophic hormone; *CRH*, corticotrophin-releasing hormone.

Congenital adrenal hyperplasia

In congenital adrenal hyperplasia (CAH), an inherited enzyme defect in corticosteroid biosynthesis means that the adrenals cannot secrete cortisol and some other steroids. Severe hyponatraemia and hyperkalaemia may result from lack of mineralocorticoid activity and can be fatal in the neonatal period if the condition is not diagnosed quickly.

Because of lack of cortisol, negative feedback to the pituitary is absent; ACTH secretion continues to drive the biosynthesis of cortisol precursors proximal

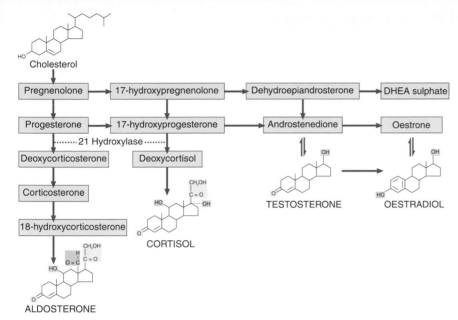

Fig. 47.3 Pathways of steroid metabolism. *DHEA*, Dehydroepiandrosterone.

to the block (see Fig. 47.3). The diverted pathways produce metabolites which can be used to diagnose CAH, and androgens, which cause many of its clinical features. For example, 21-hydroxylase is the deficient enzyme in 95% of cases of CAH. Here, elevated plasma concentrations of 17-hydroxyprogesterone (proximal to the block) are diagnostic as early as 2 days after birth, and increased stimulation of adrenal androgen production can cause virilisation in baby girls and precocious puberty in boys. A milder variant (late-onset CAH) is the result of a partial enzyme defect and presents as menstrual irregularity and hirsutism in young women.

Relationship of adrenal cortex and medulla

For a multicellular organism to survive, it is essential that the extracellular fluid bathing the tissues is continually circulating so that nutrients may be supplied to cells and waste products removed. The adrenal medulla and the two separate hormone systems of the adrenal cortex act together to ensure that this occurs. Adrenaline (epinephrine) and noradrenaline (norepinephrine), through inotropic effects on the heart and their vasoconstrictor actions on arterioles, maintain blood pressure and tissue perfusion. Cortisol facilitates the synthesis of adrenaline and potentiates its vasopressor effects. Cortisol is also required for efficient excretion of water in the kidney. Aldosterone, through its action on sodium reabsorption, maintains the extracellular volume.

Adrenocortical pathophysiology

- The adrenal glands comprise three histologically separate zones and hormone systems:
  - the zona glomerulosa (aldosterone)
  - the zonae fasciculata and reticularis (cortisol and the adrenal androgens)
  - the adrenal medulla (adrenaline).
- Steroids with cortisol-like activity are known as glucocorticoids; they are potent metabolic regulators and immunosuppressants.
- Steroids with aldosterone-like activity are called mineralocorticoids; they promote renal retention of sodium and water.
- Adrenal steroid concentrations fluctuate widely. Single ('random') measurements are of limited value, and dynamic tests are widely used in diagnosis.
- Congenital adrenal hyperplasia (CAH) is an inherited enzyme defect in corticosteroid biosynthesis that can prove fatal unless diagnosed early.
- 21-hydroxylase deficiency is the most commonly encountered form of CAH. The finding of a raised plasma 17-hydroxyprogesterone confirms the diagnosis.

Case history 35

A 40-year old man was investigated for severe skeletal muscle pains. The following biochemical results in a serum sample were unexpected:

Na⁺	K⁺	Cl⁻	HCO₃⁻	Urea	Creatinine
		mmol/L			µmol/L
130	6.1	90	17	7.6	150

- Suggest a likely diagnosis.
- What other biochemistry tests might be helpful in the investigation of this patient?
  Comment in Case history comments.

Want to know more?

Pihlajoki M, Dörner J, Cochran RS, Heikinheimo M, Wilson DB. Adrenocortical zonation, renewal, and remodeling. *Front Endocrinol (Lausanne).* 2015;6:27. http://journal.frontiersin.org/article/10.3389/fendo.2015.00027/full

This interesting paper not only describes adrenocortical hormone synthesis but also discusses the renewal and regeneration of the zones of the adrenal cortex based on physiological demand.

48 | Hypofunction of the adrenal cortex

Adrenal insufficiency

Acute adrenal insufficiency is rare but potentially fatal. Precisely because of its rarity, it is often overlooked. It is moreover relatively simple to treat once diagnosed, and patients can lead a normal life. Thus it is imperative to be able to recognise its clinical features.

Clinical features

The clinical features of adrenal insufficiency are shown in Fig. 48.1. Some are quite nonspecific, i.e. many patients may present with similar symptoms and signs. Others, e.g. hypotension and dehydration, also are seen in other conditions but are characteristic of severe adrenal insufficiency; the alert clinician will recognise the need to exclude it. The finding of pigmentation as well, or of hyponatraemia and dehydration together, should prompt urgent investigation.

Pathogenesis

The basic problem in adrenal insufficiency is the inability to synthesise steroid hormones. The specific lack of mineralocorticoid activity means that sodium cannot be retained in the kidneys and therefore is lost from the extracellular fluid (ECF), along with water. This explains many of the clinical and biochemical features. Reduced ECF volume results in dehydration and hypotension, with resultant dizzy spells and lethargy. Excess pigmentation reflects excess pituitary adrenocorticotrophic hormone (ACTH) due to reduced negative feedback. The amino acid sequence for melanocyte-stimulating hormone (MSH) lies within the ACTH molecule; degradation of ACTH by proteases eventually exposes MSH, which then acts on skin and mucous membranes. Finally, the absence of mineralocorticoid activity also explains the hyponatraemia and hyperkalaemia. (If bicarbonate is measured, it is low, reflecting retention of H^+ in addition to K^+.) In addition, a high urea may reflect dehydration.

Hyponatraemia is exacerbated by the secretion of arginine vasopressin, stimulated by hypovolaemia and hypotension, causing compensatory retention of pure water. The ability of the kidneys to excrete water is further impaired without cortisol. Despite these mechanisms, there is net loss of body water (due to the obligatory loss of water with sodium), best judged by dehydration.

Diagnosis

If a patient is suspected to be suffering from adrenal insufficiency, it is essential to ensure sodium intake is adequate whilst investigations proceed. Patients with adrenal insufficiency are not able to retain sodium effectively; sodium requirements will be higher than normal.

Random cortisol

Random cortisol measurements are not without value in the evaluation of suspected adrenal insufficiency, but results must be interpreted with caution. A very low or very high result is most useful.

Synacthen tests

Formal diagnosis or exclusion of adrenal insufficiency requires a short Synacthen test (SST). Synacthen is a synthetic 1-24 analogue of ACTH and is administered intravenously at a dose of 250 µg. Cortisol is measured at 0, 30 and sometimes 60 minutes. The criteria for a normal response are shown in Fig. 48.2. Equivocal or inadequate responses to an SST may require a long Synacthen test (LST) (see Chapter 41) in order to establish whether adrenal insufficiency is primary or is secondary to pituitary or hypothalamic disease. Synacthen (1 mg) is given intramuscularly daily for 3 days and the SST repeated on the fourth; a normal response excludes primary adrenal insufficiency. Measurement of ACTH may obviate the need for an LST – unequivocally elevated ACTH in the presence of an impaired response to Synacthen confirms the diagnosis of primary adrenal failure.

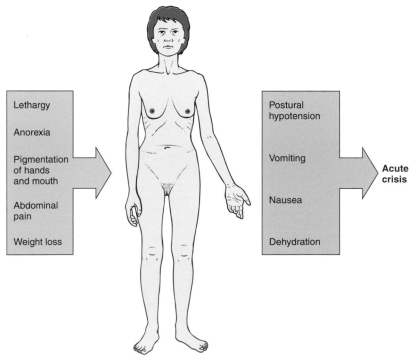

Fig. 48.1 Features of adrenocortical insufficiency.

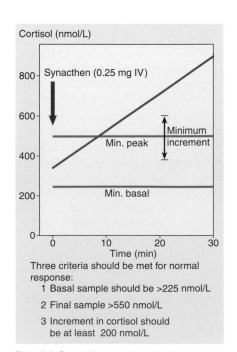

Fig. 48.2 Synacthen test responses.
Synacthen is given intravenously after a basal blood sample have been taken.

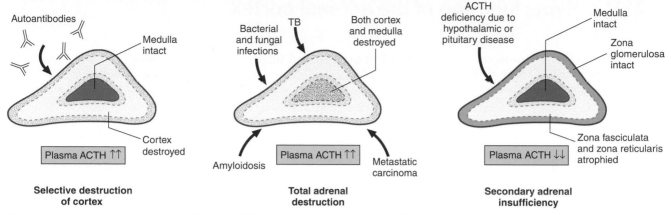

Fig. 48.3 Causes of adrenocortical insufficiency. *ACTH*, Adrenocorticotrophic hormone; *TB;* tuberculosis.

Causes of adrenal insufficiency

Adrenal insufficiency can be primary or secondary. Primary adrenal insufficiency is also known as *Addison's disease*. Secondary adrenal insufficiency is more common, because the therapeutic administration of corticosteroids is widespread and results in suppression of the entire hypothalamic–pituitary–adrenocortical (HPA) axis. In developed countries, autoimmune disease is the main cause of primary adrenal failure. In areas where tuberculosis is endemic, this may cause adrenal gland destruction. Both cortisol and aldosterone production may be affected. The causes of adrenal insufficiency are summarised in Fig. 48.3.

Relative adrenal insufficiency

Inability to mount an adequate cortisol response is well recognised in acutely ill patients. Such 'relative adrenal insufficiency' carries a poor prognosis. Cortisol levels are high in absolute terms, but there is a flat response to Synacthen.

Clinical note

Primary adrenal insufficiency may have an insidious onset. Pallor is a characteristic feature, as is dry flaky skin with pigmentation, especially in palmar creases and pressure points (Fig. 48.4). Patients may present asymptomatically with apparently isolated hyperkalaemia or hyponatraemia. Addison's disease must always be considered as a possible diagnosis in patients with raised serum potassium, especially if they do not have renal failure.

Hypofunction of the adrenal cortex

- Adrenocortical insufficiency is rare, but life-threatening.
- Failure of the adrenal cortex to produce cortisol and aldosterone may be due to autoimmune, infective or infiltrative diseases. Suppression of the hypothalamic–pituitary–adrenocortical (HPA) axis by prescribed corticosteroids is much commoner.
- The Synacthen test is used in diagnosis of primary adrenocortical failure.
- The long Synacthen test may be used to distinguish primary and secondary failure of the adrenal cortex. Pigmentation is a useful clinical feature seen only in primary adrenal insufficiency.
- The mainstay of therapy is appropriate hormone replacement and maintenance of sodium intake.

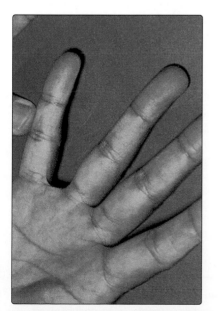

Fig. 48.4 Pigmented skin creases in patient with primary adrenal insufficiency.

Case history 36

A 31-year-old woman was admitted to a surgical ward with a 2-day history of abdominal pain and vomiting. Her blood pressure was 110/65 mmHg and her pulse 88 beats/min and regular. A provisional diagnosis of intestinal obstruction was made. On admission, tests showed:

Na⁺	K⁺	Cl⁻	HCO₃⁻	Urea	Creatinine
			mmol/L		μmol/L
128	6.1	92	18	10.8	180

She was given 1.5 L of 0.9% saline intravenously overnight, and the following morning her symptoms had resolved. Her serum sodium had increased to 134 mmol/L, and her serum potassium had fallen to 4.8 mmol/L. On reviewing her history, it was found she had been unwell for a number of months with weight loss and anorexia. She was noted to be pigmented.

A short Synacthen test was performed, and the serum cortisol was less than 60 nmol/L both before and after an intravenous injection of 0.25 mg of Synacthen.

- Suggest the diagnosis.
- How could the changes in her sodium and potassium be explained? *Comment in Case history comments.*

Want to know more?

Michels A, Michels N. Addison disease: early detection and treatment principles. *Am Fam Physician.* 2014;89(7):563–568.

http://www.aafp.org/afp/2014/0401/p563.pdf

This paper reviews early detection and treatment principles of Addison's disease.

49 | Hyperfunction of the adrenal cortex

Hyperfunction of the adrenal cortex can be conveniently discussed in terms of the overproduction of the three main products:
- cortisol
- adrenal androgens
- aldosterone.

Cortisol excess

Prolonged exposure of body tissues to cortisol or other glucocorticoids gives rise to the clinical features collectively known as *Cushing's syndrome* (Fig. 49.1), after the American neurosurgeon Harvey Cushing. It most often results from prolonged use of steroid medications (iatrogenic). Much less frequently, it is caused by tumours that secrete either cortisol or adrenocorticotrophic hormone (ACTH) (see later); these can sometimes be difficult to diagnose.

In any investigation of Cushing's syndrome the clinician should ask two questions:
- 'Does the patient actually have Cushing's syndrome?' Obese or hypertensive patients may sometimes appear 'Cushingoid', prompting investigations to exclude Cushing's syndrome.
- If the diagnosis of Cushing's syndrome is established, this raises a second question: 'What is the cause of the excess cortisol secretion?' Tests used in teasing out the differential diagnosis are different from those used to confirm the presence of cortisol overproduction.

Confirming overproduction

Iatrogenic Cushing's syndrome is usually obvious – the patient is on steroids (oral, inhaled or topical). Iatrogenic Cushing's is not a diagnostic dilemma and is not considered further here.

Overnight dexamethasone suppression test

Dexamethasone is a synthetic steroid which suppresses the hypothalamic–pituitary–adrenocortical axis. It can be given in various doses. The screening dexamethasone suppression test (DST) is done overnight, usually in primary care. If 1 mg dexamethasone taken at 23:00 fully suppresses the serum cortisol (to less than 50 nmol/L) at 09:00 the following morning, further investigation is not required. Failure to suppress fully usually prompts more detailed investigations.

Early morning urine cortisol:creatinine ratio in a 'spot' urine specimen (i.e. a small aliquot) is another way of investigating suspected Cushing's syndrome. Excess cortisol exceeds the capacity of the binding protein, cortisol-binding globulin; unbound cortisol appears in urine. Equivocal or high results may be confirmed by a full 24-hour collection for urinary free cortisol. Increased urinary excretion of cortisol is sufficient evidence to proceed with further investigations.

Cortisol concentrations normally show a circadian rhythm (lower in the evening). Patients with Cushing's syndrome usually have high cortisol all the time. However, loss of circadian rhythm is not widely used any more to decide on the need for further investigations.

Insulin-induced hypoglycaemia is a specialist endocrine investigation normally performed to assess pituitary reserve. In normal individuals hypoglycaemia (glucose <2.2 mmol/L) normally stimulates a rise in serum cortisol of more than 200 nmol/L. This may not be seen in Cushing's syndrome.

Determining the cause

Possible causes of Cushing's syndrome are illustrated in Fig. 49.2. These include:
- pituitary adenoma secreting ACTH
- malignant tumour secreting ectopic ACTH
- adrenal adenoma secreting steroids
- adrenal carcinoma secreting steroids.

Plasma ACTH

Classically, ACTH is undetectable in patients with adrenal tumours because of negative feedback from the secreted steroids. In patients with pituitary-dependent Cushing's syndrome (confusingly known as Cushing's *disease*), ACTH is, inappropriately, not suppressed (it may be within the reference range or modestly elevated). ACTH is very high in patients with ectopic ACTH production.

High-dose dexamethasone suppression test

Higher doses of dexamethasone may be used to distinguish causes of Cushing's syndrome from each other. Dexamethasone 2.0 mg four times daily is given for 2 days. In patients with Cushing's disease, serum or urine cortisol will be partially suppressed (Fig. 49.3). Failure to suppress suggests either ectopic ACTH production or the autonomous secretion of cortisol by an adrenal tumour.

Biochemical investigations are complemented by computed tomography scans or magnetic resonance imaging of the pituitary. These may help detect a pituitary adenoma in patients with Cushing's disease. In difficult cases, selective venous sampling with ACTH measurement is sometimes carried out to locate the ACTH source.

Androgen excess

Adrenocortical tumours, particularly adrenal carcinomas, may produce excess androgens (dehydroepiandrosterone (DHEA), androstenedione and testosterone) causing hirsutism and/or virilisation in females (see Chapter 50). This is not always

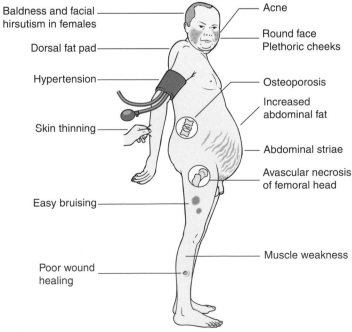

Baldness and facial hirsutism in females
Dorsal fat pad
Hypertension
Skin thinning
Easy bruising
Poor wound healing

Acne
Round face
Plethoric cheeks
Osteoporosis
Increased abdominal fat
Abdominal striae
Avascular necrosis of femoral head
Muscle weakness

Fig. 49.1 Some clinical features of Cushing's syndrome.

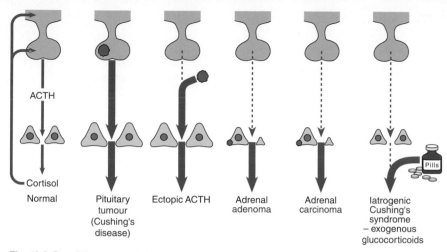

Fig. 49.2 Possible causes of Cushing's syndrome. *ACTH*, Adrenocorticotrophic hormone.

Normal / Pituitary tumour (Cushing's disease) / Ectopic ACTH / Adrenal adenoma / Adrenal carcinoma / Iatrogenic Cushing's syndrome – exogenous glucocorticoids

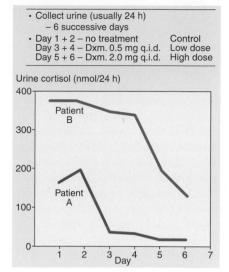

- Collect urine (usually 24 h)
  – 6 successive days
- Day 1 + 2 – no treatment   Control
  Day 3 + 4 – Dxm. 0.5 mg q.i.d.   Low dose
  Day 5 + 6 – Dxm. 2.0 mg q.i.d.   High dose

Fig. 49.3 The dexamethasone suppression test. Patient A showed a greater than 75% fall in urinary cortisol excretion on the low dose. This is a *normal response*. Patient B showed some suppression of cortisol secretion on the high dose. This is typical of *Cushing's disease*. *Dxm*, Dexamethasone; *q.i.d.*, four times daily.

accompanied by cortisol excess, so signs of Cushing's syndrome may be absent. Patients with congenital adrenal hyperplasia also may present with signs of increased androgen production. Excess androgens may be produced by ovarian tumours. In female patients, DHEA (or its sulphated metabolite DHEAS) is sometimes used to establish whether excess androgen production is adrenal or ovarian – if high, it indicates an adrenal source.

Aldosterone excess

Primary hyperaldosteronism (*Conn's syndrome*), usually due to a single adrenocortical adenoma, is rare. Patients classically present with hypertension and hypokalaemia. Symptoms include polydipsia and polyuria, weakness, paraesthesiae and tetany, all of which are attributable to potassium depletion.

Preliminary investigations must include determination of serum and urine electrolytes over several days, with adequate sodium intake. Serum potassium is low, and urinary potassium excretion is inappropriately elevated. Aldosterone and renin are often required to confirm the diagnosis. The diagnosis of hyperaldosteronism may be made in the hypokalaemic patient if the serum aldosterone level exceeds the upper limit of normal or if the level is persistently inappropriate to the serum potassium. In primary hyperaldosteronism, where the excess aldosterone arises from an adrenal adenoma, the levels of plasma renin will be low.

Secondary (compensatory) hyperaldosteronism is common and is associated with renal, heart and liver disease.

Clinical note

Excessive alcohol intake can cause pseudo-Cushing's syndrome when patients may present with hypertension, truncal obesity, plethora or acne. Preliminary investigations may demonstrate hypercortisolism, which may fail to suppress fully with 1 mg overnight dexamethasone. The biochemical features of Cushing's syndrome will resolve after 2 or 3 weeks of abstinence from alcohol.

Hyperfunction of the adrenal cortex

- In Cushing's syndrome, serum cortisol does not suppress overnight in response to 1 mg dexamethasone; the early morning urinary cortisol:creatinine ratio will be elevated.

- The cause of Cushing's syndrome can be established by the high-dose dexamethasone suppression test and by measuring adrenocorticotrophic hormone (ACTH).

- Clinical evidence of androgen excess should prompt a search for the source. Adrenal androgens include dehydroepiandrosterone (DHEA) and androstenedione.

- Primary excess of aldosterone is rare and usually due to an adenoma (Conn's syndrome).

Case history 37

A 31-year-old woman presented with a 3-month history of weight gain, hirsutism, amenorrhoea and hypertension. Her urine cortisol:creatinine ratio was increased, and serum cortisol diurnal rhythm was absent. Treatment with 0.5 mg of dexamethasone q.i.d. did not suppress her cortisol, and insulin-induced hypoglycaemia did not cause her serum cortisol to rise.

- What investigations should now be carried out?
  Comment in Case history comments.

Want to know more?

Sharma ST, Nieman LK, Feelders RA. Cushing's syndrome: epidemiology and developments in disease management. *Clin Epidemiol*. 2015;7:281–293. https://www.ncbi.nlm.nih.gov/pmc/articles/PMC4407747/pdf/clep-7-281.pdf

This paper discusses the epidemiology and updates on management of Cushing's syndrome.

50 | Gonadal function

Sex steroid hormones

Testosterone is the principal androgen and is synthesised by the testes in the male. Oestradiol, which is secreted by the ovaries, varies widely in concentration in plasma throughout the female menstrual cycle. Steroids with oestradiol-like actions are called *oestrogens*. Progesterone is also a product of the ovary and is secreted when a corpus luteum forms after ovulation. Normal female plasma also contains a low concentration of testosterone, about half of which comes from the ovary and half from peripheral conversion of androstenedione and dehydroepiandrosterone sulphate (DHEAS), which are secreted by the adrenal cortex. Some oestradiol is present in low concentration in normal male plasma.

Testosterone and oestradiol circulate in plasma mostly bound to plasma proteins, particularly sex hormone-binding globulin (SHBG). The plasma concentration of SHBG in females is twice that in males. In both sexes the effect of an increase in SHBG is to increase oestradiol-like effects, whereas a decrease in SHBG increases androgenic effects.

In females, testosterone and SHBG concentrations are sometimes reported by the laboratory as a ratio (the free androgen index), which gives a clearer indication of androgen status than does serum testosterone alone. In males, calculated free testosterone (calculated using testosterone, SHBG and albumin concentrations) is a more reliable indicator than measured total testosterone; free androgen index is not useful.

Hypothalamic–pituitary–gonadal axis

The episodic secretion of the hypothalamic hormone, gonadotrophin-releasing hormone (GnRH) stimulates synthesis and release of the gonadotrophins, luteinising hormone (LH) and follicle-stimulating hormone (FSH) from the anterior pituitary. Despite the names, both gonadotrophins act cooperatively on the ovaries in the woman and the testes in the man to stimulate sex hormone secretion and reproductive processes.

Male gonadal function

The testes secrete testosterone and manufacture spermatozoa. Before puberty, gonadotrophin and testosterone concentrations in plasma are very low. The development of the Leydig cells and their secretion of testosterone is influenced by LH, whereas Sertoli cell function is influenced by FSH (Fig. 50.1). Testosterone is responsible for the development of the male secondary sex characteristics, e.g. hair growth, deep voice and characteristic musculature.

Disorders of male sex hormones

Hypogonadism may result in deficient sperm production and decreased testosterone secretion. This may be due to a testicular deficiency (primary disorders or *hyper*gonadotrophic hypogonadism) or a defect in the hypothalamus or pituitary (secondary disorders or *hypo*gonadotrophic hypogonadism). In hypogonadotrophic hypogonadism, both gonadotrophins, or only LH, may be reduced. There may be a generalised failure of pituitary function.

Causes of primary hypogonadism include:
- congenital defects, e.g. Klinefelter's syndrome or testicular agenesis
- acquired defects due to testicular infections (e.g. mumps), trauma, irradiation or cytotoxic drugs.

Causes of secondary hypogonadism include:
- pituitary tumours
- hypothalamic disorders, e.g. Kallmann syndrome.

Dynamic tests such as stimulation with GnRH may help establish the cause of the hypogonadism in some patients.

Disorders of male sexual differentiation

Disorders of male sexual differentiation are rare. Testosterone production may be impaired. In the androgen resistance syndrome, androgen receptors are inactive from birth, and target tissues cannot respond to stimulation by circulating testosterone, leading to a female phenotype.

Female gonadal function

Oestradiol is responsible for:
- female secondary sex characteristics
- stimulation of follicular growth
- development of the endometrium.

Concentrations are low before puberty, but then rise rapidly and fluctuate cyclically during reproductive life. After menopause, plasma oestradiol concentrations fall despite high circulating concentrations of the gonadotrophins.

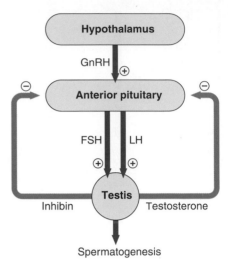

Fig. 50.1 Control of testicular function by the gonadotrophins. *FSH*, Follicle-stimulating hormone; *GnRH*, gonadotrophin-releasing hormone; *LH*, luteinising hormone.

The normal hormonal control of the menstrual cycle is shown in Fig. 50.2. At the beginning of the cycle, FSH is released and initiates follicular growth. At mid-cycle a surge of LH triggers ovulation. The ruptured follicle differentiates into the corpus luteum that secretes progesterone and oestradiol, the target of which is the endometrium, which they prepare for implantation.

Disorders of female sex hormones

Disorders of female sex hormones include:
- *Subfertility, amenorrhoea and oligomenorrhoea* (see Chapter 51).
- *Hirsutism.* This is an increase in body hair with male pattern distribution. It may be idiopathic, but the commonest pathological cause is obesity (causing insulin resistance), often in association with polycystic ovary syndrome. It is essential when investigating women with hirsutism that serious disease is excluded. A diagnostic decision chart for the investigation of hirsutism is shown in Fig. 50.3.
- *Virilism.* Although uncommon, it is a sign of serious disease. Testosterone concentrations are markedly elevated in the virilised patient and there is evidence of excessive androgen action such as clitoral enlargement, hair growth in a male pattern, deepening of the voice and breast atrophy. Tumours of the ovary or of the adrenal are often implicated.

The androgen screen in women

The observation of elevated testosterone in a woman always should be investigated

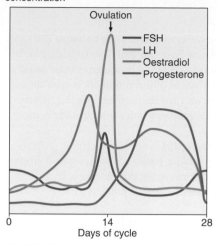

Fig. 50.2 Plasma hormone concentrations throughout the female menstrual cycle. *FSH*, Follicle-stimulating hormone; *LH*, luteinising hormone.

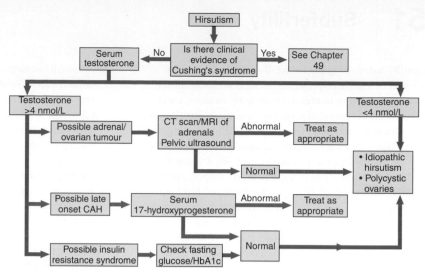

Fig. 50.3 Diagnostic decision chart for the investigation of hirsutism. *CAH*, Congenital adrenal hyperplasia, *CT*, computed tomography; *MRI*, magnetic resonance imaging.

further. A decreased SHBG concentration is usually evidence of elevated androgen, as the synthesis of this protein in the liver is depressed by testosterone. By measuring the concentration of other androgens such as androstenedione and DHEAS (an 'androgen screen'), the source of the testosterone can be pinpointed (Fig. 50.4). An elevated DHEAS suggests that the adrenal, or an adrenal tumour, is overproducing androgens. If the ovary is the source, then only androstenedione will be raised.

Clinical note

Low sex hormone-binding globulin (SHBG) (and raised free androgen index) is often found in people with obesity where it usually reflects obesity-associated insulin resistance (insulin depresses SHBG production). This explains why female patients with obesity have a tendency towards hirsutism. The patient's body mass index (BMI) is therefore relevant to the assessment of their androgen status.

Gonadal function

- Testosterone is the main hormone secreted by the testes in the male and is regulated by pituitary luteinising hormone (LH). Testosterone is responsible for the male secondary sex characteristics.

- Oestradiol is the main product of the ovary and is responsible for the female secondary sex characteristics, development of the ovarian follicle and proliferation of the uterine epithelium.

- Hypogonadism in the male may be primary (where the cause is a failure of testosterone synthesis or of spermatogenesis in the testes) or secondary (where the problem is in the hypothalamus or pituitary).

- Gonadal dysfunction in women may present as primary or secondary amenorrhoea, infertility, hirsutism or virilism.

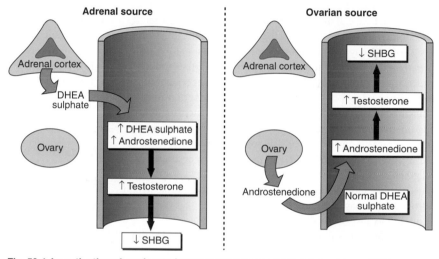

Fig. 50.4 Investigation of an elevated testosterone concentration in a woman. *DHEA*, Dehydroepiandrosterone; *SHBG*, sex hormone-binding globulin.

Case history 38

A 29-year-old woman complained of acne and irregular periods. On examination she had an increased body mass index and moderate hirsutism.

Initial investigations showed a slightly elevated testosterone of 3.7 nmol/L and reduced sex hormone-binding globulin (SHBG) of 19 nmol/L. Luteinising hormone (LH) was 15 U/L and follicle-stimulating hormone (FSH) 5.6 U/L.

- What other investigations should be undertaken to make a diagnosis in this patient? *Comment in Case history comments.*

Want to know more?

Martin KA, Anderson RR, Chang RJ, et al. Evaluation and treatment of hirsutism in premenopausal women: an Endocrine Society clinical practice guideline. *J Clin Endocrinol Metab.* 2018;103(4):1233–1257.

https://doi.org/10.1210/jc.2018-00241

Hirsutism can be a difficult symptom to manage. A practical approach to its investigation and management is provided in this clinical guideline from the Endocrine Society.

http://issam.ch/freetesto.html

This online free and bioavailable testosterone calculator uses testosterone, sex hormone-binding globulin (SHBG) and albumin concentrations to calculate free and bioavailable testosterone in male patients.

51 | Subfertility

Subfertility is defined as the failure of a couple to conceive after 1 year of regular, unprotected intercourse. A full clinical history obtained prior to physical examinations should seek information about previous pregnancies, contraceptive practice, serious illnesses, past chemotherapy or radiotherapy, congenital abnormalities, smoking habits, drug usage, sexually transmitted infections and the frequency of intercourse. Physical examination should look for indications of hypothalamic–pituitary or thyroid disorders, Cushing's syndrome, galactorrhoea and hirsutism. In males, semen analysis should detail volume, sperm density, motility and the presence of abnormal spermatozoa.

In females, endocrine abnormalities are found in one-third of patients. Hormone dysfunction is a very rare cause of male subfertility. In some couples, no cause can be identified.

Endocrine investigations in the subfertile woman

The investigation of infertile females depends on the phase of the menstrual cycle. If there is a regular menstrual cycle, serum progesterone should be measured in the middle of the luteal phase (day 21 of a 28-day cycle). If progesterone is high (>30 nmol/L), the patient has ovulated and there is no need for further endocrine investigations. Other causes of subfertility should be sought. If progesterone is low (<10 nmol/L), ovulation has not occurred.

In women who present with irregular or absent menstruation (oligomenorrhoea or amenorrhoea) or who are not ovulating, hormone measurements may be diagnostic. A protocol for investigation is shown in Fig. 51.1. Measurement of oestradiol and gonadotrophin concentrations may detect primary ovarian failure or polycystic ovarian disease. Measurement of prolactin and androgens also may assist.

Endocrine causes of subfertility in women include:

- *Excessive androgen secretion* by the ovaries in response to insulin resistance. This is commonly a feature of central obesity.
- *Primary ovarian failure.* This is indicated by elevated gonadotrophins and low oestradiol concentration (the postmenopausal pattern). Hormone replacement therapy assists libido and prevents osteoporosis but does not restore fertility.
- *Hyperprolactinaemia* (Chapter 42).

- Although not diagnostic, elevated luteinising hormone (LH) and normal follicle-stimulating hormone (FSH) are consistent with polycystic ovarian disease. Oestradiol measurements are usually unhelpful. Hirsutism, a feature of this condition, is associated with raised testosterone and low sex hormone-binding protein concentrations, with free androgen index consequently being increased.
- *Cushing's syndrome* (Chapter 49).
- *Hypogonadotrophic hypogonadism.* Rarely, subnormal gonadotrophin and oestradiol concentrations suggest the presence of a hypothalamic–pituitary lesion such as a pituitary tumour.

Endocrine investigations in the subfertile man

In eugonadal males with normal sperm analysis, no endocrine investigations are required. In the hypogonadal male, testosterone and the gonadotrophins should be measured first (Fig. 51.2). Causes of subfertility in males include:

- *Primary testicular failure.* Where both the interstitial cells and tubules are damaged, FSH and LH will be elevated and testosterone reduced. Where tubular function only is impaired, FSH is selectively increased and androgen levels may be normal.
- *Hypothalamic–pituitary disease.* Decreased testosterone with low or normal gonadotrophins suggests hypogonadotrophic hypogonadism.
- *Hyperprolactinaemia.* This is a rare cause of subfertility in males.

Subfertility

- Endocrine problems are a common cause of subfertility in females but are rare in males.
- An elevated serum progesterone in a specimen at day 21 of the menstrual cycle confirms that ovulation has occurred.
- In both men and women a serum follicle-stimulating hormone (FSH) concentration greater than 25 U/L indicates primary gonadal failure.
- Hyperprolactinaemia is a common cause of female subfertility.

Want to know more?

National Institute for Health and Care Excellence. Fertility problems: assessment and treatment; 2013 [Clinical Guideline 156]. https://www.nice.org.uk/guidance/cg156/resources/fertility-problems-assessment-and-treatment-35109634660549.

This 2013 NICE guideline makes recommendations for investigation and management of people with fertility problems, from initial advice through investigation to treatment.

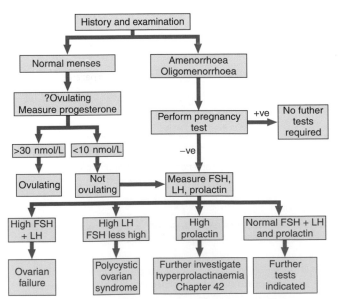

Fig. 51.1 Diagnostic approach to subfertility in the woman. *FSH,* Follicle-stimulating hormone; *LH,* luteinising hormone.

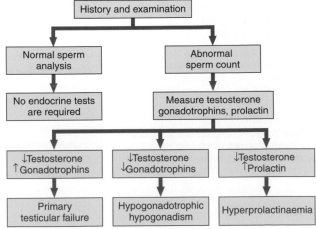

Fig. 51.2 Diagnostic approach to subfertility in the man.

Specialised investigations

4

52 | Nutritional assessment

Malnutrition is a common problem worldwide, and in developed countries it is associated particularly with social deprivation and alcohol. It is also encountered among patients in hospitals. Various studies have shown that patients may have evidence not only of protein-calorie malnutrition but also of vitamin and mineral deficiencies, especially after major surgery or chronic illness.

Malnutrition to the lay person usually means starvation, but the term has a much wider meaning encompassing both the inadequacy of any nutrient in the diet and *excess* food intake. The pathogenesis of malnutrition is shown in Fig. 52.1.

Malnutrition related to surgery or following severe injury occurs because of the extensive metabolic changes that accompany these events: the metabolic response to injury (Chapter 55).

The assessment of a patient suspected of suffering from malnutrition is based on:
- history
- examination
- laboratory investigations, including biochemistry.

History

Medical history may point to changes in weight, poor wound healing or increased susceptibility to infection. The ability to take a good *dietary* history is one of the most important parts of a full nutritional assessment. Taking a dietary history may involve recording in detail the food and drink intake of the patient over a 7-day period. Usually, however, a few simple questions may yield a lot of useful information about a person's diet. Depending on the background to the problem, different questions will be appropriate. For example, in some patients, questions about appetite and general food intake may suggest an eating disorder such as anorexia nervosa, but in the patient presenting with a skin rash, details of the specific food groups eaten will be required to help exclude a dietary cause. In the patient at increased risk of coronary heart disease, questions on saturated fat intake may be most revealing.

Examination

Simple anthropometric measurements will include height, weight, arm circumference and skin-fold thickness.

Body mass index (BMI), weight in kilograms divided by the height in metres squared, is a reasonable indicator of nutritional state, except when the patient is oedematous. Arm circumference is an indicator of skeletal muscle mass, and skin-fold thickness reflects subcutaneous fat stores. In addition, general physical examination may reveal signs of malnutrition in the skin, nails, hair, teeth and mucous membranes. Fig. 52.2 shows some features to consider when deciding if a patient may need nutritional support.

Biochemistry

A number of biochemical tests are used to complement the history and examination in assessing the general nutritional status of a patient. None are completely satisfactory, and they should never be used in isolation. The most common tests include:
- *Protein*. In the vast majority of cases, serum albumin is not useful as a marker of nutritional status. It is affected by many factors other than nutrition, e.g. hepatic and renal diseases and the hydration of the patient. Serum albumin concentration rapidly falls as part of the metabolic response to injury, and the decrease may be mistakenly attributed to malnutrition.
- *Blood glucose concentration*. This will be maintained even in the face of prolonged starvation. Ketosis develops during starvation and carbohydrate deficiency. Hyperglycaemia is frequently encountered as part of the metabolic response to injury, reflecting stress.
- *Lipids*. Fasting plasma triglyceride levels provide some indication of fat metabolism but are again affected by a variety of metabolic processes.

Unlike the assessment of overall status, biochemical measurements play a key role in identifying excesses or deficiencies of specific components of the diet. Both blood and urine results may be of value. Such assays include:
- *Vitamins*. These organic compounds are vital for normal metabolism. Usually they are classified by their solubility; they are listed in Table 52.1, and their average adult daily requirements are shown in Fig. 52.3. Some assays are

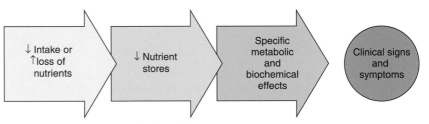

Fig. 52.1 The development of malnutrition.

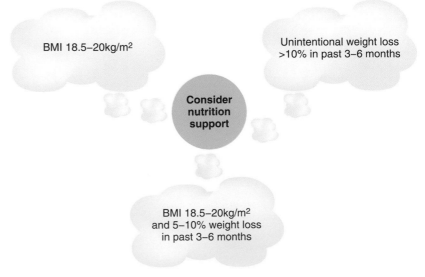

Fig. 52.2 Selection of patients for nutritional support. *BMI*, Body mass index.

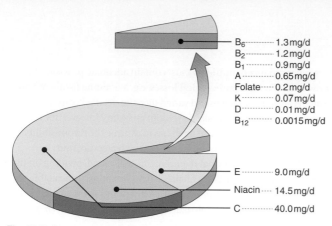

Fig. 52.3 **Average adult daily requirements of vitamins.**

B6 .... 1.3 mg/d
B2 .... 1.2 mg/d
B1 .... 0.9 mg/d
A .... 0.65 mg/d
Folate ..... 0.2 mg/d
K .... 0.07 mg/d
D .... 0.01 mg/d
B12 .... 0.0015 mg/d

E .... 9.0 mg/d
Niacin .... 14.5 mg/d
C .... 40.0 mg/d

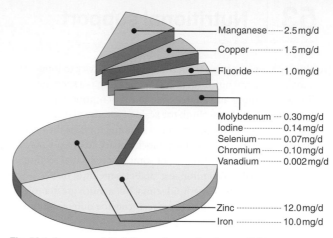

Manganese ... 2.5 mg/d
Copper ...... 1.5 mg/d
Fluoride .... 1.0 mg/d

Molybdenum ... 0.30 mg/d
Iodine .... 0.14 mg/d
Selenium ..... 0.07 mg/d
Chromium ..... 0.10 mg/d
Vanadium ..... 0.002 mg/d

Zinc .... 12.0 mg/d
Iron .... 10.0 mg/d

Fig. 52.4 **Average adult daily requirements of essential trace elements.**

Table 52.1 Classification of vitamins

Vitamins	Deficiency state	Laboratory assessment
Water-soluble		
C (Ascorbate)	Scurvy	Plasma levels
B₁ (Thiamine)	Beriberi	Red blood cell (RBC) levels
B₂ (Riboflavin)	Rarely single deficiency	RBC levels
B₆ (Pyridoxine)	Dermatitis/Anaemia	RBC levels
B₁₂ (Cobalamin)	Pernicious anaemia, neurological problems	Serum B₁₂
Folate	Megaloblastic anaemia	Serum folate, RBC folate, full blood count
Niacin	Pellagra	Urinary niacin metabolites (not commonly available)
Fat-soluble		
A (Retinol)	Blindness	Serum vitamin A
D (Cholecalciferol)	Osteomalacia/rickets	Serum 25-hydroxycholecalciferol
E (Tocopherol)	Anaemia/neuropathy	Serum vitamin E
K (Phytomenadione)	Defective clotting	Serum vitamin K, prothrombin time

available to measure the blood levels of vitamins directly, but often functional assays that utilise the fact that many vitamins are enzyme cofactors are used. These latter assays may help identify gross abnormalities. However, to detect subtle deficiencies and the increasing problem of excess intake, quantitative measurements are required.

- *Major minerals.* These inorganic elements are present in the body in quantities greater than 5 g. The main nutrients in this category are sodium, potassium, chloride, calcium, phosphorus and magnesium. All of these are readily measurable in blood, and their levels may in part reflect dietary intake, although abnormalities in these parameters usually are due to pathology rather than dietary intake
- *Trace elements.* Inorganic elements present in the body in quantities less than 5 g are often found in complexes with proteins.

The essential trace elements are shown in Fig. 52.4.

Preoperative nutritional assessment

Nutritional assessment is not only necessary following surgical procedures. Patients need to be in good nutritional condition before an operation, and the assessment should be done well in advance to allow build-up of reserves before surgery where necessary (see Fig. 52.2).

Clinical note

The 'Malnutrition Universal Screening Tool' (MUST) is commonly used to identify people who are at risk of malnutrition. It uses the easily recorded parameters of body mass index (BMI), unintentional weight loss and the effect of acute illness to quantify risk of malnutrition as low, medium or high.

Nutritional assessment

- Nutritional assessment is important in every patient.
- Malnutrition is common and usually reflects the inadequacy of a nutrient or nutrients in the diet.
- History, examination and laboratory investigations are complementary.
- Patients do not always present with 'textbook' symptoms – e.g. people with vitamin B₁₂ deficiency often present with non-textbook fluctuant symptoms including 'brain fog' and 'jelly-legs'.
- A variety of biochemical investigations may assist in the diagnosis of nutritional deficiencies and in the monitoring of patients undergoing nutritional support.

Case history 39

A 68-year-old man with motor neurone disease is admitted because of severe anorexia and weight loss. Suspecting malnutrition, the junior doctor requests a battery of biochemical tests, including serum vitamin E and selenium.

- How useful will these be in the management of this patient?
Comment in Case history comments.

Want to know more?

http://www.bapen.org.uk/pdfs/must/must-full.pdf

MUST stands for Malnutrition Universal Screening Tool (MUST), developed by the British Association for Parenteral and Enteral Nutrition (BAPEN). This useful resource gives step-by-step instructions on how to identify patients at risk of malnutrition.

http://www.trace-elements.co.uk

This source gives detailed advice on laboratory aspects of nutritional assessment (how to request and interpret results of trace element and micronutrient measurements).

53 | Nutritional support

Nutritional support ranges from simple dietary advice to long-term total parenteral nutrition (TPN). In between is a spectrum of clinical conditions and appropriate forms of nutritional support (Fig. 53.1). As we climb the scale of severity of disease, we increase the level of support and in so doing increase the need for laboratory support. The clinical biochemistry laboratory plays an important role in the diagnosis of some disorders that require specific nutritional intervention, e.g. diabetes mellitus, iron-deficiency anaemia and hyperlipidaemia, but a much greater role is played in the monitoring of patients receiving the different forms of nutritional support.

What do patients need?

Assessing the dietary nutritional requirements of some patients is a highly specialised task. Fig. 53.2 outlines details to consider when contemplating referring a patient for nutrition support.

A balanced mix of nutrients must contain adequate provision for growth, healing and pathological losses, e.g. a draining fistula. Where patients are able to eat a mixed varied diet, the detailed consideration of their specific dietary intakes is seldom an issue. However, for those patients in whom the clinical team has to assume the responsibility of providing the balance of nutrients, much greater care must be taken. Individual nutritional requirements will vary depending on the phase of injury/recovery. Several predictive equations are available for estimating adult energy requirements. Activity and stress factors also must be considered when calculating requirements and will change depending on clinical status.

Energy

Several equations have been proposed over the years to predict energy requirements. The most commonly applied equations at present are those published by C. J. K. Henry in 2005. These equations use age, weight and sex to predict basal metabolic rate.

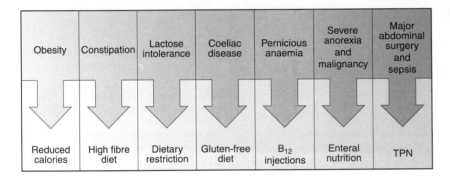

Fig. 53.1 The spectrum of nutritional support.
TPN, Total parenteral nutrition.

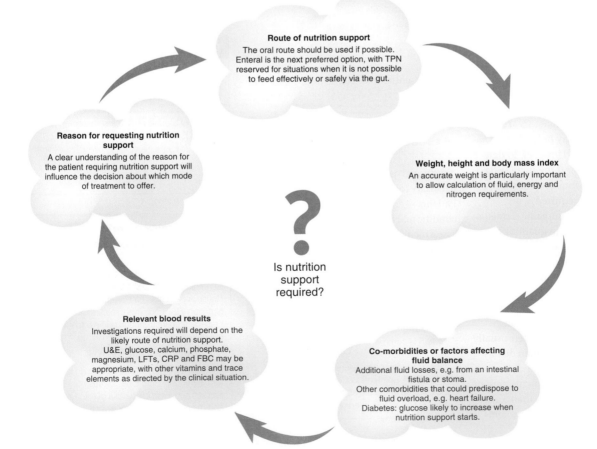

Fig. 53.2 Issues to consider when referring a patient for nutrition support. *CRP*, C-reactive protein; *FBC*, full blood count; *LFT*, liver function test; *TPN*, total parenteral nutrition; *U&E*, urea and electrolytes.

Adjustments are then made based on metabolic stress and physical activity. A further adjustment can be made in metabolically stable patients who are aiming to gain weight. For people who are not severely ill or injured, and are not at risk of refeeding syndrome (Chapter 54), energy requirements can be estimated as 25–35 kcal/kg/day. The principal energy sources in the diet are carbohydrates and fats. Glucose provides 4 kcal/g, and fat provides 9 kcal/g. The entire calorie load may be administered using carbohydrates, but prescribing a mixture of carbohydrates and lipids is more physiological and reduces the volume of the diet. This is important in both enteral tube feeding and parenteral nutrition.

Nitrogen

Recommended protein intake is 0.8–1.5 g protein/kg body weight/day. This equates to a nitrogen requirement of 0.13 to 0.24 g/kg body weight/day, with 1 g of nitrogen being equal to 6.25 g of protein.

Fluid

Basic fluid requirements are 35 mL/kg body weight for patients under 60 years old and 30 mL/kg body weight for patients over 60 years old. This amount should be increased if the patient has additional fluid losses, e.g. from an intestinal fistula or stoma, and reduced if the patient is likely to be unable to cope with significant fluid volumes, e.g. because of heart failure.

Vitamins and trace elements

Vitamins and trace elements are collectively described as *micronutrients*, not because they are of limited importance, but because they are required in relatively small amounts. Reference nutrient intakes (RNIs) have been defined for most nutrients, and these are used in the make-up of artificial diets.

How should patients receive nutrition?

Care must be exercised to prevent over- and underfeeding. Patients may be fed in the following ways:

- oral feeding
- tube feeding into the gut (enteral)
- feeding that bypasses the gut (parenteral).

Oral feeding should be used whenever possible. Tube feeding (Fig. 53.3) involves the use of small-bore nasogastric, nasoduodenal or gastrostomy tubes. Defined diets of homogeneous composition can be continually administered. Tube feeding in this way bypasses problems with oral pathology, swallowing difficulties (e.g. after a stroke) and anorexia. Even patients who have had gastric surgery can be tube fed postoperatively if a feeding jejunostomy is fashioned during the operation distal to the lesion. However, tube feeding also presents mechanical problems in terms of blockage or oesophageal erosion. Gastrointestinal problems, e.g. vomiting and diarrhoea, and metabolic problems can be minimised by the gradual introduction of the feeds and are rarely contraindications to enteral feeding. The problems associated with parenteral nutrition are even more challenging and are discussed in Chapter 54. It should be noted, however, that the vast majority of patients can be fed successfully either orally or with enteral tube feeds.

Monitoring patients

Clinical and biochemical monitoring should always go hand in hand with the assessment of any form of nutritional support. In some circumstances the contribution of the laboratory may be the simple measurement of blood glucose, whereas in other situations the measurements and advice provided by the laboratory may dictate the regimen in a patient receiving parenteral nutrition.

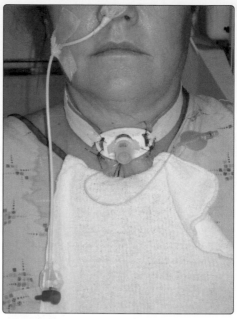

Fig. 53.3 Patient on tube feeding in the intensive care unit. Note this patient is also being ventilated via a tracheostomy and has a central line in place. *(From Groher M.E., Crary M.A.* Dysphagia: Clinical Management in Adults and Children. *St. Louis, MO: Elsevier; 2010.)*

Clinical note

By far the most effective route of supplying nutrients to a patient is via the gut. Use of nasogastric tubes and electively inserted stoma tubes to the stomach or small intestine ensures that only a small minority of patients will require parenteral feeding.

Nutritional support

- Nutritional support is required in a wide spectrum of conditions.
- It consists of a variety of approaches, from simple dietary advice to total parenteral nutrition (TPN).
- The route of first choice for nutritional support is oral, followed by enteral and then by parenteral.
- Careful clinical and laboratory monitoring is required to some extent in all forms of nutritional support.
- Most laboratory support is needed for those patients receiving parenteral nutrition.

Case history 40

A patient with pernicious anaemia is being treated with parenteral vitamin B_{12}. Because she has recently been feeling tired and 'run down', her physician sends a blood sample to the clinical biochemistry laboratory requesting a serum B_{12} level.

- Is this the most appropriate way to monitor the patient?
  Comment in Case history comments.

Want to know more?

https://www.nice.org.uk/guidance/cg32/

This 2006 National Institute for Health and Care Excellence (NICE) clinical guideline provides comprehensive guidance on all aspects of nutrition support. Issues addressed include how to identify patients who require nutrition support, how to select the most appropriate mode of nutrition support and how to decide on the composition of preparations.

54 | Parenteral nutrition

The provision of nutrients to the body's cells is a highly complex physiological process involving many endocrine, exocrine and other metabolic functions. Total parenteral nutrition (TPN) completely bypasses the gastrointestinal tract, delivering processed nutrients directly into the venous blood. It is more physiological to feed patients enterally, and parenteral nutrition should be considered only once other possibilities have been deemed unsuitable. The institution of TPN is never an emergency, and there always should be time for consultation and for baseline measurements to be performed. A team approach is best practice (Fig. 54.1) and is followed in most hospitals.

Indications for parenteral nutrition

Patients who do not have a working, accessible gastrointestinal tract should be considered for parenteral nutrition. The circumstances in which this occurs include:
- inflammatory bowel disease, e.g. Crohn's disease
- postoperative ileus
- short bowel syndrome, e.g. mesenteric artery infarction.

Route of administration

Parenteral nutrition may be given in the following ways:
- *Via peripheral veins*. This route may be successfully used for a short period of 1 to 2 weeks. Only certain parenteral nutrition preparations have a low enough osmolality to be given peripherally.
- *Via a central venous catheter*. This route is used where long-term intravenous feeding is anticipated. Central vein catheters may remain patent for years if cared for properly.

Although most recipients of TPN are in-patients, many individuals who require long-term TPN successfully manage to administer TPN in the home. These patients have permanent central catheters through which prepackaged nutrition fluids are administered, usually at night.

Components of TPN

TPN should, as its name suggests, provide complete artificial nutrition. An appropriate volume of fluid will contain a source of calories, amino acids, vitamins and trace elements (Fig. 54.2). The calorie source is a mixture of glucose and lipid. Many patients who receive TPN are given standard proprietary regimens and prepackaged solutions. These have made TPN much easier, but as with any such approach in medicine, some patients require more tailored regimens.

Complications

TPN is the most extreme form of nutritional support and can give rise to considerable difficulties. In order to pre-empt these, consistent careful nursing care and biochemical monitoring are required.

Catheter site sepsis is a constant fear in these patients. The nutrient-containing infusion fluids are, of course, also excellent bacterial and fungal growth media, and risk of infection is further heightened by the presence of a foreign body, the catheter. Strict attention to aseptic technique both in the siting of a catheter and in its maintenance will avoid many of these problems.

Misplacement of a catheter and infusion of nutrient solutions extravascularly can be very serious. Central catheters should be placed under X-ray control. The possibility of embolism, either thrombotic or air, should be easily avoided as long as their potential is recognised.

The most common metabolic complication is hyperglycaemia. Against a background of increased stress hormones, especially if there is infection, there may be marked insulin resistance and consequently an increased glucose concentration. The

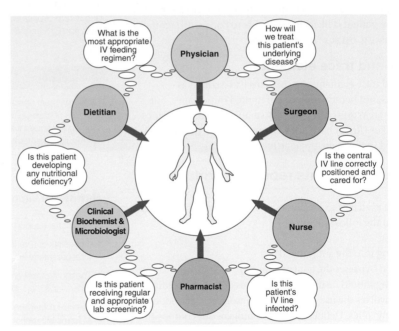

Fig. 54.1 Team approach to total parenteral nutrition.

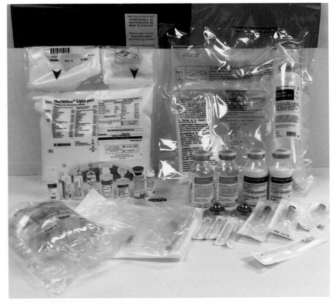

Fig. 54.2 Total parenteral nutrition preparations.

use of insulin to correct these metabolic effects is best avoided. The composition of the intravenous regimen should be adjusted if metabolic disorders occur. Many other biochemical abnormalities have been reported in association with TPN. These include:

- hypokalaemia
- hypomagnesaemia
- hypophosphataemia
- hypercalcaemia
- acid–base disorders
- hyperlipidaemia.

An acute form of metabolic disturbance is the *refeeding syndrome*. Patients who have been malnourished for a significant period of time before initiation of TPN are most at risk, especially those with chronic alcohol-related health problems. In the undernourished state, the metabolic and cellular processes are slowed. As soon as nutrition is supplied, there is activation of these processes and increased utilisation of minerals and micronutrients. This may result in dangerously low plasma levels of some minerals, trace elements and vitamins, especially inorganic phosphate, magnesium and vitamin B_1. Refeeding syndrome is preventable by prescribing TPN at half or even a quarter of total calculated requirements over the initial few days and gradually increasing it as a metabolically stable state is achieved. Thiamine should be given (usually as part of an intravenous vitamin B preparation) before and during the initial stages of treatment with TPN if there is a risk of refeeding syndrome.

With proper patient assessment and biochemical and clinical monitoring, these complications can be minimised.

Monitoring patients on TPN

In addition to baseline assessment of patients receiving TPN, there should be a strict policy for careful clinical and biochemical monitoring of these patients (Fig. 54.3). This is especially important if the duration of TPN is medium to long term. The tests described in Fig. 53.2 have particular relevance here.

Special attention must be paid to the micronutrients in patients receiving long-term TPN, as any imbalance here may result in a single-nutrient deficiency state. Such situations are increasingly rare, except in patients relying solely on artificial diets for their nutrients.

Because biochemical changes may precede the development of any clinical manifestation of a nutritional deficiency, careful laboratory monitoring should be instituted. However, measurement of trace elements and vitamins is often affected by the acute phase response and care needs to be taken in interpretation.

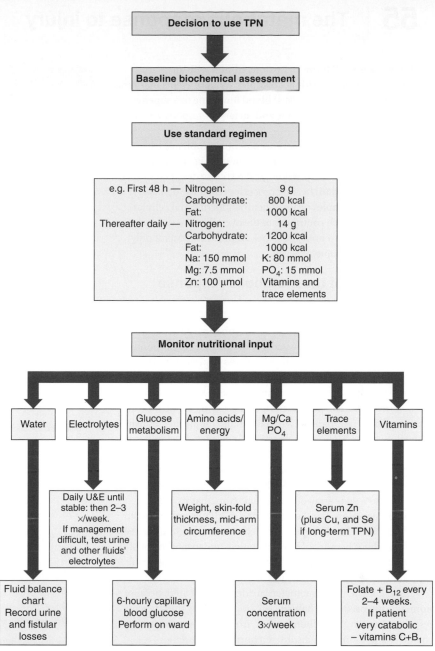

Fig. 54.3 Intravenous nutrition and its monitoring. *TPN*, Total parenteral nutrition; *U&E*, urea and electrolytes.

Clinical note

Patients often receive lipid emulsions as part of their intravenous regimen. Visible lipaemia in a blood sample usually suggests that the patient is unable to clear the lipid from the plasma.

Parenteral nutrition

- Total parenteral nutrition (TPN) is never an emergency procedure and should be carefully planned.
- A multidisciplinary team approach to TPN is the most effective.
- The main problems are due to sepsis and mechanical and metabolic complications.
- The use of commercial preparations has made the incidence of deficiency states much less common.
- Patients receiving TPN require careful clinical and biochemical monitoring.

Case history 41

A 54-year-old man was admitted with a superior mesenteric artery thrombosis. He had gross bowel ischaemia and necrosis. Subsequently he had only 15 cm of viable small bowel.

- What form of feeding would be appropriate in this man?
- What assessment should be made before commencing treatment?
  Comment in Case history comments.

Want to know more?

http://www.sas-centre.org/assays/trace-elements

This very useful website is hosted by the Supra-Regional Assay Service – the laboratories across the UK that measure trace elements. It provides a list of elements (and associated supplementary assays) that are measured and relevant information.

55 | The metabolic response to injury

The body reacts to all forms of noxious stimuli with an inflammatory response. This is a complex series of events that varies from mild hyperaemia (increased blood flow) due to a superficial scratch, to major haemodynamic and metabolic responses to a severe injury.

Trauma is associated with various potential problems, listed in Box 55.1. The metabolic response to injury (Fig. 55.1) can be thought of as a protective physiological response designed to keep the individual alive until healing processes repair the damage. It is mediated by a complex series of neuroendocrine and cellular processes, all of which contribute to the overall goal – survival. The metabolic response to injury becomes clinically important only when the degree of injury is severe.

The phases of the metabolic response to injury

The metabolic response to injury has two phases: *ebb* and *flow* (Fig. 55.2). The ebb phase is usually short and may correspond to clinical shock, resulting from reduced tissue perfusion. The physiological changes that occur here are designed to restore adequate vascular volume and maintain essential tissue perfusion. The severity of the ebb phase determines the clinical outcome. If it is mild or moderate, patients will have an uncomplicated transition to the flow phase. However, if severe, patients may develop *systemic inflammatory response syndrome* (SIRS), the features of which are shown in Box 55.2. Patients who meet two or more of these criteria may be classified as having SIRS. This complex pathophysiological state involves a wide array of inflammatory mediators and hormonal regulators, but the underlying mechanisms have yet to be fully clarified. No therapeutic strategies have been found to be helpful, perhaps because of our incomplete understanding of SIRS. However, a proportion of patients will recover with intensive life support, including ventilation and dialysis.

Various biochemical parameters are deranged in SIRS, because normal homeostatic mechanisms are overridden by the stress response. Low levels of albumin, zinc, iron and selenium are characteristic, along with disordered hormonal regulation, e.g. low triiodothyronine (T_3), thyroid-stimulating hormone and thyroxine (T_4). Nearly all of these patients develop the syndrome of inappropriate diuresis (see Chapter 9).

The flow phase may last for days to weeks depending on the extent of the injury. In this phase, metabolism is altered to ensure that energy is available for dependent tissues at the expense of muscle and fat stores (Table 55.1).

The acute phase protein response

The acute phase protein response leads to greatly increased *de novo* synthesis (principally by the liver) of a number of plasma proteins, along with a decrease in the plasma concentration of others. This response is stimulated by the release of cytokines, e.g. interleukin-1 and interleukin-6 and tumour necrosis factor α, and raised concentrations of the 'stress' hormones cortisol and glucagon. The major human acute phase proteins are listed in Table 55.2.

The acute phase protein response is an adaptive response to disease. Its role is not fully understood, but certain aspects can be seen to be of benefit to the individual. The increases in C-reactive protein (CRP) and complement contain and eliminate infection; increased coagulation factors prevent excess blood loss; protease inhibitors prevent spread of tissue necrosis when lysosomal enzymes are released by damaged cells at the site

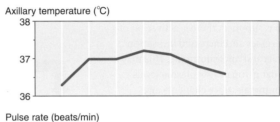
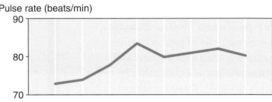
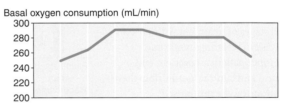
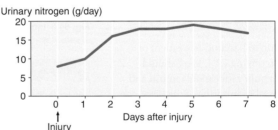

Fig. 55.1 The changes in body temperature, pulse rate, oxygen consumption and urinary nitrogen excretion which accompany injury.

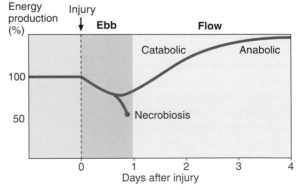

Fig. 55.2 The phases of the metabolic response to injury.

Table 55.1 Biochemical changes in the metabolic response to injury

Metabolic Change	Consequence
Increased glycogenolysis	Leads to increased circulating blood glucose to be used as an energy substrate
Increased gluconeogenesis	Leads to increased circulating blood glucose to be used as an energy substrate
Increased lipolysis	Leads to increased free fatty acids which are used to provide energy and increased glycerol which may be converted to glucose
Increased proteolysis	Leads to increased amino acids which may be catabolised to provide energy or used for tissue synthesis and wound healing

Table 55.2 The acute phase protein response

Protein Types	Increased	Decreased
Protease inhibitors	α_1-antitrypsin α_2-macroglobulin	
Coagulation proteins	Fibrinogen Prothrombin Factor VIII Plasminogen	
Complement proteins	C1s C2, B C3, C4, C5 C56 C1 INH	Properdin
Miscellaneous	Haptoglobin Caeruloplasmin C-reactive protein Serum amyloid A protein	Albumin HDL LDL

HDL, High-density lipoprotein; *LDL*, low-density lipoprotein.

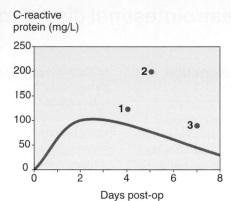

C-reactive protein (mg/L)

— Normal CRP response to cholecystectomy
1 Abnormally high CRP in patient 4 days post-op with fever
2 Patient's condition deteriorating, wound re-opened and abscess drained on day 5
3 CRP level falling and patient making good recovery

Days post-op

Fig. 55.3 C-reactive protein *(CRP)* concentrations in a patient who developed an abscess following abdominal surgery.

Starvation and the metabolic response to injury

The metabolic responses to injury and to starvation are quite different. After injury the body is at war, defences are mobilised, metabolic activity increases and resources are directed to the site of action. In starvation, the body is in a state of famine, resources are rationed and metabolic activity is limited to the absolute minimum necessary for survival. Hypoalbuminaemia is often erroneously perceived as an index of nutritional status. In starvation not associated with inflammation, the serum albumin is characteristically within the reference interval. In clinical practice a low serum albumin concentration is almost invariably caused by the inflammatory response; it results from redistribution of the albumin from the intravascular to the interstitial fluid compartment due to increased capillary permeability.

Clinical note

Antibiotic therapy for an infection, perhaps indicated by increased C-reactive protein (CRP) concentration, should be started only after appropriate specimens have been taken for bacteriological investigation.

of injury. The precise role of other proteins in this response such as caeruloplasmin and serum amyloid A remains to be established.

Clinical uses

The acute phase response is widely used to monitor the course of inflammatory processes. This is done in two ways:
- *By measuring serum CRP.* CRP concentrations change very rapidly and can be used to monitor changes on a daily basis (Fig. 55.3).
- *By monitoring the erythrocyte sedimentation rate (ESR).* This partly reflects fibrinogen and immunoglobulin concentration. ESR changes slowly and is used to monitor the inflammatory process over weeks rather than days. (See also the clinical note in Chapter 25).

In neonates and immunocompromised patients, bacterial infection can be difficult to diagnose in its early stages. This includes patients with AIDS. Failure to make the diagnosis may have fatal consequences. In practice, a serum CRP concentration greater than 100 mg/L (normal is <3 mg/L) is frequently taken to indicate the presence of bacterial infection.

The metabolic response to injury

- The metabolic response to injury is a protective physiological response.
- The ebb phase may progress to recovery or to systemic inflammatory response syndrome (SIRS).
- The flow phase involves changes in metabolism to ensure that energy is made available to dependent tissues.
- The flow phase persists until the inflammatory response provides for tissue healing and/or eradication of infection.
- C-reactive protein (CRP) and albumin measurements are useful in monitoring day-to-day changes in the inflammatory response.

Case history 42

A 28-year-old man was admitted to the intensive care unit after a road traffic accident in which he sustained multiple injuries. After initial resuscitation and surgery for his injuries, he was considered stable but in a coma.

- What is the role of biochemical measurements in this patient's management?
Comment in Case history comments.

Want to know more?

Marik PE, Taeb AM. SIRS, qSOFA and new sepsis definition. *J Thorac Dis.* 2017;9(4):943–945. doi: 10.21037/jtd.2017.03.

This editorial discusses and compares the different definitions and criteria to define sepsis.

56 | Gastrointestinal disorders

Physiology of digestion and absorption

Cooking food kills bacteria and other pathogens; neutralises toxins, e.g. in some beans; and breaks down food. Chewing breaks down food, further increasing the surface area and thus facilitating enzymatic digestion. Major nutrients (carbohydrate, protein and fat) are broken down enzymatically to low-molecular-weight compounds. Digestive enzymes are secreted by the salivary glands, stomach, pancreas and small intestine.

Absorption refers to the transport of products of digestion into gut epithelial cells and from there to the portal blood. Absorption of some nutrients is passive, whereas others require energy-dependent active transport.

Malabsorption

The term *malabsorption* describes impairment of the absorptive mechanisms, but in practice also encompasses failure of digestion (maldigestion). Malabsorption can occur at any stage of life, from a variety of causes (Fig. 56.1).

The clinical effects of malabsorption result from failure to absorb nutrients. The major consequences of generalised malabsorption arise from inadequate energy intake, resulting in weight loss in adults and growth failure ('failure to thrive') in children.

In suspected malabsorption, a detailed dietary history is essential to establish eating patterns and habits. Provided dietary input is adequate, the presence of malabsorption often will be indicated by diarrhoea and changes in the appearance and consistency of the faeces.

Fig. 56.2 illustrates how the normal mucosal structure is designed to maximise absorptive capacity. Although mucosal surface enzymes play an important role in digestion, the most important source of digestive enzymes is the exocrine pancreas. As with many other organs in the body, there is more than 50% reserve capacity in both the small intestine and exocrine pancreas. Thus, disorders in these organs are usually quite advanced before malabsorption can be detected by functional tests or is clinically manifest. As a result, the role of functional tests of malabsorption has diminished and they have largely been abandoned.

Endoscopy and biopsy are the most important tools available for investigation of gastrointestinal disorders. They allow both macroscopic and microscopic investigation of the gut. Radiological investigations are important when detecting abnormal anatomy of the bowel and motility.

In the case of fat malabsorption, the faeces will contain unabsorbed fat. When present in large quantities it often gives rise to typical greenish-yellow 'greasy' appearance and is exceptionally foul-smelling. This is referred to as steatorrhoea. Qualitative or quantitative faecal fat analysis has essentially been discarded as a test. Where small molecules such as monosaccharides or disaccharides are not absorbed, they exert an osmotic effect in the large intestine, giving rise to a large volume of watery stools.

Laxative abuse is an important diagnosis that may be missed. In cases of suspected abuse a urine laxative screen can be performed.

Gastrointestinal disorders

Gastro-oesophageal

The gastric mucosa secretes pepsinogen (converted to the active enzyme pepsin by hydrochloric acid) and intrinsic factor, which is essential for vitamin B_{12} absorption in the terminal ileum. Gastric acid may be tested qualitatively, but quantifying gastric acid secretion has effectively been dropped in practice.

Dyspepsia is a common symptom. Oesophageal reflux, peptic ulcer disease,

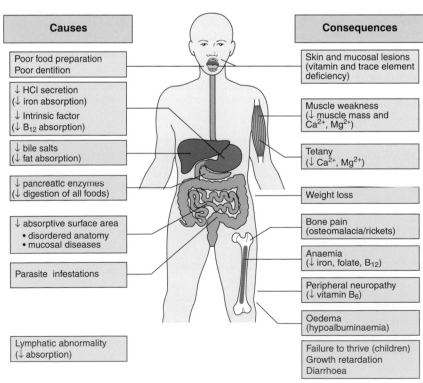

Fig. 56.1 Causes and consequences of malabsorption.

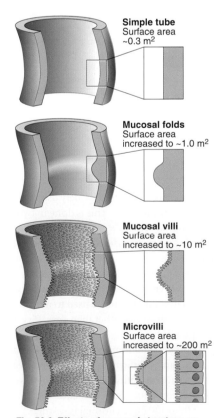

Fig. 56.2 Effects of mucosal structure on absorptive surface area of the small intestine.

gastritis or gastric malignancy are diagnosed by endoscopy and biopsy. Peptic ulcer disease is usually due to *Helicobacter pylori* infection. Excessive acid secretion due to gastrin-secreting tumours *gastrinomas* is very rare. Gastrin and other 'gut hormones' can be tested for in specialist laboratories, but appropriate sample collection is imperative to avoid potentially misleading results.

Pancreas

The pancreas plays a major role in digestion and is the subject of a separate chapter (Chapter 57).

Small intestine

The absorption of nutrients, which occurs at the mucosal microvillous surface of the enterocytes, is the major role of the small intestine (see Fig. 56.2).

Mucosal disease is diagnosed by biopsy. Coeliac disease is the commonest cause of villous atrophy. The presence of autoantibodies (Table 56.1) may indicate a likely diagnosis of coeliac disease, but confirmation is made by biopsy.

Inflammatory bowel disease

Inflammatory bowel diseases (IBDs) include Crohn's disease and ulcerative colitis. The former can affect any section of the gastrointestinal tract from the mouth to the anus and is characterised by inflammation affecting all layers of the gut. The latter is confined to the superficial mucosa of the large bowel. The clinical presentation of both diseases— typically an increase in frequency with blood and/or mucus in the stool— will usually indicate the presence of inflammatory bowel disorders. They are usually diagnosed by a combination of endoscopy, biopsy and radiology. The aetiology of these disorders is unknown, and frequently there can be difficulties in making a definitive histological diagnosis. In all inflammatory bowel disorders, faecal calprotectin concentration will be increased when the diseases are active. IBD must not be confused with irritable bowel syndrome (IBS).

Malignant disease

The small intestine contains a large amount of lymphoid tissue. Mucosa-associated lymphoid tumours (MALT

tumours) can cause malabsorption. Their presentation is variable, and they are diagnosed histologically.

Colon cancer is a major cause of mortality and morbidity. In its early stages it is asymptomatic, hence the introduction of national screening for the condition in those over 50 years of age. Faecal immunochemical tests (FIT) detect very small quantities of haemoglobin in a stool sample and may be used in the investigation of symptomatic patients, or in population screening, allowing selection of patients for colonoscopy and biopsy, for early detection of colon cancer.

Table 56.1 Laboratory investigations used in the investigation of gastrointestinal disorders

Disorder	Investigations
Peptic ulcer	Serum anti-*Helicobacter pylori* antibody titre. Urea breath test. Endoscopic biopsy with subsequent testing for urease activity, culture and histology is the most reliable investigation.
Pernicious anaemia	Serum anti-intrinsic factor antibody titre. Serum antiparietal cell antibody titre. The classical Schilling test is no longer widely used.
Coeliac disease	Immunoglobulin A (IgA) anti-endomysial antibody titre; antitissue transglutaminase titre. Patients should, at the same time, be screened for IgA deficiency as this can cause false negative results. Duodenal biopsy is the definitive investigation but is invasive.
Small bowel bacterial overgrowth	Hydrogen breath test—this test is also used in combination with oral doses of lactose or fructose to diagnose malabsorption of these sugars.
Inflammatory bowel disease	Faecal calprotectin concentration. Patients will also have a high serum C-reactive protein and white blood cell count. Patients with high faecal calprotectin must undergo endoscopy and biopsy to make a specific diagnosis.
Exocrine pancreatic insufficiency	Faecal pancreatic elastase-1 (E1) concentration. Faecal chymotrypsin is less reliable as it is prone to some degradation in the gut.

Clinical note

Many patients with malabsorption recognise that certain things in their diet, usually fatty foods, cause diarrhoea. They avoid these foods and reduce their fat intake. As a result, faecal fat excretion may be normal.

Gastrointestinal disorders

• In suspected malabsorption, a detailed dietary history is essential to establish eating patterns and habits.

• Endoscopy and biopsy are the most important diagnostic tools.

• Laboratory tests in the investigation of gastrointestinal disorders fall into one of two groups: tests of malabsorption or tests of pancreatic function.

Case history 43

A 69-year-old woman, who had made an excellent recovery after local excision of a breast tumour 8 years previously, presented with weight loss, bone tenderness and weakness. Her symptoms had developed over a number of months. Her family was concerned that she was not caring for herself or eating adequately. There was no clinical evidence of recurrence of breast cancer. Liver function tests showed only an elevated alkaline phosphatase (430 U/L).

• What other biochemical tests would be of assistance in making a diagnosis? *Comment in Case history comments.*

Want to know more?

https://en.wikipedia.org/wiki/Helicobacter_pylori#cite_note-118

That *Helicobacter pylori* causes peptic ulcer disease is now universally accepted. Yet until the 1980s it was believed that the acid environment of the stomach prevented bacterial growth. The work of two Australians in proving that this was not the case was rewarded with the 2005 Nobel Prize for Physiology or Medicine. The History section of this excellent wiki provides an accessible account of their discoveries.

57 | Disorders of the pancreas

Structure

Functionally and anatomically, the pancreas is a complex gland. It is about 30 cm long, mostly retroperitoneal and is in close anatomical relation with the stomach, small intestine (especially the duodenum), transverse colon and the spleen. Externally it comprises of a head, neck, body and tail. Internally, the main pancreatic duct (of Wirsung) traverses its entire length and connects with the common bile duct in the head of the pancreas. This forms a small prominence called the *ampulla of Vater*, which opens into the descending part of the duodenum. Flow through the ampulla occurs via a smooth muscular *sphincter of Oddi*, which stops duodenal contents from entering the pancreatic duct. There is also an accessory pancreatic duct which has separate openings in the duodenum (Fig. 57.1).

Exocrine function

The pancreas plays an important role in the digestive process. Approximately 2 L of pancreatic fluid is secreted every day into the duodenum. It contains digestive enzymes which help to break down proteins, carbohydrates and fats. The enzymes are secreted in an inactive form as proenzymes. When they come in contact with an enterokinase in the mucosal lining of the duodenum, a cleavage process is initiated which converts the proenzymes into activated enzymes. Table 57.1 lists these enzymes and their digestive functions. The pancreatic fluid is also rich in bicarbonate, which helps to counter the acidity of the gastric contents entering the duodenum (due to gastric acid) and aids in digestion of food.

Endocrine function

Fig. 57.2 details various cell types in the *islets of Langerhans* in the pancreas and the corresponding hormones secreted. The main endocrine function of the pancreas is regulation of blood glucose concentration. High blood glucose stimulates insulin secretion from the β cells, which results in increased cellular glucose uptake and a reduction in blood glucose. Conversely, low blood glucose stimulates secretion of glucagon from the α cells which raises blood glucose by reducing its uptake in muscles and adipose tissue, and also by means of gluconeogenesis and glycogenolysis. Delta cells produce

somatostatin which reduces the secretion of both insulin and glucagon. Maintenance of blood glucose is complex, and other factors involved include amino acids, thyroid hormones, growth hormone, corticosteroids and the autonomic nervous system. Pancreatic polypeptide has multiple roles including influencing appetite, energy expenditure and gastric motility.

Acute pancreatitis

Acute pancreatitis refers to inflammation of the pancreas. In most patients it runs a mild clinical course and recovery occurs within a few days. At the other end of the spectrum, the inflammation is associated with widespread destruction of pancreatic tissue (the full histopathological term is *acute haemorrhagic pancreatic necrosis*) leading to clinical shock and requiring intensive

haemodynamic support. In this scenario, mortality can be as high as 20%.

The commonest presenting clinical feature is abdominal pain, often with vomiting. In the classic presentation, the pain is epigastric and radiates to the back, with abdominal tenderness and guarding. Turner and Cullen signs (haemorrhagic discolouration of the flanks and umbilicus, respectively), if present, signify severe disease (Fig. 57.3).

The biochemical hallmark of acute pancreatitis is marked elevation in activities of some of the pancreatic digestive enzymes, notably *amylase* and *lipase*. Of these two, lipase is diagnostically superior, but amylase is long-established and remains the first-line diagnostic test in many hospital laboratory services.

Usually, the diagnosis is clear from the clinical and biochemical picture.

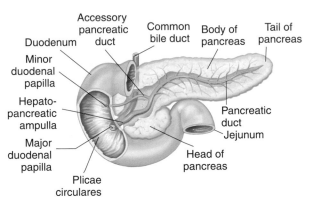

Fig. 57.1 Anatomical relations of the pancreas. *(From Patton KT, Thibodeau GA. Anatomy and Physiology. 9th ed. St Louis, MO: Mosby; 2016.)*

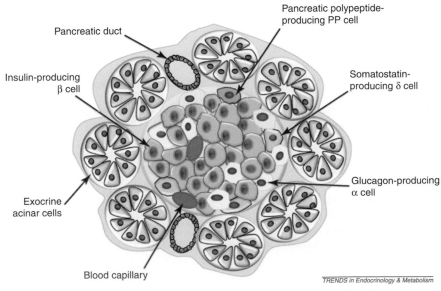

Fig. 57.2 Anatomy of the islets of Langerhans. *PP*, Pancreatic polypeptide. *(From Efrat S, Russ HA. Making β cells from adult tissues.* Trends in Endocrinol Metabol. *2012;23(6):278–285.)*

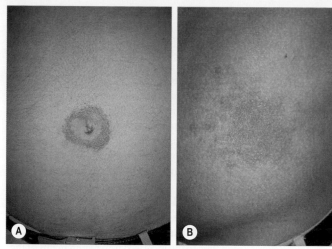

Fig. 57.3 Clinical findings of intraabdominal haemorrhage. (A) Cullen sign and **(B)** Turner sign. *(With permission from Chauhan S, Gupta M, Sachdev A, D'Cruz S, Kaur I. Cullen's and Turner's sign associated with portal hypertension. Lancet. 2008;372(9632):54.)*

Abdominal imaging (CT scan if available) may be indicated when the diagnosis remains in doubt. Other acute abdominal conditions (e.g. acute cholecystitis, perforated peptic ulcer, mesenteric artery thrombosis) may also present in a similar way. The principles of management are mostly supportive: intravenous fluids, pain relief and adequate nutrition whilst awaiting recovery. Table 57.2 outlines various causes and precipitating factors of acute pancreatitis, although it should be noted that in many cases the cause may not be obvious.

Chronic pancreatitis and pancreatic insufficiency

Chronic pancreatitis refers to long-standing inflammation of the pancreas, often resulting from repeated episodes of acute pancreatitis. Eventually the cumulative damage alters the structure and both exocrine and endocrine function of the pancreas. Chronic alcohol consumption remains the commonest aetiological factor.

Chronic pancreatitis typically presents with recurrent abdominal pain, often post-prandially, as well as vomiting, steatorrhoea and malabsorption, leading to nutritional deficiencies and weight loss. Damage to pancreatic islets may lead to diabetes. Faecal elastase can be used to screen for exocrine insufficiency and abdominal imaging may be used to look for structural damage and glandular calcification. Treatment involves pain relief, enzyme replacement therapy and surgery.

Cystic fibrosis, although much less common, is associated with pancreatic insufficiency in a large majority of cases.

Table 57.1 Pancreatic enzymes and their functions

Enzymes	Function
Chymotrypsin and trypsin	Breakdown of proteins and peptides to amino acids
Pancreatic lipases, phospholipases and cholesterol esterase	Breakdown of triglycerides and cholesterol esters
Amylase	Breakdown of starches and other carbohydrates
Nucleases	Breakdown of nucleotides of DNA and RNA

Table 57.2 Causes of acute pancreatitis

Cause	Example
Mechanical obstruction of pancreatic ducts	Gallstones Trauma Postoperative
Metabolic/toxic causes	Alcohol Drugs, e.g. corticosteroids. thiazide diuretics, azathioprine Hypercalcaemia Hyperlipidaemia
Vascular/poor perfusion	Shock Atherosclerosis Hypothermia Polyarteritis nodosa
Infections	Mumps

(Adapted from Xiu, Philip. *Crash Course: Pathology*, 4th edn, 2012.)

Clinical note

Acute pancreatitis may be diagnosed when two of the following three criteria are present: typical abdominal pain, raised enzyme levels, or appearances of pancreatitis on computer tomography. Computed tomography also has a role in the assessment of the severity of acute pancreatitis if the illness fails to resolve within 1 week.

Pancreatic disorders

- Sometimes it can be difficult to clinically differentiate between acute pancreatitis and inferior myocardial infarction.
- Pancreatic pseudocyst may be a sequelae of acute or chronic pancreatitis, resulting in persistence of symptoms and chronic elevation of serum amylase.
- In severe haemorrhagic pancreatitis the serum amylase peak may be missed, in which case urine amylase or serum lipase may offer a larger diagnostic window.
- The commonest type of pancreatic cancer is an adenocarcinoma accounting for about 90% of all cases.

Case history 44

A 45-year-old man presented to the emergency department with severe unrelenting epigastric pain, not relieved by proton pump inhibitors. The pain had fluctuated over the previous few months but had significantly worsened recently. He had also had chronic diarrhoea over the same period and had lost about 5 kg weight.

a) What is the likely clinical diagnosis?
b) How may biochemical tests help to establish the cause of his symptoms?

Comment in Case history comments.

Want to know more?

2019 WSES guidelines for the management of severe acute pancreatitis | World Journal of Emergency Surgery | Full Text (biomedcentral.com).

58 | Iron

Iron is an essential element in humans, being the central ion in haem, the nonprotein component of haemoglobin, myoglobin and the cytochromes (Fig. 58.1). Iron deficiency causes a failure in haem synthesis, and since haemoglobin is required for delivery of oxygen to the tissues, this leads to anaemia and tissue hypoxia. Conversely, free iron is highly toxic to cells and must be bound to protein at all times.

Iron physiology

Iron levels are controlled by regulating iron uptake, since there is no mechanism for controlling its excretion. There are 50 to 70 mmol (3–4 g) of iron in the body. Dietary intake of iron is about 0.35 mmol (20 mg) per day, of which only 5% to 10% is absorbed and the rest is excreted in faeces along with the shedding of the intestinal mucosal cells. Tissue iron is bound to the iron storage proteins ferritin (soluble) and haemosiderin (insoluble). The 1% of body iron in the plasma is associated with the iron-binding glycoprotein, transferrin, each molecule of which binds two Fe^{2+} ions. Fig. 58.2 summarises iron distribution and metabolism.

Iron concentrations differ with age and sex. Normal adult concentrations are 5 to 32 μmol/L. There is a marked circadian rhythm (up to 50%) in serum iron concentrations (higher in the morning, lower in the evening).

Laboratory investigation of iron disorders

- *Serum iron determinations* are of limited routine value, being of most assistance in the diagnosis of iron overload and acute iron poisoning.

- *Transferrin* can be measured directly, or indirectly as the *total iron-binding capacity (TIBC)*. Normally transferrin is about 30% saturated with iron. When saturation falls to 15%, iron deficiency is likely and some degree of clinical effect can be expected. A higher percentage saturation indicates iron overload. Transferrin and, therefore, also total serum iron, is decreased as part of the acute phase response. Protein energy malnutrition decreases transferrin synthesis and hence its serum concentration.

- *Serum ferritin* is the best indicator of body iron stores; less than 15 μg/L indicates significant iron deficiency. The acute phase response can result in increases in serum ferritin, making the diagnosis of marginal iron deficiency difficult or impossible in these circumstances.

- *Zinc protoporphyrin* (ZPP), a precursor of haem is markedly increased in iron deficiency and is sometimes used as a screening test in children; it is expressed as μmol ZPP/mol haem and is usually less than 60. ZPP is also increased following chronic exposure to lead, though in children the rise is late and lead levels are more reliable. For a full investigation of suspected iron deficiency, haemoglobin concentration and a blood film for red cell morphology are required.

Iron deficiency

Iron-deficiency anaemia is the commonest single-nutrient deficiency, causing seriously impaired quality of life. Principal causes are chronic blood loss and poor dietary intake of bioavailable iron. Uptake of iron can be decreased by a number of dietary constituents, e.g. phytates (beans, seeds, nuts and grains are high in phytates), and can also occur in malabsorptive conditions, such as coeliac disease. In iron-deficiency anaemia it is important to diagnose the underlying condition, especially malignant disease, the presence of intestinal parasites or any other intestinal pathology that may cause chronic blood loss. Even well-nourished women may develop iron deficiency during pregnancy due to the increased iron requirements of the developing fetus.

Iron-deficiency anaemia develops in three stages:
1. *Depletion of iron stores:* confirmed by low serum ferritin levels.
2. *Deficient erythropoiesis:* marked by a fall in serum iron concentration and increased synthesis of transferrin, both of which result in decreased percentage saturation. Although haemoglobin is normal, ZPP is increased.
3. *Iron-deficiency anaemia:* both iron and haemoglobin are low, and there is a microcytic, hypochromic anaemia (Fig. 58.3). Low stainable iron is seen in the bone marrow.

Treatment

Oral iron salts or glycine chelates or intramuscular injection of sodium ferric gluconate are used to treat deficiency. It can take up to 6 months to replete the body stores. With oral treatment, compliance may be a problem due to nausea, diarrhoea and other intestinal complaints. These are all lessened if the iron salts are taken with food.

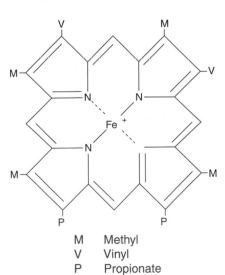

M — Methyl
V — Vinyl
P — Propionate

Fig. 58.1 Structure of haem.

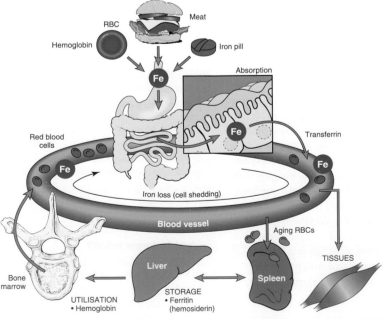

Fig. 58.2 Iron metabolism. *RBC*, Red blood cells. *(From Damjanov I, Perry A, Perry, K. Pathology for the Health Professions. 6th ed; Elsevier, 2022.)*

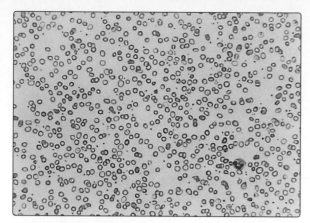

Fig. 58.3 An iron-deficient blood film.

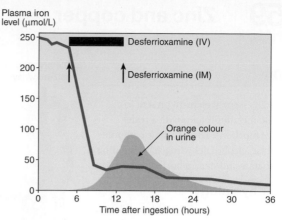

Fig. 58.4 The effect of desferrioxamine on iron excretion in overdose. *IM*, Intramuscular; *IV*, intravenous.

Iron overload

Iron overload may be caused by chronic blood transfusions and where there is ineffective haematopoiesis, as in renal failure. Other important causes of iron overload are haemochromatosis and iron poisoning (see later). It has also been reported in children on long-term parenteral nutrition. Since there is no major mechanism for excretion of iron except by cell desquamation and occult blood loss, iron overload is also a possibility when iron therapy is prescribed. In iron overload the serum ferritin concentrations may rise to 500 to 5000 µg/L.

Haemochromatosis

This is a relatively common inherited disease characterised by increased iron absorption (2–3× normal) that leads to iron deposition in various organs. Whole body iron content may be increased tenfold. The excess iron leads to free radical generation, fibrosis and organ failure. The commonest mutation (C282Y) in the *HFE* gene results in decreased production of hepcidin, the main regulator of iron absorption and distribution. This small peptide targets ferroportin, a transmembrane protein present in intestinal cells that binds to absorbed iron. Hepcidin binds to ferroportin and induces its internalisation and degradation, thereby retaining the iron within the cells; this iron is subsequently lost with cellular desquamation. Low hepcidin production leads to excessive iron absorption. The clinical presentation varies widely depending upon dietary iron uptake, alcohol abuse or the presence of hepatotoxins. Women are less severely affected than men, being protected by physiological iron loss during menstruation and in pregnancy.

Clinical features include chronic fatigue and, in extreme cases, skin pigmentation, diabetes mellitus, cardiomyopathy, hepatic cirrhosis and hepatoma. Serum iron is increased, with almost complete saturation of transferrin. Transferrin saturation is the test with the greatest sensitivity and specificity for haemochromatosis, but serum ferritin is also increased to greater than 500 µg/L. Hereditary haemochromatosis may be confirmed by genotyping. Liver biopsy also may be used to confirm iron overload but is rarely performed. Chronic iron overload is usually treated by regular venesection; removal of 500 mL blood accounts for approximately 250 mg iron. In chronic treatment, ferritin levels should be maintained below 100 µg/L.

Iron poisoning

Iron poisoning in children is relatively common and may be life-threatening.

Iron is present in various 'tonics' and supplements, and iron tablets are particularly attractive to children as they look like sweets (candy). Symptoms include nausea and vomiting, abdominal pain and haematemesis, or, in severe cases, hypotension and coma. Serum iron and transferrin saturation is increased. Treatment is by chelation of iron in the plasma with desferrioxamine. Chelated iron is excreted in the urine as a deep orange-coloured complex (Fig. 58.4).

> **Clinical note**
>
> A microcytic hypochromic anaemia, and the absence of stainable iron in a bone marrow biopsy, are the best diagnostic indices of established iron deficiency.

> **Iron**
>
> - Iron deficiency is commonly caused by the combination of blood loss and low dietary intake.
> - Iron deficiency can be diagnosed by finding a hypochromic microcytic anaemia.
> - Serum ferritin is the most reliable single biochemical test of iron deficiency.
> - Iron overload may arise following repeated blood transfusions.
> - Iron overload is diagnosed by finding an increased serum iron concentration and percentage transferrin saturation, and increased serum ferritin.
> - Accidental iron poisoning in children is an important medical emergency.

> **Case history 45**
>
> A 42-year-old woman presented with a history of increasing lethargy, dizziness and breathlessness. She had brittle hair and nails. She complained of heart palpitation on exercise and reported particularly heavy periods. Biochemical investigation revealed the following results:
>
> | | |
> |---|---|
> | Serum iron | 4 µmol/L |
> | Transferrin saturation | 10% |
> | Ferritin | <5 µg/L |
>
> - What is the diagnosis and what other investigations should have been done first?
>   *Comment in Case history comments*.

> **Want to know more?**
>
> Siah CW, Ombiga J, Adams LA, Trinder D, Olynyk JK. Normal iron metabolism and the pathophysi- ology of iron overload disorders. *Clin Biochem Rev*. 2006;27(1):5–16. https://www.ncbi.nlm.nih.gov/ pmc/articles/PMC1390789/pdf/cbr27_1p005.pdf
>
> This article provides a more detailed insight into the physiology of iron metabolism and iron overload.

59 | Zinc and copper

Zinc

Zinc is an essential element present in over 200 metalloproteins with a wide range of functions. These include carbonic anhydrase, alcohol dehydrogenase, alkaline phosphatase and steroid hormone receptors.

Zinc physiology

Zinc deficiency is a major health problem in the poorer nations of the world. The daily requirement, which varies with age and sex and during pregnancy, is about 150 µmol (10 mg) (Fig. 59.1). Zinc is present in all protein-rich foods, and approximately 30% is absorbed. Phytates (the principal storage form of phosphorus in many plant tissues, especially bran and seeds) are indigestible in humans; when consumed in large quantities, they bind calcium, iron and zinc, and reduce their absorption. In the liver, zinc is incorporated into metalloenzymes, whereas in blood most zinc is contained in erythrocytes. In plasma, 90% of zinc is bound to albumin and 10% to α_2-macroglobulin. Zinc reserves in the body are located mainly in muscle and bone. Zinc is excreted in urine, bile, pancreatic fluid and milk in lactating mothers.

Zinc deficiency

In children who survive famine, the rate of growth during rehabilitation from starvation has been clearly related to the dietary supply of bioavailable zinc. Zinc deficiency is known to occur in patients on parenteral nutrition and causes a characteristic skin rash (Fig. 59.2) and hair loss. Wound breakdown and delayed healing are other complications. *Acrodermatitis enteropathica*, a rare inherited disorder of zinc metabolism, manifests in infancy as a skin rash; other clinical features include diarrhoea, alopecia and nail dystrophy. Untreated, the prognosis is poor, but oral zinc therapy leads to complete remission. Cadmium displaces zinc from metalloproteins, and zinc deficiency can be a consequence of chronic cadmium poisoning. (Cadmium exposure may occur during the production of batteries and some plastics, and in the smelting of metals.)

Zinc toxicity

Zinc toxicity is uncommon. It is usually due to exposure to high levels of zinc fumes. It is difficult to induce toxicity by dietary means. However, in cases of self-poisoning with zinc salts, symptoms include fever, vomiting, stomach cramps and diarrhoea.

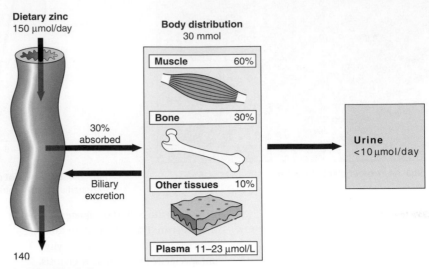

Dietary zinc
150 µmol/day

Body distribution
30 mmol

Muscle 60%

Bone 30%

30% absorbed

Biliary excretion

Other tissues 10%

Urine <10 µmol/day

140

Plasma 11–23 µmol/L

Fig. 59.1 Zinc balance.

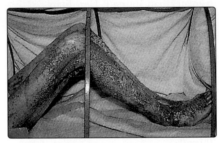

Fig. 59.2 Skin lesions in zinc deficiency.

Laboratory assessment

The concentration of zinc in plasma decreases as part of the metabolic response in inflammation; when C-reactive protein (CRP) is greater than 20 mg/L, plasma zinc is an unreliable indicator of zinc status. The repeated finding of a plasma zinc less than 5 µmol/L is suggestive of impending zinc deficiency and merits further investigation.

Marginal zinc deficiency is best demonstrated by a positive clinical response to supplementation. Oral or intravenous zinc reverses the signs and symptoms of zinc deficiency within weeks.

Copper

Copper, an essential trace metal, is a component of a wide range of intracellular metalloenzymes, including cytochrome oxidase, superoxide dismutase, tyrosinase, dopamine hydroxylase and lysyl oxidase.

Copper physiology

About 50% of the average daily dietary copper of around 25 µmol (1.5 mg) is absorbed from the stomach and the small intestine (Fig. 59.3). There is evidence that not all modern diets contain sufficient copper, especially when large amounts of refined carbohydrate are consumed. Copper absorption is facilitated by cation

transport enzymes in the mucosal cells. A high zinc intake blocks absorption of copper by inducing metallothionein in the mucosal cells; copper has high affinity for metallothionein and is lost when the mucosal cells are shed in the faeces. This relatively rare condition of zinc-induced copper deficiency may occur when patients are left on zinc supplementation for prolonged periods of time. Absorbed copper is transported to the liver bound to albumin, where it is incorporated into caeruloplasmin, which contains six copper atoms per molecule, and exported into the circulation (Fig. 59.4).

Copper is present in all metabolically active tissue. The highest concentrations are found in the liver and the kidneys, with significant amounts in cardiac and skeletal muscle and in bone. The liver contains 10% of the total body content of 1200 µmol (80 mg). Excess copper is excreted in bile into the gut.

Copper deficiency

Children and adults can develop symptomatic copper deficiency. Premature infants are most susceptible since copper stores in the liver are laid down in the third trimester of pregnancy. In adults, deficiency is usually found following intestinal resection, bypass surgery or inappropriate oral zinc supplementation. Deficiency usually presents as refractory anaemia or leucopenia. Neurological consequences, e.g. spasticity or neuropathy, are later complications.

Copper toxicity

Copper toxicity is uncommon and is most often due to administration of copper sulphate solutions. Oral copper sulphate may lead to gastric perforation. Serum copper concentrations may be greatly elevated. Treatment is by chelation with penicillamine.

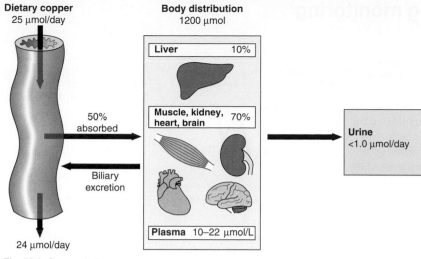

Dietary copper
25 µmol/day

Body distribution
1200 µmol

Liver 10%

50% absorbed

Muscle, kidney, heart, brain 70%

Biliary excretion

Urine
<1.0 µmol/day

Plasma 10–22 µmol/L

24 µmol/day

Fig. 59.3 Copper balance.

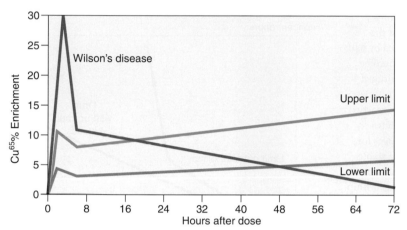

Fig. 59.4 Cu⁶⁵ uptake test. The most abundant stable isotope of copper is Cu^{63}. A standard dose of Cu^{65}, another naturally occurring stable isotope, is given orally. The initial increase in enrichment is followed by a decrease at 6 h, representing liver uptake. The later increase represents the export of caeruloplasmin from the liver. In Wilson's disease the initial increase in Cu^{65} is exaggerated, typically five times normal, with subsequent diminished export from the liver. In Cu malabsorption, due to disease or Zn-induced mucosal block, the initial increase is blunted but the subsequent export from the liver is normal.

Table 59.1 **Typical biochemistry in patients with Wilson's disease**

Investigation	Normal adult	Wilson's disease
Serum copper µmol/L	10–22	<10
Caeruloplasmin g/L	0.15–0.6	<0.15
Urinary copper µmol/24 h	<1	5–15
Liver copper µg/g dry weight	20–50	>250

Clinical note

Prolonged inappropriate zinc supplementation is a potentially serious and avoidable cause of copper deficiency. Patients with unexplained marrow suppression and/or neuropathy should be asked about their use of dietary supplements.

Zinc and copper

- Adequate zinc is needed for growth in children.

- Symptomatic zinc deficiency in the adult causes dermatitis, hair loss and poor wound healing.

- Serum zinc concentrations persistently below 5 µmol/L warn of impending clinical deficiency.

- Diagnosis of severe copper deficiency can be made by measurement of serum copper. Values of less than 10 µmol/L in adults and of less than 5.0 µmol/L in neonates require investigation.

- The major inborn error of copper metabolism is Wilson's disease.

- Wilson's disease is treatable and requires prompt diagnosis.

Case history 46

A 15-year-old girl presented with abdominal pain and diarrhoea for 3 days. She became jaundiced and a presumptive diagnosis of infective hepatitis was made, but serological tests were negative. She subsequently died of fulminant liver failure. At postmortem examination, her liver copper concentration was found to be grossly increased.

- What investigations should be carried out on this patient's younger sister?
Comment in Case history comments.

Want to know more?

Osredkar J, Sustar N. Copper and zinc: biological role and significance of copper/zinc imbalance. *J Clin Toxicol.* 2011;S3:001. https://www.omicsonline.org/copper-and-zinc-biological-role-and-significance-of-copper-zincimbalance-2161-0495.S3-001.pdf

This article provides more information on the biology and significance of zinc and copper imbalance.

Laboratory assessment

- *Serum copper.* 90% is bound to caeruloplasmin. Total copper concentration may vary due to changes in copper itself or changes in the concentration of caeruloplasmin.
- *Serum caeruloplasmin.* Increases greatly in the acute phase reaction, when it may reach concentrations 5 to 20 times normal levels.
- *Urinary copper.* Normal excretion is less than 1.0 µmol/24 hours.

The oral Cu⁶⁵ absorption test (see Fig. 59.4) is a useful tool in the investigation of patients found to have a low plasma copper.

Inborn errors of copper metabolism

Wilson's disease and the much rarer Menke's syndrome are the main inborn errors of copper metabolism.

Wilson's disease

All adolescents or young adults with otherwise unexplained neurological or hepatic disease should be investigated for Wilson's disease. Symptoms result from copper deposition in the liver, brain and kidneys. Copper deposits in the eye can sometimes be seen as a brown pigment around the iris (*Kayser–Fleischer rings*). These are pathognomonic, i.e. if present, Wilson's disease can be diagnosed.

Wilson's disease is caused by a mutation in the gene *ATP7B* that codes for an enzyme involved in copper transport. Urinary free copper excretion is high and total serum concentrations are low (Table 59.1). Confirmation is by measurement of copper in a liver biopsy, which is usually greater than 250 µg/g dry weight in patients with the disease. The noninvasive Cu⁶⁵ oral uptake test is a reliable test for the diagnosis of Wilson's disease and available in some specialist laboratories.

Treatment is by administration of a chelating agent, penicillamine, to promote urinary copper excretion. Patients are maintained on oral penicillamine for life. Liver transplantation may be considered, particularly in young patients with severe disease.

60 | Therapeutic drug monitoring

Most drug therapy is assessed by observing the change in the patient's clinical state, i.e. how the patient responds in terms of what the drug does. Therapeutic drug monitoring (TDM) is a useful adjunct to clinical assessment. It refers to the measurement of drug concentrations (usually in blood) as a means of assessing the adequacy of dosage. TDM is not necessary where there is a clear and measurable clinical effect, such as with antihypertensive or hypoglycaemic drugs, but is important with those drugs for which there is no good objective measurement of effectiveness and/or there is a serious risk of toxicity. *For TDM to be of value there must be a proven relationship between the plasma drug concentration and the clinical effect.*

Following the administration of a drug, the graph of plasma concentration against time, plotted on semi-logarithmic graph paper, will look like that in Fig. 60.1. Analysis of such graphs can allow an estimate of the half-life of the drug and the volume of distribution. The *half-life* is the period of time required for the concentration or amount of drug in the body to be reduced by half. The *volume of distribution* is the theoretical volume that would be required to contain the total amount of an administered drug at the observed plasma concentration. These can be used to estimate the correct dose to give. After several doses a steady state is reached, at which point the plasma drug concentration oscillates between a peak and a trough level. It usually takes about five half-lives for the steady state to be attained. In the steady state there is a stable relationship between the dose and the effect, and decisions can be made with confidence. For most drugs there is a linear relationship between dose and plasma concentration. However, some drugs, e.g. phenytoin show nonlinear kinetics (Fig. 60.2).

Sampling for TDM

The concentration of drug in plasma or saliva changes constantly over the period of treatment, and in order to compare one treatment with another, standardisation must be introduced. When taking a sample for TDM, it is important to:
- ask the patient about compliance
- check for interacting drugs (including over-the-counter complementary/herbal therapies)
- note the dose and the time since last dose
- take the sample at an appropriate time, e.g. pre dose.

Interpretation of drug levels

Where drug concentrations are lower than expected, the most likely cause is noncompliance. Higher than expected concentrations, in the absence of an increase in dose, indicate that a change has taken place either in other drug therapy or in hepatic or renal function. Cumulative reporting allows comparisons between drug concentrations. The therapeutic range for each drug indicates broadly the limits within which most patients will show maximum therapeutic effect with minimum toxicity. However, a concentration that is therapeutic in one patient may give rise to toxicity in another (Fig. 60.3). The most likely reasons for the plasma drug concentration to fall above or below the therapeutic range are given in Table 60.1.

Although many drugs *can* be measured in specialist laboratories, only a few drugs are *required* to be measured in most laboratories. Examples of drugs for which TDM is appropriate, and the reasons why, are shown in Table 60.2. Many of these drugs have a low therapeutic index. This means that the concentration at which

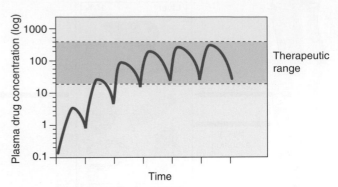

Fig. 60.1 Plasma drug concentration shown after a series of identical doses equally spaced. After approximately 5 half-lives, steady state is achieved.

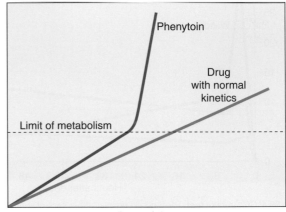

Fig. 60.2 Nonlinear (saturation) kinetics of phenytoin.

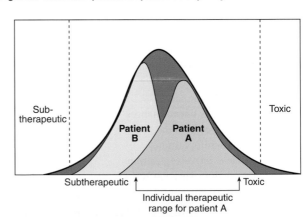

Fig. 60.3 A population therapeutic range for a common drug.

Table 60.1 **Common reasons for subtherapeutic or toxic levels**
Subtherapeutic Levels
Noncompliance
Dose too low
Malabsorption
Rapid metabolism
Toxic Levels
Overdose
Dose too high
Dose too frequent
Impaired renal function
Reduced hepatic metabolism

toxicity occurs is not much higher than that required for therapeutic effect. It should be noted that some drugs are highly bound to albumin. In patients with low albumin concentrations, the total drug concentration may be low but the effective (free) level may be adequate.

Drug interactions

Some drugs interfere with the metabolism and excretion of others, and as a result the addition of one drug will alter the plasma concentration of another (Fig. 60.4). In such circumstances, rather than attempt to establish a new steady state, it may be appropriate, when a patient is receiving a short course of a drug such as an antibiotic, temporarily to change the dose of the drug it affects. Drug interactions are particularly problematic where several drugs must be coprescribed, as in treatment of tuberculosis, HIV and cancer.

Pharmacokinetics

Although there is considerable variation between patients and the rate at which they metabolise and excrete drugs, predictions can be made based on population averages. These allow the calculation of doses that are usually better than the rough guidance given by the manufacturers. Once a patient with good compliance has been stabilised and the plasma drug concentration at steady state has been measured, it is possible to control the plasma concentrations accurately over a long period by small dosage adjustments.

Therapeutic drug monitoring

- Therapeutic drug monitoring (TDM) is only of use where the plasma concentration of a drug relates to its clinical effect.
- TDM samples should be taken at the correct time in relation to the dose.
- For a correct interpretation of a drug level, full details of the patient's dosing history should be obtained.
- Poor compliance is the commonest cause of subtherapeutic drug concentrations.
- Used correctly, TDM can identify noncompliance and can avoid iatrogenic toxicity.

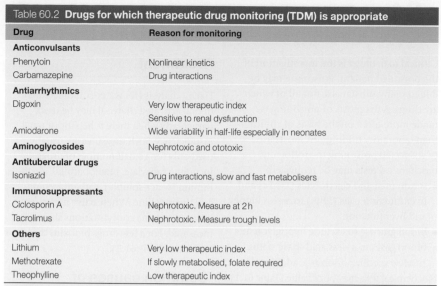

Table 60.2 Drugs for which therapeutic drug monitoring (TDM) is appropriate

Drug	Reason for monitoring
Anticonvulsants	
Phenytoin	Nonlinear kinetics
Carbamazepine	Drug interactions
Antiarrhythmics	
Digoxin	Very low therapeutic index
	Sensitive to renal dysfunction
Amiodarone	Wide variability in half-life especially in neonates
Aminoglycosides	Nephrotoxic and ototoxic
Antitubercular drugs	
Isoniazid	Drug interactions, slow and fast metabolisers
Immunosuppressants	
Ciclosporin A	Nephrotoxic. Measure at 2 h
Tacrolimus	Nephrotoxic. Measure trough levels
Others	
Lithium	Very low therapeutic index
Methotrexate	If slowly metabolised, folate required
Theophylline	Low therapeutic index

Note. Significant drug interactions between antiretroviral drugs and the antibiotics used in patients with HIV/AIDS indicate that TDM of these drugs may be required in certain clinical scenarios—although TDM of antiretroviral drugs is not routinely required.

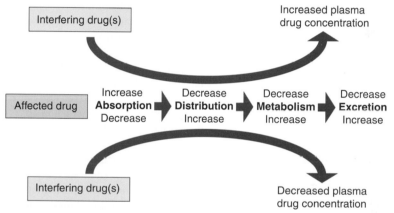

Fig. 60.4 Common mechanisms of drug interactions.

Case history 47

A patient with chronic asthma, well controlled on theophylline, developed a severe chest infection. She was prescribed clarithromycin and later presented to her general practitioner complaining of tachycardia and dizziness. Her plasma theophylline concentration was found to be 140 μmol/L, much higher than the therapeutic range of 55 to 110 μmol/L.

- Explain the theophylline result.
  Comment in Case history comments.

Want to know more?

https://www.sps.nhs.uk/home/tools/drug-monitoring/

This guidance advises on appropriate monitoring of patients on a range of drugs, when to measure drug concentrations (and when not to), as well as on other laboratory tests required in monitoring patients on particular drugs.

61 | Toxicology

Clinical toxicology is the investigation of the poisoned patient. Poisoning may be due to many substances, not all of which are drugs. A diagnosis of poisoning is made more often on the basis of clinical than laboratory findings. In most cases of suspected poisoning the following biochemical tests may be requested:

- serum urea and electrolytes (U&Es) and liver function tests (LFTs) to assess kidney and liver function
- blood glucose to exclude hypoglycaemia
- blood gases to assess acid–base status.

In a few specific poisonings, additional biochemical tests may be of value (Table 61.1).

Confirming poisoning

Few of the clinical signs or symptoms that may be present, including coma, are specific for any one drug or poison. A limited toxicology screen in urine can be carried out in many laboratories, but a positive finding indicates only that a toxin has been taken and not the severity of the overdose.

Measurement of drug levels

Sometimes knowledge of the plasma concentration of a drug or toxin alters the treatment of the patient. Drugs for which measurement is useful include paracetamol, salicylate, theophylline, lithium, iron, phenytoin, quinine, phenobarbital and carbon monoxide. *Quantitative* analysis will give an indication of the severity of the poisoning and serial analyses provide a guide to the length of time that will elapse before the effects begin to resolve (Fig. 61.1).

Qualitative drug analysis simply indicates if a drug is present or not. Reasons for qualitative drug analysis include:

- differential diagnosis of coma
- confirmation of brain death
- monitoring of drug abuse
- investigation of suspected nonaccidental poisoning (e.g. in children).

Treatment

Haemodialysis (for water-soluble toxins) or oral activated charcoal may be used, particularly when there is hepatic or renal insufficiency. Such measures are usually used only for a small number of drugs, including salicylate, phenobarbital, alcohols, lithium (water-soluble), carbamazepine and theophylline. When active measures are used, plasma concentrations should be measured. For a few drugs or toxins there are antidotes (Table 61.2).

Common causes of poisoning

Poisonings in which patients may present with few clinical features are salicylate, paracetamol, theophylline, ethylene glycol and methanol. If rapid action is not taken in such cases, the consequence can be severe or fatal illness.

- *Salicylate* toxicity can result in severe metabolic acidosis, from which the patient may not recover. It can also cause a respiratory alkalosis by its action on the respiratory centre in the brain, and occasionally causes both at the same time, i.e. a mixed acid–base picture (metabolic acidosis and respiratory alkalosis). The treatment for salicylate toxicity is forced alkaline diuresis, which both enhances excretion and helps correct the acidosis (Fig. 61.2).
- *Paracetamol (acetaminophen)* toxicity has the potential to cause serious hepatocellular damage, and severely affected patients may die of liver failure. In cases of paracetamol overdose, the serum paracetamol concentration, related to time of ingestion, is widely used to decide on the administration of antidote (Fig. 61.3). A specific therapy, *N*-acetylcysteine, given intravenously, can prevent all of the hepatotoxic and nephrotoxic effects of paracetamol. Therapy should be started

no later than 12 hours of ingestion and hopefully before any clinical symptoms or biochemical changes develop. Patients who consume excess alcohol are at particular risk from paracetamol toxicity. This relates to the induction of metabolising enzymes by alcohol. (Paracetamol is not toxic itself – it gets metabolised to toxic metabolites that overwhelm the antioxidant capacity of the liver.)

- Slow-release *theophylline* preparations in overdose can lead to late development of severe arrhythmias, hypokalaemia and death. In cases of suspected poisoning, the serum theophylline concentration should be measured and its rise or fall monitored. Measures to aid elimination are of limited effect.

Table 61.1 Toxins for which biochemical tests are potentially useful

Toxin	Additional biochemical tests
Amphetamine and ecstasy	Creatine kinase, aspartate aminotransferase
Carbon monoxide	Carboxyhaemoglobin
Cocaine	Creatine kinase, potassium
Digoxin/cardiac glycosides	Potassium
Ethylene glycol	Serum osmolality, bicarbonate, calcium
Fluoride	Calcium and magnesium
Insulin	Glucose, C-peptide
Iron	Iron, glucose
Lead (chronic)	Lead, zinc protoporphyrin (Basophilic stippling on a blood film is a useful pointer if lead poisoning is suspected)
Organophosphates	Cholinesterase
Dapsone/oxidising agents	Methaemoglobin
Paracetamol	Paracetamol
Salicylate	Salicylate
Theophylline	Glucose
Warfarin	International normalised ratio (prothrombin time)

Table 61.2 Commonly used antidotes

Toxin	Antidote
Atropine/hyoscyamine	Physostigmine
Benzodiazepines	Flumazenil
Carbon monoxide	Oxygen
Cyanide	Dicobalt edetate
Digoxin/cardiac glycosides	Neutralising antibodies
Ethylene glycol/ methanol	Ethanol/fomepizole
Heavy metals	Chelating agents
Nitrates/dapsone	Methylene blue
Opiates	Naloxone
Organophosphates	Atropine/pralidoxime
Paracetamol	*N*-Acetylcysteine
Salicylate	Sodium bicarbonate
Warfarin	Vitamin K

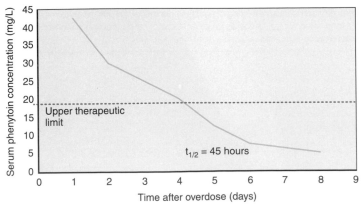

Fig. 61.1 Elimination of phenytoin from serum.

Plasma [HCO₃⁻] and [H⁺]   Plasma salicylate

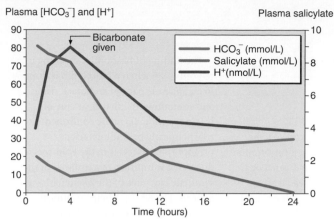

Fig. 61.2 Bicarbonate administration in salicylate overdose.

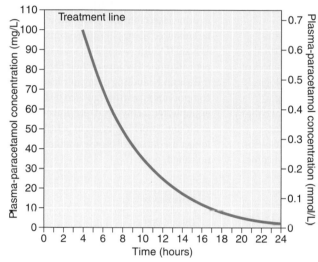

Fig. 61.3 Treatment chart for paracetamol poisoning. *(From MHRA Drug Safety Update, September 2012, Crown Copyright 2012.)*

Other serious poisonings are:

- *Organophosphate and carbamate pesticides*, in which cholinergic symptoms persist for some time. Cholinesterase should be monitored.
- *Atropine*, causing anticholinergic features, e.g. hallucinations with dry mouth, dry hot skin and dilated pupils. Cases occur most often from ingestion of herbal medicines.
- *Opiates*, where overdose leads to pin-point pupils that rapidly dilate on treatment with naloxone.
- *Cardiac glycosides*, both pharmaceutical (e.g. digoxin) and herbal, give rise to severe bradycardia.
- *Ethylene glycol and methanol* poisoning are occasionally encountered. Usually, but not invariably, there is a history of ingestion or suspected ingestion. These *toxic alcohols* are metabolised to oxalic acid and formic acid, respectively. Patients develop a severe metabolic acidosis and, in the case of ethylene glycol, hypocalcaemia. Measuring the serum osmolality and calculating the osmolal gap can be useful here. In the absence of the preferred treatment (fomepizole), patients may be treated with intravenous ethanol to a plasma concentration of around

92 mg/dL. The ethanol is preferentially metabolised, and the unchanged toxic alcohols are gradually eliminated in the urine. (Fomepizole works the same way, i.e. it blocks metabolism.). For reasons that are unclear, methanol (but not ethylene glycol) is toxic to the optic nerve, and visual disturbances may be a presenting feature.

Chronic poisoning

Chronic poisoning occurs when there is a gradual build-up in drug concentration over a period of time. Patients may present with a history of taking only their usual medication. In such cases, plasma drug concentrations can be of assistance in confirming the cause of the symptoms. The drug should be withdrawn and treatment with a lower dose reinstated once the plasma concentrations fall.

Poisoning due to the interaction of drugs whose effect is additive is not uncommon. An example is that of alcohol and benzodiazepines. These are not usually lethal when taken separately, but can be fatal when taken together in overdose. It is important to be aware that patients also may be taking over-the-counter drugs or herbal remedies that may contain pharmacologically active compounds.

Clinical note

If the plasma drug concentration is rising, the drug is still being absorbed. The most likely causes are:

- the presence of a bolus of drug in the gastrointestinal tract
- correction of hypotension has led to increased absorption via the portal system.

Toxicology

- Diagnosis of poisoning is often made clinically. Symptoms may be specific or nonspecific.
- Serum urea and electrolytes (U&Es), blood glucose, blood gases and liver function tests (LFTs) should be requested in every suspected poisoning.
- For paracetamol, salicylate and theophylline, serum drug concentrations are used in prognosis and should always be requested.
- Poisoning may require general supportive therapy or specific treatment.

Case history 48

A 38-year-old man presented at the accident and emergency department late one afternoon, claiming to have taken 100 aspirin tablets early in the day. He was hyperventilating and complaining of ringing in his ears. He felt anxious, but his pupils were of normal size and no other abnormalities were observed. He was given gastric lavage, and blood was taken for measurement of salicylate, urea and electrolytes, and blood gases. The results were as follows:

Na⁺	K⁺	Cl⁻	HCO₃⁻	Urea	Creatinine	H⁺	PCO₂	PO₂
	mmol/L			*μmol/L*		*nmol/L*	*kPa*	*kPa*
140	3.7	102	20	8.1	110	35	3.7	13.3

Salicylate 635 mg/L

- Comment on these results.
- What other information would be useful in determining treatment? *Comment in Case history comments.*

Want to know more?

https://www.nlm.nih.gov/pubs/factsheets/toxnetfs.html

TOXNET is a comprehensive resource of information on all matters toxicological. This fact sheet orientates the uninitiated reader.

62 | Metal poisoning

Poisoning with metals is one of the oldest forms of toxicity known to man. However, it is only recently that some of the mechanisms of toxicity have been established. More importantly, the means of diagnosis and treatment are now available. Symptoms of poisoning are related to the amount ingested or absorbed and the duration of exposure. In general, elemental metals are less toxic than their salts. Organic compounds, in which the metal is covalently bound to carbon compounds, e.g. methyl or ethyl groups, are highly toxic. Patients with metal poisoning should be investigated and managed in specialist units.

Metals associated with poisoning

The metals that give rise to clinical symptoms in humans are shown in Table 62.1. Although some metal poisoning is intentional, e.g. suicide or murder, most cases of poisoning reflect environmental contamination or administration of drugs, remedies or cosmetics that contain metal salts. There are three main clinical effects of exposure to toxic metals – renal tubular damage, gastrointestinal erosions and neurological damage.

Diagnosis

Clinicians rely heavily on biochemical measurements to confirm or refute their clinical suspicion of metal poisoning. Diagnosis may be made by measuring:
- plasma or blood levels of the metal
- urinary excretion of metals
- an associated biochemical abnormality related to the toxicity.

Blood, plasma, serum and urine all can be used for measurement, and in some cases, it also may be helpful to measure the metal concentration in other tissues, e.g. hair. The action limits for metals in plasma and urine are shown in Table 62.1.

Treatment

As with most poisons, treatment consists of removal of the source of the metal and increasing the elimination from the body, while correcting deranged physiological or biological parameters. Removal of the source may require that a person be removed from a contaminated site or workplace or that the use of a medication or cosmetic be discontinued. Elimination of heavy metals is achieved by treatment with chelating agents that bind the ions

and allow their excretion in the urine (Fig. 62.1).

Lead

Inorganic lead has long been known to be toxic, but acute lead poisoning is uncommon. Chronic toxicity is related to industrial or other work-related exposure, lead leached from (old) water pipes, or the eating of lead-containing paints or dirt by children (pica). Only 5% to 10% of lead is absorbed from the gastrointestinal tract in adults, but the proportion is higher in children.

Lead poisoning causes anaemia as well as hepatic, renal and neurological sequelae. In general, the consequences of organic lead poisoning are neurological, whereas inorganic lead poisoning results in constipation, abdominal colic, anaemia and peripheral and motor neuron deficiencies. Severe cases develop encephalopathy with seizures and coma.

The finding of basophilic stippling in red cells seen when a blood film is done in an anaemic patient is characteristic, and sometimes the first clear clue of lead poisoning. It can be confirmed biochemically by finding raised protoporphyrin levels in the erythrocytes due to the inhibition of a number of the synthetic enzymes of the haem pathway by lead (Fig. 62.2). A helpful clinical sign is the appearance of a blue line on the gums.

Lead is measured in whole blood or in urine (see Table 62.1). Excretion can be enhanced using chelating agents such as NaEDTA, dimercaprol or N-acetyl-penicillamine. Because of their high toxicity, the use and handling of organic lead compounds is strictly regulated by law. For example, tetra-ethyl-lead, previously used as an 'anti-knocking' agent in petrol, is no longer used – petrol is only available in unleaded form.

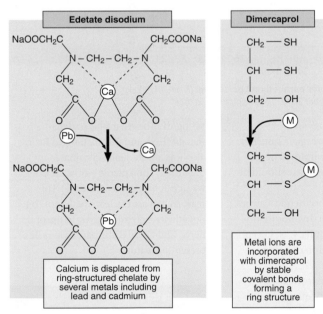

Fig. 62.1 Structures and actions of chelating agents.

Table 62.1 Reference and action limits for toxic metals		
Metal	**Action limits/indices of toxicity**	**Clinical sequelae**
Arsenic	>0.5 µg/g hair	Diarrhoea, polyneuropathy, gastrointestinal pain, vomiting, shock, coma, renal failure
Aluminium	>3 µmol/L in plasma – chronic >10 µmol/L in plasma – acute	Encephalopathy, osteodystrophy
Cadmium	>90 nmol/L in blood or >90 nmol/24 h in urine	Renal tubular damage, bone disease, hepatocellular damage
Lead	>50 µg/100 mL (2.41 µmol/L) adults >25 µg/100 mL (1.21 µmol/L) females in reproductive years >40 µg/100 mL (1.93 µmol/L) those under 18 y	Acute: colic, seizures and coma Chronic: anaemia, encephalopathy
Mercury	>20 nmol/mmol creatinine in urine	Nausea and vomiting, nephrotoxicity, neurological dysfunction

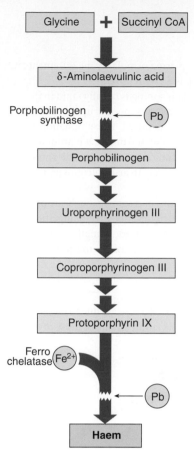

Fig. 62.2 Effects of lead on haem synthesis.
Lead (Pb) inhibits porphobilinogen synthase and separately Fe^{2+} incorporation into haem, resulting in increased levels of δ-aminolaevulinic acid and coproporphyrin in urine and protoporphyrin in erythrocytes.

Mercury

Mercury poisoning may be acute or chronic and is related to exposure to elemental mercury vapour, inorganic salts or organic forms such as methylmercury. Metallic mercury is relatively nontoxic if ingested, but mercury vapour can give rise to acute toxicity. The symptoms are respiratory distress and a metallic taste in the mouth.

Mercurous salts, notably calomel, have been known to cause chronic toxicity following skin absorption from powders and other forms, but are less toxic than mercuric salts, notably mercuric chloride. This is highly toxic when ingested. The symptoms are nausea and vomiting, muscular tremors, central nervous system symptoms and renal damage.

Diagnosis is by estimation of blood and urine mercury concentrations (see Table 62.1). Long-term monitoring of exposure, such as may be necessary with those working with dental amalgam, may be carried out using hair or nail clippings.

Organic mercury compounds are very toxic. The methylmercury concentration in the flesh of marine life increases the further up the food chain. The concentration in,

for example, tuna is such that organisations such as UK Food Standards Agency advise pregnant women to limit their intake.

Aluminium

Aluminium is very poorly absorbed from the gastrointestinal tract. Aluminium sulphate is used as a flocculating agent in the treatment of drinking water, and aluminium hydroxide is used therapeutically as a phosphate-binding agent and an antacid.

Aluminium levels in water supplies are variable and may contain from less than 50 to more than 1000 µg/L. This is a potential hazard to patients on renal dialysis when the aluminium can enter the body across the dialysis membrane, thus bypassing intestinal absorption. The water used in dialysis is now treated to remove contaminating metals. Acute aluminium toxicity is extremely rare. Aluminium toxicity in patients with renal dysfunction causes bone disease (aluminium osteodystrophy) and gradually failing cerebral function (dialysis dementia).

Diagnosis is by measurement of aluminium in blood (see Table 62.1). Aluminium content of bone biopsy material is also used, with levels greater than 100 µg/g dry weight indicating accumulation.

Treatment of aluminium toxicity is by prevention. In cases of toxicity, aluminium excretion may be enhanced by using the chelating agent desferrioxamine.

Arsenic

Arsenic never occurs as the free element, but as the ions As^{3+} and As^{5+}, and may be found in some insecticides. Acute ingestion gives rise to violent gastrointestinal pain and vomiting, with clinical shock. Chronic ingestion is associated with diarrhoea, dermatitis and polyneuropathy. Paradoxically, arsenic is sometimes used to treat colitis, and this is the most frequent exposure. Urine arsenic measurement is widely used to assess the extent of recent or current exposure. The best indicator of chronic arsenic exposure is hair analysis. The arsenic content will vary with time along the length of the hair. A level of more than 0.5 µg/g arsenic in hair indicates significant exposure.

Cadmium

Chronic cadmium toxicity occurs in industrial workers exposed to cadmium fumes. The symptoms are those of nephrotoxicity, bone disease and, to a lesser extent, hepatotoxicity. Renal stone formation may be increased.

In diagnosis, indicators of renal damage, in particular β_2-microglobulin in urine, can be used to monitor the effects. Blood and urine cadmium estimates (see Table 62.1) will give an objective index of the degree of exposure, and, in some cases, the cadmium content of renal biopsy tissue may be useful.

Treatment of chronic cadmium toxicity is by removal from exposure. The use of chelating agents is not recommended because mobilisation of cadmium may cause renal damage.

The major source of cadmium exposure in the general population is tobacco smoke, with smokers having blood cadmium levels twice that of nonsmokers.

Cobalt and chromium

Metal prostheses are widely used in orthopaedics. There is a lot of concern that cobalt and chromium released from 'metal-on-metal' units may result in toxicity. Thus some agencies, e.g. the UK Medicines and Healthcare Products Regulatory Agency (MHRA), have issued guidance recommending that cobalt and chromium should be measured in the blood of patients with some prostheses to detect potential toxicity.

Clinical note

Often associated in the past with murders, arsenic poisoning may still be encountered as an industrial disease. The features are abdominal pain, headache, confusion, peripheral neuropathy and coma.

Metal poisoning

- Heavy metals are an insidious cause of gastrointestinal, renal and neurological disease.

- Measurement of blood and urine levels is used in diagnosis of poisoning.

- Treatment of acute exposure is with chelating agents.

Case history 49

A 12-year-old girl presents with nausea and vomiting and non-localising neurological signs. She has been using brightly coloured facial cosmetics obtained abroad.

- What biochemical investigations would be appropriate?
  Comment in Case history comments.

Want to know more?

http://www.trace-elements.co.uk

Details of reference intervals and action limits for all of the metals discussed here can be obtained from the Scottish Trace Element and Micronutrient Diagnostic and Research Laboratory website.

63 | Alcohol

Abuse of alcohol (ethanol) is a major contributor to morbidity and mortality, far outstripping other drugs in its effects on the individual and on society. Alcohol is a drug with no receptor. The mechanisms by which it exerts its detrimental effect on cells and organs are not well understood, but the effects are summarised in Table 63.1.

For clinical purposes, alcohol consumption is estimated in arbitrary 'units' – 1 unit representing 8 g of pure ethanol. The ethanol content of some common drinks is shown in Fig. 63.1. The legal limit for driving in England, Wales and Northern Ireland is a blood alcohol level of 80 mg/dL (17.4 mmol/L); in Scotland the limit is lower, at 50 mg/dL.

Metabolism of ethanol

Ethanol is sometimes described as a 'selfish' molecule, i.e. it is metabolised in preference to other substrates. (This can be exploited – see clinical note). It is metabolised to acetaldehyde by two main pathways (Fig. 63.2). The alcohol dehydrogenase route operates when the blood alcohol concentration is up to approximately 25 mg/dL. Above this most of the ethanol is metabolised via the microsomal P450 system. Although the end-product in both cases is acetaldehyde, the side-effects of induced P450 can be significant. Ethanol metabolism and excretion in a normal 70-kg man is summarised in Fig. 63.3.

Acute alcohol poisoning

The effects of ethanol excess fall into two categories:
- those that are directly related to the blood alcohol concentration at the time, e.g. coma
- those that are caused by the metabolic effects of continued high ethanol concentrations.

The relative contribution of ethanol in cases of coma, especially where other drugs and/or head injury are present, may be difficult to distinguish. Blood ethanol determinations are the best guide.

Table 63.1 **Effects of ethanol on organ systems**

System	Condition	Effect
CNS	Acute	Disorientation → coma
	Chronic	Memory loss, psychoses
	Withdrawal	Seizures, delirium tremens
Cardiovascular	Chronic	Cardiomyopathy
Skeletal muscle	Chronic	Myopathies
Gastric mucosa	Acute	Irritation, gastritis
	Chronic	Ulceration
Liver	Chronic	Fatty liver → cirrhosis, decreased tolerance to xenobiotics
Kidney	Acute	Diuresis
Blood	Chronic	Anaemia, thrombocytopenia
Testes	Chronic	Impotence

CNS, Central nervous system.

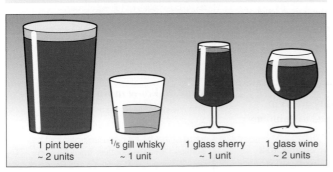

Fig. 63.1 **Alcohol content of common drinks.**

1 pint beer ~ 2 units | 1/5 gill whisky ~ 1 unit | 1 glass sherry ~ 1 unit | 1 glass wine ~ 2 units

Where these are not available, plasma osmolality measurement and calculation of the osmolal gap is a useful proxy.

Recovery from acute alcohol poisoning is usually rapid in the absence of renal or hepatic failure and is speeded up if hepatic blood flow and oxygenation are maximised. The elimination rate of ethanol is dose-related; at a level of 460 mg/dL it is around 460 to 690 mg/hour. Ethanol concentrations in a group of alcohol-dependent people admitted in coma with acute alcohol poisoning are shown in Fig. 63.4.

Alcohol inhibits gluconeogenesis, and some patients are prone to develop hypoglycaemia 6 to 36 hours after alcohol ingestion, especially if they are malnourished or fasted. A small number of these malnourished patients develop alcoholic ketoacidosis.

Chronic alcohol abuse

Many of the effects of chronic alcohol abuse are due to either the toxicity of acetaldehyde and/or the failure of one or more of the

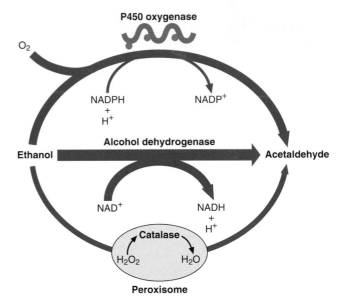

Fig. 63.2 **The metabolism of ethanol.**

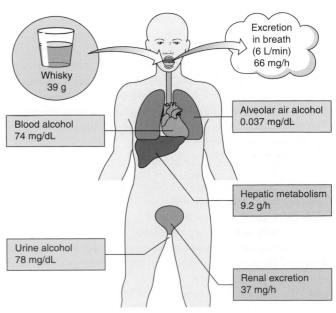

Fig. 63.3 **Metabolism and excretion of alcohol.**

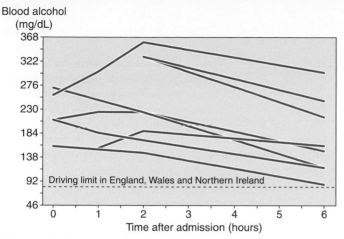

Fig. 63.4 **Alcohol concentrations in patients admitted in a coma.**

many homeostatic and synthetic mechanisms in the liver. One of the earliest signs of chronic alcohol abuse is hepatomegaly. This results from the accumulation of triglyceride due to increased synthesis from the carbohydrate load and reduced protein synthesis. Continued high ethanol intake may cause the following sequelae:

- impaired glucose tolerance and diabetes mellitus
- hypertriglyceridaemia
- cirrhosis of the liver with resultant decreased serum albumin concentration
- portal hypertension with resultant oesophageal varices
- coagulation defects
- cardiomyopathy
- peripheral neuropathy.

Diagnosis of chronic alcohol abuse

Chronic alcohol abuse is usually determined from the patient's history. However, in some, the suspicion persists despite the patient's denial, and in this group an objective marker of chronic ethanol ingestion would be helpful. Although there is no definitive (i.e. sufficiently sensitive and specific) marker, a number of blood components are altered and these can give an indication of chronic alcohol ingestion. The most commonly used are:

- Elevated gamma-glutamyl transpeptidase (GGT). This enzyme is increased in 80% of people who consume excess alcohol. It is not a specific indicator as it is increased in all forms of liver disease and is induced by drugs such as phenytoin and phenobarbital.
- Elevated serum triglyceride.
- Raised mean cell volume (MCV).
- Hyperuricaemia.

There are a number of other potentially useful markers, notably isoforms of transferrin that are deficient in the carbohydrate linked to the protein. This carbohydrate-deficient transferrin is present in more than 90% of patients with chronic alcohol abuse.

Once the diagnosis of chronic alcohol abuse is made, these markers are of use in monitoring behaviour, since even a single 'binge' may lead to their derangement. GGT is used regularly in this manner.

Chronic alcohol abuse exposes the individual to increased risk of damage from other substances. Long-term alcohol excess is associated with higher rates of smoking-related disease and poisoning with hepatotoxic substances. Chronic alcoholic patients also have different rates of metabolism of therapeutic drugs, and care needs to be taken in treating them with drugs that are metabolised by the cytochrome P450 system.

Admission rates to hospital with alcohol-related diseases are high (Fig. 63.5).

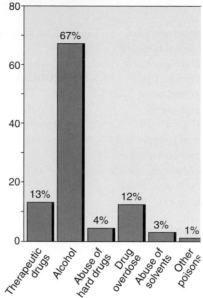

Fig. 63.5 **Admissions of drug-related problems to one UK hospital.**

Clinical note

Ethylene glycol and methanol are both metabolised by alcohol dehydrogenase to oxalic and formic acids, which are toxic. In order to prevent this metabolism, ethanol may be infused, since it is metabolised in preference, until the toxic alcohols are excreted unchanged. Ethylene glycol is the more commonly encountered of the two. It is found in antifreeze, and patients sometimes drink this in suicide or parasuicide attempts.

Alcohol

- Health-related effects of ethanol consumption are common clinical problems.
- An elevated serum osmolality and an increased osmolal gap can be of diagnostic value in acute ethanol toxicity.
- Chronic ethanol abuse can be difficult to detect.
- Serum gamma-glutamyl transpeptidase (GGT) is of limited value for diagnosis of ethanol abuse but good for monitoring abstinence.
- The effects of chronic alcohol abuse are not limited to the liver.

Case history 50

A 16-year-old boy whose epilepsy had recently become poorly controlled was found to have an elevated GGT of 82 U/L. Because of his troublesome behaviour, his parents suspected he was drinking.

- How might alcohol abuse be confirmed or excluded?
- His serum alkaline phosphatase was 520 U/L. Does this support a diagnosis of alcoholic liver disease?
  Comment in Case history comments.

Want to know more?

https://www.nice.org.uk/guidance/cg115

This is quite a useful starting point for specific National Institute for Health and Care Excellence (NICE) guidance on various aspects of alcohol and its effect on health.

64 | Ascites

Ascites refers to the presence of abnormal amounts of fluid in the peritoneal space. It is classically detected by 'shifting dullness' on clinical examination (Fig. 64.1). Its pathogenesis is complex; contributory factors include increased pressure in the circulation that drains blood from abdominal viscera to the liver (portal hypertension), reduced albumin and other proteins resulting in reduced plasma oncotic pressure (Chapter 25), as well as secondary hyperaldosteronism (Chapter 10).

Abdominal paracentesis

Laboratory analyses can help to establish the cause of ascites and, in patients with ascites and peritonitis, tell whether the peritonitis is likely to be secondary to an abdominal source of infection. Less frequently, they can help establish if ascites is related to the presence of malignancy. These investigations require the collection of peritoneal (ascitic) fluid. The procedure whereby a needle is inserted into the peritoneal cavity (Fig. 64.2) is known as abdominal paracentesis (or, more colloquially, an *ascitic tap*).

Ascites accumulates continually in patients with advanced cirrhosis, causing progressive abdominal distension and discomfort. Such patients require the ascitic fluid to be removed periodically. Clinicians performing such *therapeutic drainage* often send the ascitic fluid for analysis even though there may not be a clear diagnostic question.

Differential diagnosis of ascites

The traditional classification of body fluids into transudates and exudates on the basis of the fluid total protein concentration (see Chapter 65) is relevant to ascites, but the ability of ascitic total protein to reflect pathogenesis is limited, and it is not widely used in this context. The most widely used parameter is the serum ascites albumin gradient (SAAG).

The SAAG is the serum albumin concentration minus the ascitic fluid albumin concentration. Its main value lies in the fact that it correlates with the portal pressure; a wide gradient (≥11 g/L) signifies portal hypertension and is seen in, for example, cirrhosis or congestive cardiac failure. Not surprisingly, wide gradients are also associated with other sequelae of portal hypertension, e.g. oesophageal varices. Narrow gradients (<11 g/L) are seen in nephrotic syndrome, for example, where the plasma oncotic pressure is reduced. Fig. 64.3

summarises key causes of wide and narrow gradients.

Peritonitis

A minority of cirrhotic patients with ascites develop peritonitis, usually in the absence of an obvious focus of infection, in which case it is known as *spontaneous bacterial peritonitis* (SBP). Sometimes there is a clear focus of infection, e.g. intraabdominal abscess (secondary infection). Laboratory investigations can be used to predict who is likely to develop SBP, to facilitate early detection of infection and to differentiate SBP from secondary infection.

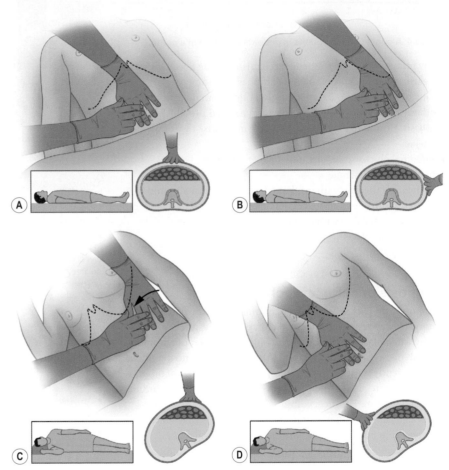

Fig. 64.1 Procedure for eliciting 'shifting dullness' on clinical examination. The percussion note changes from a resonant to a dull note due to presence of fluid underneath. When the patient moves position, the fluid is redistributed in the peritoneal cavity, and the interface between resonant and dull notes on the surface of the abdomen shifts. *(From Glynn M, Drake WM, eds. Hutchison's Clinical Methods: An Integrated Approach to Clinical Practice. 25th ed. Elsevier; 2023. Available at https://www.elsevier.com/books/hutchison's-clinical-methods/978-0-7020-8265-8.)*

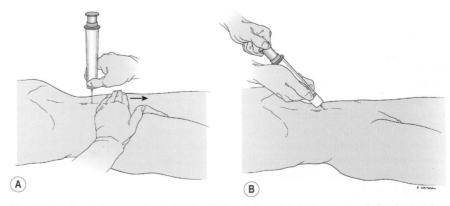

Fig. 64.2 Abdominal paracentesis. (A) The skin is pulled caudally by the non-needle-bearing hand while the needle is slowly inserted perpendicular to the skin until fluid return is observed. **(B)** The skin is then released and the needle angled caudally. *(From Roberts JR, Hedges JR, eds. Clinical Procedures in Emergency Medicine. 5th ed. Saunders, Elsevier; 2010.)*

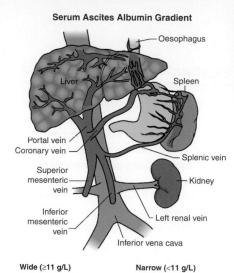

Serum Ascites Albumin Gradient

Oesophagus
Liver
Spleen
Portal vein
Coronary vein
Splenic vein
Superior mesenteric vein
Kidney
Inferior mesenteric vein
Left renal vein
Inferior vena cava

Wide (≥11 g/L)
Cirrhosis
Massive hepatic metastases
Congestive cardiac failure
Spontaneous bacterial peritonitis

Narrow (<11 g/L)
Peritoneal carcinomatosis
Nephrotic syndrome
Secondary peritonitis
Tuberculous peritonitis

Fig. 64.3 Serum ascites albumin gradient is obtained by subtracting the ascitic fluid albumin from the serum albumin. It correlates with the pressure in the portal circulation.

Prediction of SBP

When the total protein concentration in ascitic fluid falls below 10 g/L, the ability to phagocytose bacteria disappears and the patient is at increased risk of SBP. Other parameters which may help further to stratify the risk of SBP are a high serum bilirubin and a low blood platelet count.

Early detection

It is difficult to tell if a patient has developed SBP just from clinical examination. Equally, there is a significant delay before positive microbiological cultures develop; SBP is associated with low concentrations of bacteria, meaning that it may take even longer than usual. So there is a need for other parameters to 'fill the diagnostic gap' in the interim.

One of the more reliable indices of whether SBP has developed is the neutrophil count in the ascitic fluid – the higher it is the more likely that SBP has developed – so clinicians should request a differential white cell count on ascitic fluid. It has been suggested that patients whose ascitic fluid neutrophil count is $>0.5 \times 10^9$/L should be treated for SBP.

SBP or secondary infection?

The heavier bacterial loads associated with secondary peritonitis explain why it tends to be more severe than SBP. This severity is reflected in the ascitic fluid biochemistry. Ascitic fluid glucose is low, because both host neutrophils and bacteria consume glucose. Much of it is

metabolised anaerobically, resulting in lactic acidosis. Dead neutrophils shed lactate dehydrogenase and other cellular proteins, and so the ascitic fluid protein rises. Table 64.1 summarises the parameters used to differentiate SBP from secondary infection.

Ascitic fluid parameter	Spontaneous bacterial peritonitis	Secondary
Glucose (mmol/L)	>2.8	<2.8
Lactate dehydrogenase	< Upper limit of reference interval	> Upper limit of reference interval
Total protein (g/L)	<10	>10

Table 64.1 **Spontaneous bacterial peritonitis compared with secondary infection**

Microbiology

Although biochemical and haematological investigations have an important role to play in evaluating patients with peritonitis, they are additional to, rather than instead of, microbiological investigations (in the unlikely event that there is not enough specimen, microbiological analysis should get priority). However, as indicated earlier, it takes at least a couple of days for microbiological culture results to come back and during this time other investigations can help clarify the picture. The low concentrations of bacteria associated with SBP explain the observed low rates of culture positivity. If Gram stain is positive for more than one organism, or ascitic fluid cultures remain positive despite antibiotic treatment, a heavier bacterial load, and hence secondary infection, is more likely than SBP.

Malignant ascites

Ascites can develop in association with malignancy in various ways. In advanced abdominal cancer, the peritoneum can be invaded directly or 'seeded' by the tumour (peritoneal carcinomatosis). Nearly all patients with peritoneal carcinomatosis have malignant cells in the ascitic fluid. Massive liver metastases or hepatoma developing on a background of cirrhosis both cause portal hypertension and ascites, with a wide SAAG. Specific malignancies, e.g. ovarian cancer, stimulate a peritoneal reaction and ascites.

Malignant or benign?

Biochemical analysis of ascitic fluid has a limited role to play in establishing whether

ascites is benign or malignant. Clinicians occasionally request that tumour markers are measured in ascitic fluid, but this rarely adds anything to the information provided by serum measurements of the same tumour markers. Cytology may be more helpful; the finding of malignant cells in ascitic fluid indicates the presence of malignancy (but not all patients with malignant ascites have positive ascitic fluid cytology). Finally, other modalities of investigation, e.g. diagnostic imaging, may be helpful.

Other

Analysis of ascitic fluid in other clinical situations has not achieved widespread application, with the exception of chylous ascites, which may be diagnosed by comparing triglyceride concentrations in ascitic fluid and serum (Chapter 67).

Sample requirements

The laboratory analyses outlined earlier can be performed on ascitic fluid collected into a plain universal container (i.e. no preservative), unless the specimen is bloody or grossly turbid.

Clinical note

Ascites is associated with elevated serum levels of cancer antigen 125 (CA125) irrespective of the cause, i.e. in association with benign disease as well as malignant. This is not widely appreciated.

Ascites

- Ascites (excess fluid in the peritoneal space) accumulates through various mechanisms, including portal hypertension, low serum albumin and secondary hyperaldosteronism.

- The serum ascites albumin gradient (SAAG) correlates with the portal pressure. Wide SAAG is associated with portal hypertension.

- The ascitic fluid neutrophil count is a predictor of whether spontaneous bacterial peritonitis (SBP) has developed.

- Cytology is sometimes helpful in establishing if ascites is malignant.

Want to know more?

https://www.bsg.org.uk/clinical-resource/guidelines-on-the-management-of-ascites-in-cirrhosis/

This guideline provides an approach to the treatment of ascites. It provides recommendations at the end of each subsection so that the reader can read the background to each recommendation.

65 | Pleural fluid

Pleural fluid is found in the pleural cavities between the visceral and parietal pleura. Usually the amount of pleural fluid in each cavity is small (<10 mL). Larger amounts are known as *pleural effusions* (Fig. 65.1). These are most often detected either as dullness to percussion on clinical examination, or on a chest X-ray film.

Thoracentesis

As with abdominal paracentesis, the insertion of a needle into the thoracic cavity is done either for therapeutic reasons, e.g. to decompress a pneumothorax, or in order to diagnose underlying pathology. (Pneumothorax refers to the presence of air in the pleural cavity. It is potentially dangerous because it compresses the adjacent lung tissue, progressively limiting inspiratory capacity). Diagnostic thoracentesis is performed in order to try to answer the questions posed in the following sections. The procedure is illustrated in Fig. 65.2.

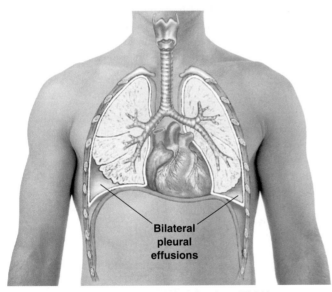

Fig. 65.1 Pleural effusion refers to the collection of fluid in one or both pleural cavities. *(From Seidel HM, Ball JW, Dains JE, Benedict GW. Mosby's Guide to Physical Examination. 5th ed. St. Louis, MO: Mosby; 2003.)*

Transudate or exudate?

Clinicians usually request pleural fluid analysis because they want to know what is causing an effusion. In some cases, a specific cause is suspected, but much more frequently the question is posed in more general terms, by asking if the effusion is a transudate or an exudate. These are defined in terms of their protein concentration; transudates have less protein than exudates (30 g/L is the usual cut-off). The underlying assumption is that fluid formed by 'exudation' from inflamed or tumour-infiltrated pleura is likely to be high in protein, whereas fluid formed by 'transudation' from normal pleura as a result of an imbalance in hydrostatic and oncotic forces is likely to be low in protein. In general terms, exudates are more likely to reflect local pathology and warrant further investigation.

Using pleural fluid protein concentration on its own to identify exudates often results in misclassification. In a seminal 1972 study, Light and colleagues found that measuring pleural fluid lactate dehydrogenase (LDH) as well as protein improved classification. A modified version of their criteria continues to be widely used (Box 65.1). Even these criteria do not always get the right answer; as a result, over the years, alternative markers have been proposed. For example, by analogy with the serum ascites albumin gradient (SAAG) (see Chapter 64), the serum effusion albumin gradient (SEAG) has been studied. In one study, all effusions with a SEAG >12 g/L were correctly identified as transudates. To date there is no single test or combination of tests which is clearly better than modified Light's criteria. However, interestingly, one meta-analysis concluded that combinations of pleural fluid measurements that included total protein, LDH and cholesterol performed as well as modified Light's criteria. This challenges the diagnostic superiority of pleural fluid:serum ratios and thus the need for blood samples.

> **Box 65.1 Modified Light's criteria for identification of an exudate**
>
> Pleural fluid is classified as an exudate if *any* of the following criteria are met:
>
> - Ratio of total protein measured in pleural fluid to total protein measured in serum is greater than 0.5.
> - Pleural fluid lactate dehydrogenase (LDH) activity is greater than two-thirds of the upper limit of the serum reference interval.
> - Ratio of LDH measured in pleural fluid to LDH measured in serum is greater than 0.6.

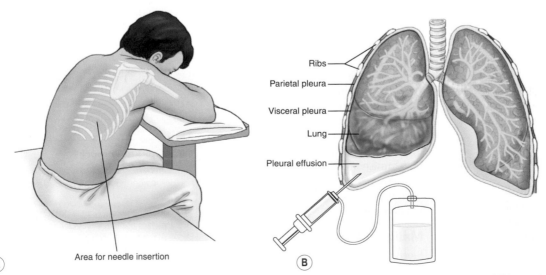

Fig. 65.2 Thoracentesis. The needle is inserted close to the base of the effusion so that gravity will help with drainage. *(With permission from ICD-10-CM/PCS Coding: Theory and Practice, 2023–2024 Edition. 1st ed. Elsevier; 2023.)*

Is it empyema?

Pneumonia (consolidation of lung tissue by an inflammatory exudate) is usually caused by bacteria. Often it affects just one lobe or lung and may be associated with an exudative pleural effusion. If this is treated successfully with antibiotics, the effusion resolves. However, if the patient is generally unwell, and/or does not respond to antibiotics, the effusion may not resolve and instead may become 'walled off' as a fibrotic, loculated collection of pus. *Empyema* refers to such a collection of pus in the pleural cavity. It sometimes may be recognised on chest X-ray film by the presence of a fluid level (Fig. 65.3). It is often resistant to antibiotics because they cannot infiltrate it and is therefore often amenable only to surgical drainage, i.e. requires a chest drain to be inserted.

Insertion of a chest drain is invasive, and clinicians will avoid this painful procedure unless it is essential. Sometimes the question of whether a chest drain is required is straightforward – if the pleural fluid being aspirated from an effusion is frankly purulent or turbid on sampling, then insertion of a chest tube is clearly indicated. However, often it is not so clear that an empyema is developing, and biochemical analysis of the aspirated pleural fluid may be helpful. We have seen in the previous chapter that secondary peritonitis and spontaneous bacterial peritonitis (SBP) can potentially be distinguished by the criteria outlined in Table 64.1. The pathology in empyema is similar. Bacteria and neutrophils consume glucose; anaerobic metabolism increases with heavier bacterial loads, resulting in the production of lactate, which correlates inversely with pH. Pleural fluid pH of less than 7.2 is the most useful predictor of empyema. This finding has been incorporated in the British Thoracic Society guidelines on the use of chest tube drainage in pleural infection.

Is it malignant?

As with ascites, finding malignant cells in pleural fluid indicates the presence of malignancy, although only 70% of patients with malignant effusions will have positive cytologic findings. Again, measurement of tumour markers in pleural fluid is rarely indicated. This in part reflects the utility of other modalities of investigation, e.g. imaging, in the diagnosis of malignancy.

Is it chyle?

Chyle is the fluid found in intestinal lymphatics during absorption of food postprandially. Chylothorax is defined as lymphatic fluid

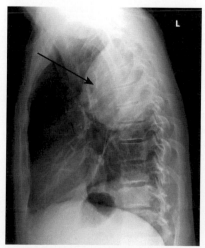

Fig. 65.3 Empyema is characterised by the presence of a collection of purulent fluid (*arrow*). *(From Garden OJ, Bradbury A, Forsythe J, Parks RW.* Principles and Practice of Surgery. *6th ed. Edinburgh: Churchill Livingstone; 2012.)*

(chyle or lymph) in the pleural space; it usually results from the leak or rupture of the thoracic duct or one of its major divisions. The role of biochemistry in the identification of chyle is dealt with in Chapter 67.

Is it tuberculosis?

In some parts of the world, pulmonary tuberculosis is rife. Tuberculous involvement of the pleural space usually arises from rupture of sub-pleural foci of caseation. *Caseation* refers to the firm, dry 'cheese-like' appearance of tissue invaded by the tubercle (Fig. 65.4). The release of tubercle resulting from such rupture stimulates a delayed hypersensitivity reaction involving lymphocytes. The finding of lymphocytes in the pleural fluid is nearly always associated with either cancer or tuberculosis. A practical problem is the fact that patients with pleurisy caused by tuberculosis often do not have positive fluid cultures. This has led to a search for alternative laboratory pointers to tuberculosis. Of these, the most promising is adenosine deaminase, an enzyme involved in purine catabolism, high activity of which is associated with lymphocyte activation.

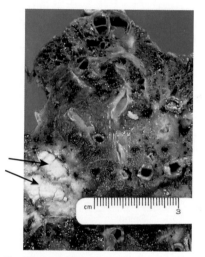

Fig. 65.4 Caseating granulomas are the histopathological hallmark of tuberculosis. *(From Husain A.* Thoracic Pathology. *Philadelphia, PA: Saunders; 2012.)*

Clinical note

Analysis of pleural fluid protein and lactate dehydrogenase (LDH) alone usually produces the same categorisation of pleural effusions as modified Light's criteria; thus a blood sample may not always be necessary.

Pleural fluid

- Modified Light's criteria involve measurement of protein and lactate dehydrogenase (LDH) in pleural fluid. They are widely used to classify pleural fluids as transudates or exudates.

- Empyema (pus in the pleural cavity) is associated with a low pleural fluid pH, which may help guide the need for chest drain insertion.

- Chylothorax may be suspected in the presence of high triglycerides and chylomicrons in aspirated pleural fluid.

- The finding of lymphocytes in the pleural fluid is nearly always associated with either cancer or tuberculosis.

Want to know more?

https://thorax.bmj.com/content/65/8/667

This guideline includes specific recommendations for biochemical measurements on pleural fluid.

66 | Cerebrospinal fluid

Cerebrospinal fluid (CSF) is produced by the choroid plexuses, partly by ultrafiltration and partly by secretion, and fills and circulates through the ventricles and spinal cord. Compared with plasma, it has less protein, and the concentrations of protein-bound components such as bilirubin are similarly reduced. Its electrolyte composition is similar to but distinct from plasma (more chloride, less potassium and calcium). Infection or the presence of blood in the CSF alters its composition. This provides the basis for biochemical analysis of CSF in the diagnosis of subarachnoid haemorrhage (SAH) and meningitis.

Lumbar puncture

Lumbar puncture (LP) is the procedure performed in order to obtain a specimen of CSF (Fig. 66.1). If signs of raised intracranial pressure such as hypertension, bradycardia and papilloedema are present, then an LP should *not* be performed.

When collecting CSF in suspected infection, e.g. meningitis, microbiological examination takes priority. If SAH is suspected, it may help to collect the CSF as several separate aliquots. These will be equally blood-stained in SAH but progressively less so if the blood in the

CSF results from damage to a blood vessel during the LP procedure (a so-called *'traumatic tap'*).

Subarachnoid haemorrhage

Bleeding into the subarachnoid space most frequently results from rupture of an aneurysm (swelling) in one or more of the arteries located within the space (Fig. 66.2). The patient typically complains of a severe headache of sudden onset ('thunderclap'), often associated with vomiting and a reduced level of consciousness. The mainstay of diagnosis is imaging by computed tomography or magnetic resonance imaging. However, in the presence of a strong clinical suspicion, negative imaging does not rule out an SAH. In these cases, LP should be performed, unless there are obvious signs of raised intracranial pressure.

Xanthochromia

Xanthochromia simply means yellow discoloration of the CSF. It results from the presence of bilirubin derived from red blood cells (RBCs) that have undergone *in vivo* lysis. *In vitro* lysis of RBCs, e.g. a traumatic LP, produces only oxyhaemoglobin and not bilirubin (which takes longer to develop). Xanthochromia can be detected by visual inspection, but this is unreliable, and where

possible, scanning spectrophotometry should be used instead. This involves measuring the absorbance of the CSF specimen across a range of wavelengths; the blood pigments have characteristic absorbance peaks (Fig. 66.3).

Meningitis

Meningitis refers to inflammation of the meninges which line the central nervous system (CNS). Bacterial meningitis presents acutely and is a medical emergency. CSF biochemistry tends to reflect the nature of the infective organism (Table 66.1) but is characteristic rather than diagnostic. Microbiological analysis should as always take priority. It is important when interpreting the relative concentrations of, for example, glucose in the CSF to take a blood sample for comparison.

Inherited metabolic disorders

CSF analysis may be helpful in the diagnosis of several inherited metabolic disorders. For example, high CSF lactate may be seen in inborn errors of metabolism affecting the mitochondrial respiratory chain, even when plasma lactate is normal or only slightly increased. This may reflect tissue specificity of electron transport chain proteins or the high-energy demand (and lactate production) of

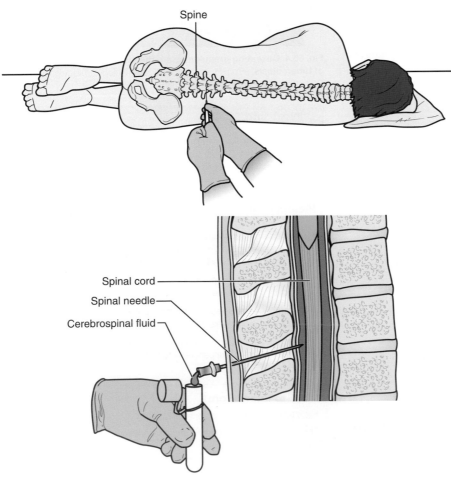

Spine

Spinal cord
Spinal needle
Cerebrospinal fluid

Fig. 66.1 Lumbar puncture. The needle is inserted in the midline between lumbar vertebrae; the patient is placed so as to facilitate access.

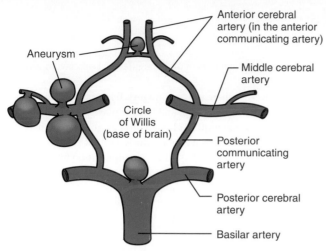

Fig. 66.2 The network of arteries at the base of the brain. Aneurysm and rupture of these arteries gives rise to subarachnoid haemorrhage (SAH).

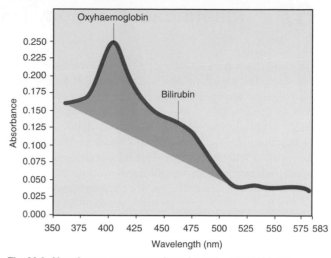

Fig. 66.3 Absorbance spectrum of cerebrospinal fluid (CSF) in subarachnoid haemorrhage (SAH). Oxyhaemoglobin and bilirubin peaks can be seen.

Table 66.1 **Cerebrospinal fluid (CSF) parameters in health and some common disorders**						
	Normal	**Subarachnoid haemorrhage**	**Acute bacterial meningitis**	**Viral meningitis**	**Tuberculous meningitis**	**Multiple sclerosis**
Pressure	50–180 mm H_2O	Increased	Normal/increasing	Normal	Normal/increased	Normal
Colour	Clear	Blood-stained; xanthochromic	Cloudy	Clear	Clear/cloudy	Clear
Red cell count	0–4/mm³	Raised	Normal	Normal	Normal	Normal
White cell count	0–4/mm³	Normal/slightly raised	1000–5000 polymorphs	10–2000 lymphocytes	50–5000 lymphocytes	0–50 lymphocytes
Glucose	>60% of blood level	Normal	Decreased	Normal	Decreased	Normal
Protein	<0.45 g/L	Increased	Increased	Normal/increased	Increased	Normal/increased
Microbiology	Sterile	Sterile	Organisms on Gram stain and/or culture	Sterile/virus detected	Ziehl–Neelsen/auramine stain or tuberculosis culture positive	Sterile
Oligoclonal bands	Negative	Negative	Can be positive	Can be positive	Can be positive	Usually positive

With permission from Haslett C, Chilvers ER, Boon NA, Colledge NR, eds. *Davidson's Principles and Practice of Medicine*. Edinburgh: Churchill Livingstone; 2002.

the brain. CSF pyruvate concentrations are also high in these conditions. CSF amino acid analysis may similarly be helpful in diagnosing various inherited disorders of amino acid metabolism; these are sometimes considered in children with unexplained seizures but are very rare.

Other conditions

Analysis of CSF may be helpful in the evaluation of a variety of nonacute conditions, but as with meningitis the findings are rarely diagnostic. Very high CSF protein concentrations may be seen where there is interruption to the circulation of CSF, e.g. spinal tumours; the mechanisms include increased capillary permeability (to plasma proteins) and CSF fluid reabsorption due to stasis. Increased capillary permeability is best revealed by CSF electrophoresis; the high-molecular-weight plasma proteins, which are not normally found in CSF, can be readily identified. This nonspecific pattern is found in many infective/inflammatory conditions involving the CNS.

CSF electrophoresis also may reveal the presence of oligoclonal bands. If these are not seen also in the serum, they reflect local (i.e. CNS) synthesis of immunoglobulin.

Of patients with multiple sclerosis (MS), 90% have these bands, but they are not specific for this condition. Thus their absence in cases of suspected MS is more diagnostically useful than their presence.

Dementia

Currently, no biochemical markers meet the criteria that would allow reliable differentiation of Alzheimer's disease from other dementias (e.g. vascular), although there are various candidates. The most promising include the ratio of a phosphorylated form of tau protein (a protein specific to CSF) to a protein known as beta-amyloid peptide 42. Recent research claims to have identified an 'Alzheimer's phenotype', based on plasma concentrations of proteins involved in intercellular communication. Though promising, these findings require replication in larger studies.

Clinical note

The commonest side effect after the removal of cerebrospinal fluid (CSF) through lumbar puncture is headache, which occurs in up to 30% of adults and up to 40% of children.

Cerebrospinal fluid

- Cerebrospinal fluid (CSF) analysis may be helpful in a number of conditions, but biochemical analysis alone is rarely diagnostic.

- When collecting CSF in suspected infection, e.g. meningitis, microbiological examination takes priority over biochemical examination.

- Xanthochromia may be due to bilirubin in the CSF from red cell lysis.

- CSF electrophoresis may reveal the presence of oligoclonal bands, which are commonly found in patients with multiple sclerosis (MS).

Want to know more?

Cruickshank A, Auld P, Beetham R, et al. Revised national guidelines for analysis of cerebrospinal fluid for bilirubin in suspected subarachnoid haemorrhage. *Ann Clin Biochem*. 2008;45(pt 3):238–244.

http://journals.sagepub.com/doi/pdf/10.1258/acb.2008.007257

This guidance on cerebrospinal fluid (CSF) analysis in suspected subarachnoid haemorrhage (SAH) is aimed squarely at laboratory professionals. Fig. 1, however, gives some idea of what patterns may be observed on spectrophotometric scanning of CSF.

67 | Identification of body fluids

The vast majority of samples analysed in biochemistry laboratories are blood or urine. As we have seen, there is a role for biochemical analysis of ascitic, pleural or cerebrospinal fluid (CSF), and samples of these are occasionally sent, but in much smaller numbers. Much less frequently, a sample is collected in which the nature of the fluid is unclear – and clinicians seek biochemical answers to the question: 'What is this?' Precisely because such scenarios occur relatively rarely, laboratory staff are often unsure on how best to advise their clinical colleagues. The purpose of this chapter is to clarify the role of biochemistry in the identification of body fluids.

Cerebrospinal fluid

Sometimes patients complain of leakage of fluid from their nose (rhinorrhoea) or ear (otorrhoea), usually after trauma or surgery to the head and neck. Clinicians may wish to establish whether this is an exudate or a transudate. Equally, they may wish to exclude the possibility that the leaking fluid is CSF; if it is, then there is a leak in the ventricular system and therefore a potential focus of pathology (e.g. infection, thrombosis, etc.). Fortunately there is a marker that is specific to the CSF, known as tau protein, an isoform of β_2-transferrin. It appears on electrophoresis as a distinct band (the tau band) (Fig. 67.1). This method of identification requires very little CSF (as little as 1 µL).

Lymph and chyle

Lymph is formed at capillary level by hydrostatic and osmotic forces. It drains into lymphatic vessels that are found throughout the body in the extracellular fluid (ECF) space. These effectively 'drain' ECF, returning it to the blood via ever-larger lymph vessels, culminating in the thoracic duct, which empties into the venous system at the junction of the jugular and subclavian veins (Fig. 67.2).

Precisely because there is a continual cycling of fluid from plasma to tissue fluid to lymph and back to plasma, there is no marker unique to lymph, although ultrafiltration leads to concentration of lymph as it ascends the lymphatic tree. However, there is one type of lymph that differs in composition from plasma. *Chyle* is the lymph found in the intestinal lymphatics during absorption of food; it appears milky because of the presence of fats. As with other sources of lymph, it drains from the intestinal lymphatic system into the thoracic duct, and from there into the venous system.

There are two main clinical scenarios in which identification of chyle is potentially useful – chylothorax and chylous ascites.

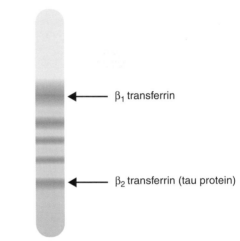

Fig. 67.1 Cerebrospinal fluid (CSF) electrophoresis and staining. Note the different mobilities of the β-transferrin isoforms. Tau protein is unique to CSF.

β_1 transferrin

β_2 transferrin (tau protein)

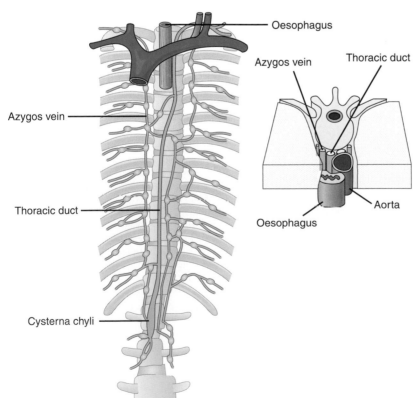

Fig. 67.2 The thoracic duct drains into the venous system, thus returning the contents of the lymphatic tree to the blood. Note its proximity to major structures in the thorax and upper abdomen.

Oesophagus

Azygos vein

Thoracic duct

Azygos vein

Thoracic duct

Aorta

Oesophagus

Cysterna chyli

Chylothorax refers to chyle in the pleural space and results from a leak of the thoracic duct or one of its major divisions (which may be damaged accidentally during thoracic surgery). *Chylous ascites* refers to chyle in the peritoneal space; it is sometimes associated with lymphatic obstruction. Chylomicrons are usually present in thoracic duct lymph, but are present in blood only postprandially, so the finding of chylomicrons in pleural or ascitic fluid usually indicates the presence of chyle. Although chylomicrons can be detected by storing spun samples in a fridge overnight, allowing the buoyant chylomicrons to rise to the top, in practice, triglycerides are easier to measure and are widely used as a screening test instead. The higher the triglyceride concentration in the fluid compared with the serum, the more likely it is that the sample is chylous.

Urine

Frequently, the question 'What is this?' is posed instead as 'Is this fluid urine, or contaminated with urine?' This sometimes arises in relation to fluid appearing in abdominal drains following surgery to the abdomen or pelvis. Urinary contamination usually can be established by comparing concentrations of creatinine or urea in the specimen, in serum and, ideally, urine; urinary concentrations of creatinine and urea exceed serum concentrations by orders of magnitude (Fig. 67.3).

Other

Amniotic fluid

Amniotic fluid is the fluid that surrounds the fetus during intrauterine life; it is released following rupture of the fetal membranes at the onset of labour. Premature rupture is associated with maternal and fetal morbidity, so it is important to recognise. Clinical diagnosis is usually easy, but occasionally it may be necessary to distinguish amniotic fluid from maternal urine, vaginal fluid, cervical mucus or blood. Side-room tests may be used – these include dipstick testing for protein and glucose (amniotic fluid is positive for both, urine is normally negative), or pH (vaginal fluid and urine are acidic, amniotic fluid neutral), or testing for 'ferning' (when amniotic fluid is dried on a glass slide, crystals appear because of its salt content, and these can be viewed under a low-power microscope resembling the branches of a fern). The protein fetal fibronectin is relatively specific to amniotic fluid; however, it is found in the cervix and vagina even when the membranes appear to be intact, meaning that it cannot reliably be used to diagnose rupture of the membranes.

Synovial fluid

Sometimes, during joint aspiration, it may be difficult to decide whether the fluid aspirated is synovial fluid, fluid from subcutaneous tissue or local anaesthetic. Mostly it is not essential to establish this, but there are two simple methods to detect synovial fluid. Both of these depend on the presence in synovial fluid of hyaluronate; synovial fluid is an ultrafiltrate of plasma combined with hyaluronate (a mucopolysaccharide) secreted by cells of the synovial membranes that line joint spaces. The mucin clot test and staining for metachromasia are straightforward, but not widely performed.

Table 67.1 summarises body fluids not normally identified by laboratory investigation and why.

Table 67.1 **Body fluids not normally identified by laboratory investigation**	
Fluid	**Comment**
Ascites	No unique marker
Bile	Usually identifiable by visual inspection
Endolymph (fluid in middle ear)	Inaccessible
Lymph	No unique marker
Pleural fluid	No unique marker
Pericardial fluid	No unique marker
Saliva	Readily accessible
Tears	Readily accessible
Vitreous humour	Identification rarely required
	Metachromatic staining could in theory be used (see text under synovial fluid)

Clinical note

The suspicion that fluid in the pleural or peritoneal space is chylous most often arises in the context of major thoracic or abdominal surgery, e.g. fluid draining the cavity.

Identification of body fluids

- Tau protein (an isoform of β_2-transferrin) is unique to cerebrospinal fluid (CSF) and is available as a supraregional assay in the UK.
- Serum triglycerides are the most convenient test for suspected chyle.
- If contamination of a sample with urine is suspected, concentrations of urea and/or creatinine should ideally be compared in the sample, serum and urine.
- When testing for synovial fluid, both the mucin clot test and metachromatic staining are readily adaptable to the clinical setting.

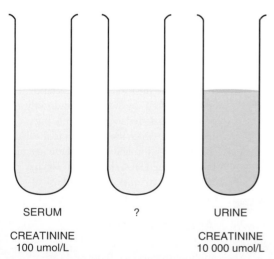

SERUM   ?   URINE

CREATININE
100 umol/L

CREATININE
10 000 umol/L

Fig. 67.3 Comparison of creatinine in serum, urine and a sample of abdominal drain fluid in a patient following abdominal surgery. Note the very large difference in typical concentrations of creatinine in serum and urine.

Want to know more?

https://acbi.ie/wp-content/uploads/2022/12/1602839709-Guidelines-of-Body-Fluids.pdf

This booklet is a useful resource for information about biochemical analysis of most body fluids.

68 | Lipoprotein metabolism

Lipoproteins solve the problem of transporting fats around the body in the aqueous environment of the blood. A lipoprotein is a complex spherical structure that has a hydrophobic core wrapped in a hydrophilic coating (Fig. 68.1). The core contains triglyceride and cholesteryl esters, and the surface contains phospholipid, free cholesterol and protein. (For clarity: in just the same way as the term 'apoenzyme' refers to the protein part of an enzyme that combines with its cofactor to form the active enzyme, so apolipoproteins are the proteins that combine with lipid components to form lipoprotein particles.) The properties of the main apolipoproteins are summarised in Table 68.1. Cholesterol is an essential component of all cell membranes and is a precursor for steroid hormone and bile acid biosynthesis. Triglyceride is central to the storage and transport of energy within the body.

Nomenclature

Several different classes of lipoproteins exist, the structure and function of which are closely related. Apart from the largest species, the chylomicron, these are named according to their density, as they were originally studied and isolated by ultracentrifugation. The four main lipoproteins and their functions are shown in Table 68.2.

Metabolism

Lipoprotein metabolism (Fig. 68.2) can be thought of as two cycles, one exogenous and one endogenous, both centred on the liver. These cycles are interconnected.

Two key enzyme systems are involved in lipoprotein metabolism:

- *Lipoprotein lipase* (LPL) is located on the vascular endothelium that lines blood vessels, especially in some tissues (see later). It releases free fatty acids and glycerol from chylomicrons and very-low-density lipoprotein (VLDL) from where they are taken up into the tissues.
- *Lecithin–cholesterol acyltransferase* (LCAT) forms cholesteryl esters from free cholesterol and fatty acids. Cholesteryl esters are more hydrophobic and can be more easily sequestered into the core of lipoprotein particles. LCAT thus facilitates cholesterol transport.

The exogenous lipid cycle

Dietary lipid is absorbed in the small intestine and incorporated into chylomicrons that are secreted into the lymphatics and reach the bloodstream via the thoracic duct. In the circulation, triglyceride is gradually removed from these lipoproteins by the action of LPL. This enzyme is present in the capillaries of a number of tissues, predominantly adipose tissue and skeletal muscle. As it loses triglyceride, the chylomicron becomes smaller and deflated, with folds of redundant surface material. These chylomicron remnants are removed by the liver. The cholesterol may be utilised by the liver to form cell membrane components or bile acids or may be excreted in the bile. The liver provides the only route by which cholesterol leaves the body in significant amounts.

The endogenous lipid cycle

The liver synthesises VLDL particles that undergo the same form of delipidation as chylomicrons, also by the action of LPL. This results in the formation of an intermediate-density lipoprotein (IDL), which becomes low-density lipoprotein (LDL) when further delipidated. LDL may be removed from the circulation by the high-affinity LDL receptor, or by other scavenger routes, used increasingly at higher LDL levels. These alternative pathways do not remove cholesterol as efficiently as the LDL receptor pathway, allowing the LDL to undergo modification, e.g. oxidation, aggregation. These modifications make the LDL more atherogenic and are a key way in which cholesterol is incorporated into atheromatous plaques.

High-density lipoprotein (HDL) particles are derived from both liver and gut. They act as cholesteryl ester shuttles, removing cholesterol from the peripheral tissues and returning it to the liver. The HDL is taken up either directly by the liver, or indirectly by being transferred to other circulating lipoproteins, which then return it to the liver. This process is thought to be antiatherogenic, and an elevated HDL cholesterol level has been shown to confer a decreased risk of coronary heart disease on an individual.

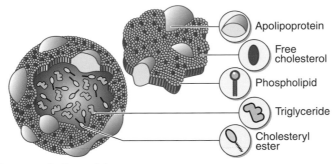

Fig. 68.1 Structure of a lipoprotein.

Apolipoprotein

Free cholesterol

Phospholipid

Triglyceride

Cholesteryl ester

Table 68.1 Properties of some human apolipoproteins

Apolipoprotein	Molecular weight	Site of synthesis	Function
A-I	28,000	Intestine, liver	Activates LCAT
A-II	17,000	Intestine, liver	–
B_{100}	549,000	Liver	Triglyceride and cholesterol transport. Binds to LDL receptor
B_{48}	264,000	Intestine	Triglyceride transport
C-I	6600	Liver	Activates LCAT
C-II	8850	Liver	Activates LPL
C-III	8800	Liver	? Inhibits LPL
E	34,000	Liver, intestine, macrophage	Binds to LDL receptor and probably also to another specific liver receptor

LCAT, Lecithin–cholesterol acyltransferase; *LDL*, low-density lipoprotein; *LPL*, lipoprotein lipase.

Table 68.2 The four main lipoproteins and their functions

Lipoprotein	Main apolipoproteins	Function
Chylomicrons	B_{48}, A-I, C-II, E	Largest lipoprotein. Synthesised by gut after a meal. Not present in normal fasting plasma. Main carrier of dietary triglyceride
Very-low-density lipoprotein (VLDL)	B_{100}, C-II, E	Synthesised in the liver. Main carrier of endogenously-produced triglyceride
Low-density lipoprotein (LDL)	B_{100}	Generated from VLDL in the circulation. Main carrier of cholesterol
High-density lipoprotein (HDL)	A-I, A-II	Smallest lipoprotein. Protective function. Takes cholesterol from extrahepatic tissues to the liver for excretion (reverse cholesterol transport)

Apolipoproteins

Apolipoproteins (see Table 68.1) are important in:

- maintaining the structural integrity of the lipoproteins
- regulating certain enzymes that act on lipoproteins
- receptor recognition.

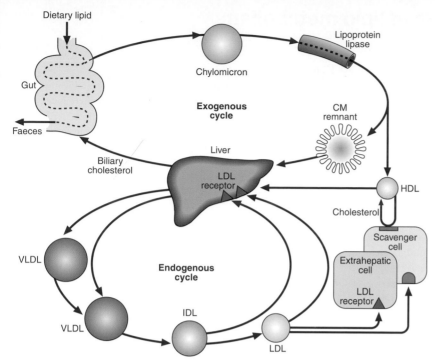

Fig. 68.2 Lipoprotein metabolism. *CM*, Chylomicron; *HDL*, High-density lipoprotein; *IDL*, intermediate-density lipoprotein; *LDL*, low-density lipoprotein; *VLDL*, very-low-density lipoprotein.

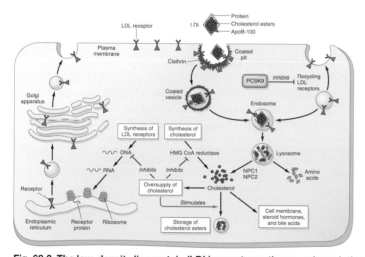

Fig. 68.3 The low-density lipoprotein (LDL) receptor pathway and regulation of cholesterol metabolism. *ApoB-100*, Apolipoprotein B-100; *HMG CoA*, 3-hydroxy-3-methylglutaryl coenzyme A; *PCSK9*, proprotein convertase subtilisin/kexin type 9. *(From Kumar V, Abbas A, Aster J.* Robbins & Cotran Pathologic Basis of Disease. *10th ed. 2020.)*

pathway are targets of lipid-lowering medications. For example, statins (HMG coenzyme A reductase inhibitors) cause upregulation of LDL receptors by inhibiting intracellular cholesterol synthesis, while PCSK9 inhibitors remove a 'brake' on LDL receptor recycling.

Inherited malfunction or absence of these receptors leads to familial hypercholesterolaemia (FH). Indeed the term FH has become an umbrella term embracing pathogenic mutations affecting the expression and/or function of the LDL receptor, apoB and PCSK9. All of them have the effect of increasing the levels of LDL cholesterol in circulation.

Clinical note

About 25% of the UK population have plasma cholesterol concentrations above the desirable level. In most cases this is the result of diet and lifestyle.

Lipoprotein metabolism

- Lipoproteins are complexes of lipid and proteins that facilitate lipid transport.

- Their metabolism can be thought of as two interconnected cycles centred on the liver.

- Lipoproteins are defined by their density and differ in composition, structure and function.

- Apolipoproteins have a functional as well as structural importance.

- Cholesterol can be excreted from the body only by way of the liver.

The LDL receptor

The LDL receptor (Fig. 68.3), a glycoprotein present on the surface of all cells, spans the cell membrane and is concentrated in special membrane recesses, called 'coated pits'. It binds to the apolipoprotein B of the LDL particles, and internalises the particles for breakdown within the cell. Receptors are then recycled to the cell surface; the rate of recycling is controlled by a protein called proprotein convertase subtilisin/kexin type 9 (PCSK9). The number and function of receptors dictate the level of circulating LDL. When the cell has sufficient cholesterol, the synthesis of receptors is down-regulated; when the cell is cholesterol depleted, the receptors increase in number. Several parts of this

Case history 51

A 3-year-old boy with a history of chronic abdominal pain was admitted as an emergency. His blood was noted to be pink in the syringe, and the serum was milky.

Serum osmolality was measured as 282 mmol/kg and amylase 1780 U/L.

His triglyceride was reported to be greater than 50 mmol/L.

Na⁺	K⁺	Cl⁻	HCO₃⁻	Urea	Glucose
			mmol/L		
103	3.8	70	20	3.1	5.2

- Why is there a discrepancy between the calculated and measured osmolality?
- What are the likely causes of the hypertriglyceridaemia?
  Comment in Case history comments.

Want to know more?

http://www.msdmanuals.com/en-gb/professional/endocrine-and-metabolic-disorders/lipid-disorders/overview-of-lipid-metabolism#v989655

There is no shortage of online material on this topic. This resource is accessible and does not go into unnecessary detail. However, it is sponsored by a pharmaceutical company (MSD), and the guidelines and recommendations reflect a US perspective.

69 | Clinical disorders of lipid metabolism

Lipoprotein disorders are some of the commonest metabolic diseases seen in clinical practice. They may present with their various sequelae, which include:

- coronary heart disease (CHD)
- acute pancreatitis
- failure to thrive and weakness
- cataracts.

Classification

Currently there is no satisfactory comprehensive classification of lipoprotein disorders. Genetic classifications have been attempted but are becoming increasingly complex as different mutations are discovered (Table 69.1). *Familial hypercholesterolaemia* (FH), which may present with xanthelasma (Fig. 69.1), tendon xanthomas, severe hypercholesterolaemia and premature CHD, may be due to any of over 500 different pathogenic mutations of the genes for the low-density lipoprotein (LDL) receptor, apolipoprotein B (apo B) or PCSK9. *Familial hyperchylomicronaemia*, which presents with recurrent abdominal pain and pancreatitis, may result from genetic mutations of the lipoprotein lipase or apo C-II genes. Eruptive xanthomas (Fig. 69.2) are characteristic of hypertriglyceridaemia.

Until gene therapy and/or specific substitution therapy become more widely available, genetic classifications, while biologically illuminating, are unlikely to prove very useful in practice. In practice, lipoprotein disorders are simplistically classified as being:

- *Primary:* when the disorder is not due to an identifiable underlying disease
- *Secondary:* when the disorder is a manifestation of some other disease

Primary

The World Health Organization (or Fredrickson) classification of primary hyperlipidaemias remains in widespread use (Fig. 69.3). It relies on the findings of ultracentrifugation of lipoprotein particles, rather than genetics. As a result, patients with the same genetic defect may fall into different groups or may change grouping as the disease progresses or is treated (see Table 69.1). The major advantage of this classification is that it is widely accepted and gives some guidance for treatment.

The six types of hyperlipoproteinaemia defined in the Fredrickson classification are not equally common. Types I and V are rare, whereas types IIa, IIb and IV are very common. Type III hyperlipoproteinaemia, also known as familial dysbetalipoproteinaemia, is intermediate in frequency, occurring in about 1 in 5000 of the population.

Secondary

Secondary hyperlipidaemia is a well-recognised feature of a number of diseases (Table 69.2) that divide broadly into two categories:

- clinically obvious diseases, e.g. renal failure, nephrotic syndrome and cirrhosis of the liver
- covert conditions that may present as hyperlipidaemia, including hypothyroidism, diabetes mellitus and alcohol abuse.

Atherogenic profiles

The causal association of certain forms of hyperlipidaemia and CHD is clearly the major stimulus for the measurement of plasma lipids and lipoproteins in clinical practice. Several lipid profiles are

Table 69.1 **Some genetic causes of dyslipidaemia**			
Disease	**Genetic defect**	**Fredrickson**	**Risk**
Familial hypercholesterolaemia	Reduced numbers of functional LDL receptors; *or* Reduced affinity of LDL receptor for apo B; *or* Altered rate of intracellular recycling of LDL receptors	IIa or IIb	CHD
Familial hypertriglyceridaemia	Possibly single gene defect	IV or V	
Familial combined hyperlipidaemia	Possibly single gene defect	IIa, IIb, IV or V	CHD
Lipoprotein lipase deficiency	Reduced levels of functional LPL	I	Pancreatitis
Apo C-II deficiency	Inability to synthesise apo C-II (cofactor for lipoprotein lipase)	I	Pancreatitis
Abetalipoproteinaemia	Inability to synthesise apo B	Normal	Fat-soluble vitamin deficiencies, neurological deficit
Analphalipoproteinaemia (Tangier disease)	Inability to synthesise apo A	Normal	Neurological deficit Cholesteryl ester storage in abnormal sites

Apo, Apolipoprotein; *CHD*, Coronary heart disease; *LDL*, low-density lipoprotein.

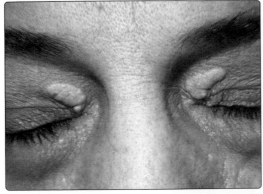

Fig. 69.1 Xanthelasmas in younger individuals (age <40 years) usually indicate hypercholesterolaemia. In the elderly they do not carry the same significance. *(From Habif T. Clinical Dermatology: A Color Guide to Diagnosis and Therapy. St. Louis, MO: Mosby; 2010.)*

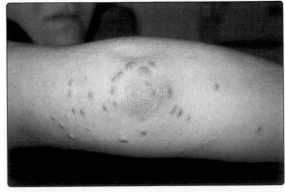

Fig. 69.2 Eruptive xanthomas in a patient with hypertriglyceridaemia. *(From Glynn M, Drake WM. Hutchison's Clinical Methods. 23rd ed. Philadelphia, PA: Saunders; 2012.)*

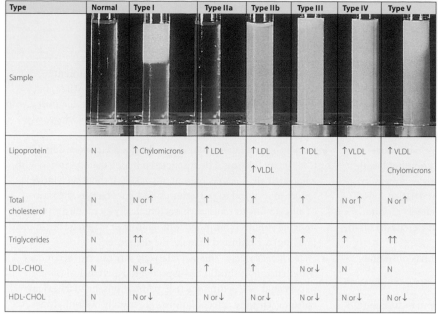

Type	Normal	Type I	Type IIa	Type IIb	Type III	Type IV	Type V
Sample							
Lipoprotein	N	↑Chylomicrons	↑LDL	↑LDL ↑VLDL	↑IDL	↑VLDL	↑VLDL Chylomicrons
Total cholesterol	N	N or ↑	↑	↑	↑	N or ↑	N or ↑
Triglycerides	N	↑↑	N	↑	↑	↑	↑↑
LDL-CHOL	N	N or ↓	↑	↑	N or ↓	N	N
HDL-CHOL	N	N or ↓	N or ↓	N or ↓	N or ↓	N or ↓	N or ↓

Fig. 69.3 WHO (Fredrickson) classification of dyslipidaemia. This is based on the appearance of a fasting plasma sample after standing for 12 hours at 4°C and analysis of its cholesterol and triglyceride content. *IDL*, Intermediate- density lipoprotein; *LDL*, low- density lipoprotein; *N*, normal; *VLDL*, very-low- density lipoprotein.

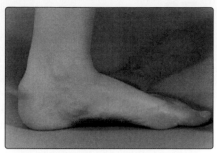

Fig. 69.5 Tendon xanthomas. These are pathognomonic of familial hypercholesterolaemia and are often first seen on the Achilles tendon as in this patient.

Table 69.2 **Common causes of secondary hyperlipidaemia**	
Disease	Usual dominant lipid abnormality
Diabetes mellitus	Increased triglyceride
Alcohol excess	Increased triglyceride
Chronic renal failure	Increased triglyceride
Drugs, e.g. thiazide diuretics	Increased triglyceride
Hypothyroidism	Increased cholesterol
Nephrotic syndrome	Increased cholesterol

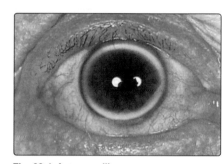

Fig. 69.4 Arcus senilis.

Clinical disorders of lipid metabolism

- The Fredrickson classification can be used to classify hyperlipoproteinaemias by phenotype.
- The genetic and environmental nature of many causes of primary hyperlipidaemia are, as yet, unclear.
- Secondary causes of hyperlipidaemia are common and include hypothyroidism, diabetes mellitus, liver disease and alcohol abuse.

linked with atherogenesis and an increased risk of CHD, including the 'classic' elevated plasma LDL cholesterol level, but also a profile which consists of low plasma high-density lipoprotein (HDL) cholesterol and hypertriglyceridaemia. This latter profile is associated with insulin resistance and so obesity is a major cause. It predisposes affected subjects to subsequent diabetes and vascular disease.

Clinical note

Most physical signs of the hyperlipidaemias are not specific for any particular disease and sometimes may be present in normolipidaemic patients, e.g. arcus senilis (Fig. 69.4). Their presence is, however, highly suggestive of raised lipids. Tendon xanthomas (Fig. 69.5) are particularly associated with familial hypercholesterolaemia.

Case history 52

A 53-year-old man was found to have the following results on a fasting blood sample:

- Total cholesterol 8.4 mmmol/L
- Triglycerides 6.8 mmol/L
- Glucose 9.8 mmol/L
- GGT 138 U/L

A nonsmoker, his blood pressure was 145/95 mmHg, and he was obese with central fat distribution.

- What other information and investigations would be helpful in this man's management?
- What treatment options would you consider in this case?
  Comment in Case history comments.

Want to know more?

http://www.assign-score.com/

When assessing whether to treat a patient with lipid-lowering therapy, the patient's overall (global) cardiovascular risk must be considered. The ASSIGN score, developed in Scotland, incorporates a range of cardiovascular risk factors (age, gender, social deprivation, family history of CHD/stroke, diabetes mellitus, rheumatoid arthritis, cigarette smoking, systolic blood pressure and total and HDL cholesterol) to estimate cardiovascular risk and guide a decision on whether treatment is required.

70 | Hypertension

Hypertension is a common clinical problem. It is defined as chronically increased systemic arterial blood pressure. The definition of hypertension has changed over the years, as more effective treatments have become available. The World Health Organization (WHO) classification of hypertension is shown in Table 70.1. It is important not to base clinical decisions on a single blood pressure reading. Some patients have 'white coat' hypertension, in which readings taken by doctors or other health professionals are misleadingly high. Ambulatory blood pressure measurement over a whole day provides the most detailed information (Fig. 70.1), although increasingly patients monitor their own blood pressure at home using monitors purchased on the high street.

If hypertension is left untreated, patients are at risk of several complications. These include:

- stroke
- left ventricular hypertrophy, leading eventually to heart failure
- chronic kidney disease
- retinopathy.

Occasionally patients present with severe hypertension, associated with a severe form of retinopathy known as papilloedema, and progressive renal failure. This is known as *malignant hypertension* and requires urgent treatment.

Causes of hypertension

Hypertension is related to genetic and environmental factors. Often it runs in families, more than would be expected simply on the basis of a shared environment; other associations include obesity, diabetes and excess alcohol consumption. In many patients, the cause is not known, and in these patients, it is referred to as 'primary' or 'essential' hypertension. So-called secondary hypertension is due to clearly identifiable causes (see later), some of which may be diagnosed or monitored biochemically. However, other modalities of investigation are at least as important in the investigation of hypertension. For example, imaging of renal arteries, or isotope renograms, may provide vital diagnostic information.

- *Renal parenchymal disease*. This is strongly suggested by the finding of a reduced estimated glomerular filtration rate (eGFR) and/or proteinuria.

- *Renal artery stenosis*. This should be suspected in refractory hypertension, especially if creatinine rises on treatment with angiotensin-converting enzyme inhibitors (ACEIs) or angiotensin receptor blockers (ARBs). This is best diagnosed with magnetic resonance angiography. It is associated with grossly elevated renin concentrations.

- *Primary hyperaldosteronism*. This is dealt with in more detail in Chapter 49. It should be suspected if hypokalaemia (often with associated alkalosis) is present, especially if there is (relative) failure to respond to potassium supplementation. The ratio of aldosterone to renin is characteristically elevated, although imaging studies (computed tomography or magnetic resonance imaging) are required to make the diagnosis.

- *Phaeochromocytoma*. This is a relatively rare cause of secondary hypertension. It should be suspected if hypertension is paroxysmal or if symptoms (e.g. palpitations, headaches) are episodic. Urinary catecholamines are usually but not always raised, and there are often false-positive results as well. Urine or, especially, plasma metadrenalines (catecholamine metabolites) are more sensitive and specific for diagnosis. Isotope (^{123}I-meta-iodobenzylguanidine) scans are very specific and help to localise the tumour. The biochemical pathways involved in the production of catecholamines are illustrated in Fig. 70.2.

- *Cushing's syndrome*. This is dealt with in more detail in Chapter 49. It is not usually a diagnostic dilemma, since the signs and symptoms of Cushing's syndrome, and the association with hypertension, are well-recognised. However, if there is doubt, a dexamethasone suppression test may be useful. Suppression of cortisol post dexamethasone to <50 nmol/L effectively excludes the diagnosis.

- *Obesity/sleep apnoea*. Obesity is an increasingly common cause of secondary hypertension, especially if it is associated with sleep apnoea. The latter is likely in the presence of an increased neck circumference.

- *Other*. Less common causes of secondary hypertension include acromegaly, hyperthyroidism and hypothyroidism, and coarctation of the aorta.

Table 70.1 **WHO classification of hypertension**	
Category	**BP (mmHg)**
Optimal blood pressure	<120/80
Normal blood pressure	<130/85
Mild hypertension	140/90–159/99
Moderate hypertension	160/100–179/109
Severe hypertension	≥180/110

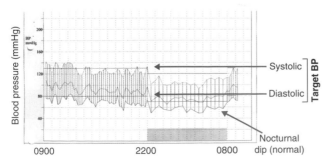

Fig. 70.1 24-hour ambulatory blood pressure monitoring.

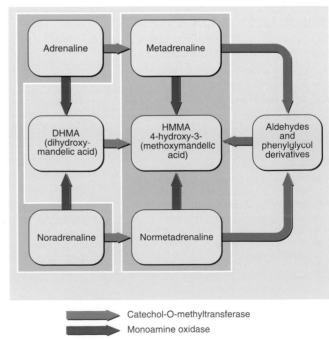

Fig. 70.2 Pathway for production of catecholamine metabolites.

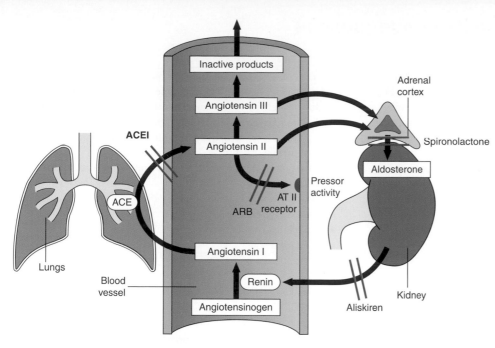

Fig. 70.3 Mechanism of some commonly used antihypertensive drugs. Sites of action are indicated by *double red lines*. See text for details. *ACEI*, Angiotensin-converting enzyme inhibitor; *ARB*, angiotensin receptor blocker.

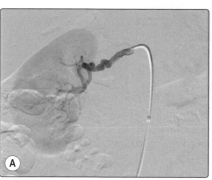

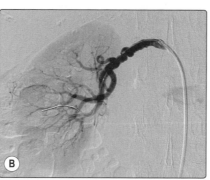

Fig. 70.4 Renal artery stenosis. (A) Pre-angioplasty and **(B)** postangioplasty. Note the substantial increase in blood flow into the kidney post procedure. The functional impact of renal artery stenosis can be assessed clinically by the response to antihypertensive treatment, and biochemically by measurement of plasma renin activity.

Treatment of hypertension

Various groups of antihypertensive drugs are used in the management of hypertension. When patients fail to respond to one or more agents, many physicians add in other drugs, on the grounds that increasing the dose of existing treatments often increases side-effects without enhancing the efficacy. Thus many patients end up on multiple drugs for their hypertension. Commonly used groups of drugs include:

- *ACEIs/ARBs*. ACEIs inhibit angiotensin-converting enzyme and so reduce production of angiotensin II (a potent vasoconstrictor) and, ultimately, aldosterone (a potent mineralocorticoid). ARBs block angiotensin receptors (Fig. 70.3). Both groups of drugs may in some patients reduce the renal damage induced by hypertension; this can be monitored by their effect on reducing proteinuria. In some patients with refractory hypertension, the introduction of ACEI/ARBs is associated with a rapid

rise in creatinine. In this scenario, the drug should be stopped and renal artery stenosis suspected (see earlier discussion; also Fig. 70.4).

- *Beta blockers*. Although these drugs now compete with more effective alternatives, they are still widely used. They act by blocking β-adrenergic receptors in the heart, kidneys and brain, thereby reducing cardiac output and renin and noradrenaline release.
- *Calcium channel blockers*. These drugs are also widely used. They reduce entry of calcium into vascular smooth muscle, thereby reducing vascular tone and peripheral arterial resistance.
- *Diuretics*. These all induce natriuresis. Thiazide diuretics, e.g. bendroflumethiazide, enhance the efficacy of other drugs and are commonly used, especially in the elderly; they may cause clinically significant hyponatraemia. Furosemide also induces natriuresis. The hypovolaemia it causes induces secondary hyperaldosteronism and absorption of sodium in the distal

tubule, in exchange for potassium, and there is therefore a risk of hypokalaemia. Spironolactone and other aldosterone antagonists (also known as potassium-sparing diuretics) are often associated with hyperkalaemia; potassium should be checked before and soon after their introduction.

- *Other drugs*. Doxazosin (an alpha-blocker) and moxonidine (centrally acting) are also used. Other drugs are reserved for specialist care.

Hypertension

- In most patients with hypertension no specific cause can be found.
- Simple biochemical tests (e.g. urea and electrolytes) are useful for monitoring the biochemical effects of treatment, e.g. hypokalaemia or hyperkalaemia.
- Biochemical tests are useful in monitoring renal damage, which can be a cause of hypertension or a manifestation of it.
- Less commonly, biochemistry may be helpful in the diagnosis of rarer causes of hypertension such as Conn's and Cushing's syndromes.

Clinical note

Serum angiotensin-converting enzyme (ACE) may be measured if noncompliance with ACE inhibitor (ACEI) treatment is suspected – an undetectable serum ACE confirms that the patient is complying.

Want to know more?

https://www.nice.org.uk/guidance/ng136

This NICE guideline provides evidence-based guidance about diagnosis and treatment of hypertension. It does not have a specifically biochemical slant.

71 | Cancer and its consequences

Cancer is the leading cause of death in Western society. The effects of tumour growth may be local or systemic (Fig. 71.1), e.g. obstruction of blood vessels, lymphatics or ducts, damage to nerves, effusions, bleeding, infection, necrosis of surrounding tissue and eventual death of the patient. The cancer cells may also secrete biochemically active molecules locally or into the general circulation. Both endocrine and nonendocrine tumours may secrete hormones or other regulatory molecules.

A tumour marker is any substance that can be related to the presence or progress of a tumour (see Chapter 72).

Local effects of tumours

Local growth of tumours causes many abnormalities in commonly requested biochemical tests. This may result from obstruction of blood vessels or ducts, e.g. blockage of bile ducts by carcinoma of the head of the pancreas causes elevated serum alkaline phosphatase and sometimes jaundice due to raised bilirubin. The symptoms that result from such local effects may be the first sign that something is wrong, but there may be no initial suspicion that there is an underlying malignancy.

Tumours often spread to other organs or tissues. Organs frequently affected by such metastatic (secondary) spread include the liver, lungs, bone and brain. Routine biochemical measurements may be the first indication of metastatic malignancy. For example, serum alkaline phosphatase may be elevated in the presence of either hepatic or bony metastases; measuring gamma-glutamyl transpeptidase (GGT) is the easiest way to tell whether it is coming from one tissue or the other. Conversely, even with significant liver involvement, there may be no biochemical abnormalities. Modest increases in alanine aminotransferase (ALT) are observed if the rate of hepatocyte destruction is increased.

Less commonly, metastatic spread of a tumour to specific glands or organs may lead to their failure. For example, destruction of the adrenal cortex by tumour causes impaired aldosterone and cortisol secretion, with potentially fatal consequences.

Rapid tumour growth gives rise to abnormal biochemistry. Leukaemia and lymphoma are often associated with elevated serum urate concentrations due to the rapid cell turnover (urate is a product of DNA breakdown). Serum lactate dehydrogenase is often elevated in these patients, reflecting the high concentration of the enzyme in the tumour and the cellular turnover; it also may be a sign of intravascular haemolysis. Large, rapidly growing tumours may not have an extensive blood supply, and tumour cells meet their energy needs via anaerobic glycolysis, causing lactic acidosis. Rarely, this can manifest as the full-blown *tumour lysis syndrome*, characterised by grossly elevated urate, potassium and phosphate, all of which are released from lysed tumour cells, and hypocalcaemia (calcium is sequestered by the excess phosphate).

Renal failure may occur in patients with malignancy for the following reasons:

- obstruction of the urinary tract
- hypercalcaemia
- Bence-Jones proteinuria
- hyperuricaemia
- nephrotoxicity of cytotoxic drugs.

Cancer cachexia

Cancer cachexia describes the characteristic wasting often seen in patients with cancer. Features include anorexia, lethargy, weight loss, muscle weakness, anaemia and pyrexia. Its development is due to many factors and is incompletely understood. Fundamentally, though, there is an imbalance between dietary calorie intake and body energy requirements. This results from a combination of factors:

- Increased energy requirement of the cancer patient. The host reaction to the tumour is similar to the metabolic response to injury, with increased metabolic rate and altered tissue metabolism.
- Competition between the host and tumour for nutrients. The growing tumour has a high metabolic rate and may deprive the body of nutrients, especially if it is large. Low plasma cholesterol in cancer patients may reflect this.
- Inadequate food intake.
- Impaired digestion and absorption.

Tumour spread may cause infection, dysphagia, persistent vomiting and diarrhoea, all of which may contribute to the overall picture seen in cancer cachexia. The observation that small tumours can have a profound effect on host metabolism suggests that cancer cells secrete or cause the release of humoral ('humoral' literally means 'relating to body fluids' – in this context, blood) agents that mediate the metabolic changes of cancer cachexia. Some of these, such as tumour necrosis factor, have been identified. This cytokine is secreted by activated macrophages and acts on a variety of tissues, including muscle, adipose tissue and liver.

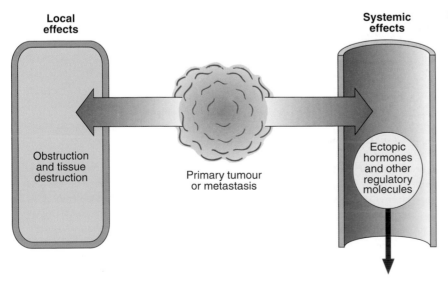

Fig. 71.1 Biochemical effects of tumour growth.

Local effects

Systemic effects

Obstruction and tissue destruction

Primary tumour or metastasis

Ectopic hormones and other regulatory molecules

Paraneoplastic syndromes and ectopic hormone production

Paraneoplastic syndromes are clinical syndromes involving nonmetastatic systemic effects of cancers. They are mediated by humoral factors or alterations in the body's immune system (Table 71.1). Some cancers secrete hormones. This is referred to as *ectopic hormone production*, meaning that the hormone is not being produced by its normal tissue of origin. Small cell carcinomas, the most aggressive of lung cancers, are the most likely to be associated with ectopic hormone production. Ectopic adrenocorticotrophic hormone (ACTH) secretion is commonest. The classic clinical features of Cushing's syndrome often are not apparent due to rapid onset; hypokalaemia and metabolic alkalosis may be the sole indicators. In practice, histochemistry provides the best proof of ectopic hormone production by a tumour (Fig. 71.2).

Patients with malignancy often develop the syndrome of inappropriate antidiuresis (SIAD), causing water retention and hyponatraemia. This is almost invariably due to *pituitary* arginine vasopressin (AVP) secretion in response to nonosmotic stimuli, rather than *ectopic* AVP secretion, which is very rare.

Some cancers cause hypercalcaemia through the secretion of parathyroid hormone–related protein (PTHrP) – so-called because of its similarity to parathyroid hormone (PTH) in structure and function. Crucially, however, PTHrP is not recognised in the immunoassay for PTH, so that when PTH is measured, it is undetectable.

Table 71.1 Examples of paraneoplastic syndromes

Paraneoplastic syndromes	Some associated cancers
Hypercalcaemia	Multiple myeloma, breast cancer, renal cell cancer
Cushing's syndrome	Small cell lung cancer, bronchial carcinoid, gastrointestinal cancer
Syndrome of inappropriate secretion of antidiuretic hormone	Small cell lung cancer, brain tumour, mesothelioma
Myasthenia gravis	Thymoma
Lambert-Eaton myasthenic syndrome	Small cell lung cancer, lymphoma
Autonomic neuropathy	Small cell lung cancer, thymoma
Sensory neuropathy	Lung cancer (usually small cell), breast cancer, ovarian cancer, Hodgkin's lymphoma
Acanthosis nigricans	Gastric adenocarcinoma
Dermatomyositis	Ovarian cancers, non-Hodgkin's lymphoma
Pemphigus	Non-Hodgkin's lymphoma, chronic lymphocytic leukaemia
Polymyalgia rheumatica	Leukaemia, lymphoma, colon cancer

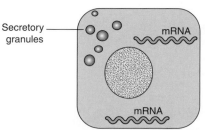

Secretory granules

mRNA

mRNA

Fig. 71.2 Histochemical demonstration of hormone in tumour cell secretory granules.

Consequences of cancer treatment

Gonadal failure arising from radiotherapy or chemotherapy is frequently encountered, as is osteopenia. Hypomagnesaemia and hypokalaemia may be a consequence of the use of platinum-based drugs, e.g. cisplatin, the effect of which on renal tubular function can last for weeks after it has been stopped. Patients treated with methotrexate may become folate deficient with resultant impact on blood cell formation.

Hyperuricaemia is a consequence of the massive cell death that occurs in the treatment of some tumours with cytotoxic drugs, particularly lymphomas and some leukaemias, and is an important component of the very rare tumour lysis syndrome.

Clinical note

Treatment with the selective oestrogen receptor modulator tamoxifen substantially reduces recurrence rates and mortality in women with receptor-positive early breast cancer. In postmenopausal women, most circulating oestrogen is produced by conversion of testosterone (from the adrenal glands) in peripheral tissues, by the enzyme aromatase. Aromatase inhibitors such as anastrozole or letrozole thus provide another therapeutic approach.

Cancer and its consequences

- Cancer may cause clinical signs and symptoms in patients by causing obstruction, exerting pressure or destroying normal tissue.
- Cancer cachexia is characterised by anorexia, lethargy, muscle wasting, weight loss and anaemia.
- Some nonendocrine tumours secrete hormones, e.g. lung cancers may secrete adrenocorticotrophic hormone (ACTH).
- Hyponatraemia, due to water retention and in turn to arginine vasopressin (AVP) secretion, is the commonest biochemical abnormality seen in patients with cancer.

Case history 53

A 37-year-old man presented to his general practitioner complaining of nocturia, frequency of micturition and polydipsia. On examination, he had mild truncal obesity, plethora and ankle oedema. He had purpura of his arms but no striae. His blood pressure was 185/115 mmHg. Biochemistry results in a serum specimen showed:

Na+	K+	Cl⁻	HCO₃⁻	Urea	Creatinine	Glucose
		mmol/L			μmol/L	mmol/L
146	2.1	96	34	7 0	135	8 5

- What is the most likely diagnosis?
- What further biochemistry tests should be requested?
  Comment in Case history comments.

Want to know more?

https://www.ncbi.nlm.nih.gov/pmc/articles/PMC2931619/pdf/mayoclin-proc_85_9_008.pdf

Review paper on paraneoplastic syndromes detailing approach to diagnosis and management.

72 | Tumour markers

A tumour marker is any substance that can be related to the presence or progress of a tumour. In practice, the clinical biochemistry laboratory measures markers that are present in blood, although the term *tumour markers* can also be applied to substances found on the surface of, or within, cells fixed in frozen or paraffin sections. A tumour marker in blood has been secreted or released by the tumour cells. Such markers are not necessarily unique products of the malignant cells, but simply may be expressed by the tumour in a greater amount than by normal cells.

Tumour markers fall into one of several groups: they may be hormones, e.g. human chorionic gonadotrophin (HCG) secreted by choriocarcinoma; or enzymes, e.g. prostate-specific antigen (PSA) in prostate carcinoma; or tumour antigens, e.g. carcinoembryonic antigen (CEA) in colorectal carcinoma.

The use of tumour markers

Tumour markers can be used in different ways. They are of most value in monitoring treatment and assessing follow-up (Fig. 72.1); their use in diagnosis, prognosis and screening for the presence of disease is more limited.

Monitoring treatment

Treatment monitoring is the area in which most tumour markers have found a useful role. The decline in concentration of the tumour marker is an indication of the success of the treatment, whether that be surgery, chemotherapy, radiotherapy or a combination of these. However, the rate of decline of marker concentration should match that predicted from knowledge of the marker's half-life. A slower than expected fall may well indicate that not all the tumour has been eliminated.

Assessing follow-up

Even when a patient has had successful treatment, it is often helpful to continue to monitor the marker long after the levels have appeared to stabilise. An increase may indicate recurrence of the malignancy, and usually prompts further investigation using other modalities, e.g. diagnostic imaging. Detection of increasing marker concentration allows therapy to be reinstituted promptly.

Diagnosis

Markers alone are rarely used to establish a diagnosis. Their detection in blood when there is clinical evidence of the tumour as well as radiological and, perhaps, biopsy evidence, often will confirm the diagnosis.

Prognosis

To be of value in prognosis, the concentration of the tumour marker in plasma should correlate with tumour mass. For example, HCG correlates well with the tumour mass in choriocarcinoma, HCG and alpha-fetoprotein (AFP) correlate with the tumour mass in testicular teratoma, and paraproteins correlate with the tumour mass in multiple myeloma.

Screening for the presence of disease

In routine clinical practice, tumour markers should not be used to screen for malignancy, however appealing this might be in theory.

The exception to this rule is the screening of specific high-risk populations. For example, the hormone calcitonin, which is increased in all patients with medullary carcinoma of thyroid, may be used to screen close relatives of patients with this form of cancer, which may run in families. Prophylactic thyroidectomy then may be advised if any are found to have elevated calcitonin concentrations.

A practical application of tumour markers

Some of the uses of tumour markers discussed previously can be illustrated with reference to Fig. 72.2. This shows how the tumour marker AFP was helpful in the management of a young man with a malignant teratoma. The presence of AFP together with the hormone HCG confirmed the diagnosis. Between 75%

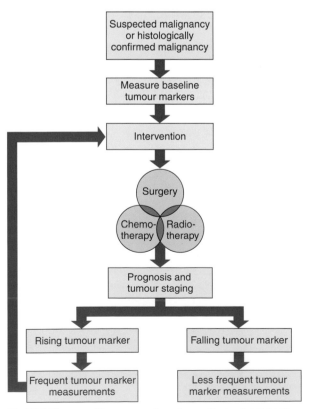

Fig. 72.1 The use of tumour markers in monitoring treatment.

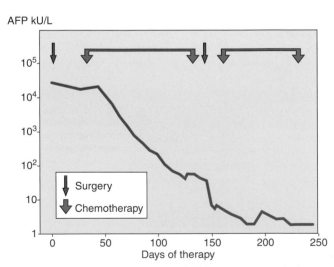

Fig. 72.2 The use of alpha-fetoprotein (AFP) measurements in the management of a patient with a testicular teratoma.

and 95% of all patients presenting with testicular teratoma have abnormalities in one or both of these markers. The very high concentration of AFP (>10,000 kU/L) indicated that the prognosis was not good and that it was likely there would be tumour recurrence after treatment. In fact, AFP concentrations fell in response to chemotherapy, and when the levels reached a plateau, surgery was performed. Thereafter, chemotherapy was continued, and AFP fell to very low levels. Continued monitoring of AFP levels in such a patient would provide early warning of tumour recurrence.

Tumour markers with established clinical value

Markers play a major role in the management of germ cell tumours and choriocarcinoma. Unfortunately, there are many cases in which markers are available but the tumours are resistant to chemotherapy, so their use is not mandatory. Table 72.1 shows which markers have gained an established place in the repertoire of tests commonly offered by the clinical biochemistry laboratory.

The future

Monoclonal antibodies raised against tumour cells and their membranes have led to the development of many new tumour marker assays, although few have as yet gained an established place in the management of patients with cancer. There is no doubt that tumour markers are an efficient and relatively cheap way to monitor treatment. The search goes on for the 'perfect' marker that could be used in population screening, diagnosis, prognosis, monitoring treatment and for follow-up of tumour recurrence. However, the capacity for tumours to alter the expression of their surface antigens may make this goal unattainable.

Table 72.1 **Clinical situations in which tumour markers have been found useful**

Marker	Tumour	Screening	Diagnosis	Prognosis	Monitoring	Follow-up
AFP	Germ cell		✔	✔	✔	✔
AFP	Hepatoma	✔	✔		✔	✔
HCG	Germ cell		✔	✔	✔	✔
HCG	Choriocarcinoma	✔	✔	✔	✔	✔
CA125	Ovarian		✔		✔	✔
Acid phosphatase	Prostate		✔		✔	✔
PSA	Prostate		✔		✔	✔
CEA	Colorectal				✔	✔
Calcitonin	Medullary carcinoma of thyroid	✔	✔		✔	✔
Hormones	Endocrine		✔		✔	✔
Paraprotein	Myeloma		✔		✔	✔

AFP, Alpha-fetoprotein; *CA125*, cancer antigen 125; *CEA*, carcinoembryonic antigen; *HCG*, human chorionic gonadotrophin; *PSA*, prostate-specific antigen.

Clinical note

Sometimes a man may be used as a negative control when his partner uses a pregnancy test kit at home. Teratoma of the testis has a peak incidence in males in their 20 s, and this tumour frequently secretes large amounts of human chorionic gonadotrophin (HCG). This will give rise to a positive pregnancy test in the man. Such a finding should be taken very seriously and followed up immediately.

Tumour markers

- The main use of tumour markers is in monitoring treatment, although they also may be of use in screening, diagnosis, prognosis and long-term follow-up.

- Calcitonin is used to screen the relatives and family of a patient with medullary carcinoma of thyroid.

- Alpha-fetoprotein (AFP), paraproteins, prostate-specific antigen (PSA) and a variety of hormones are helpful in establishing the diagnosis of certain tumours.

- AFP and human chorionic gonadotrophin (HCG) are of value in predicting the outcome of nonseminomatous germ cell tumours.

Case history 54

A 72-year-old man had complained of pains in his lower chest and abdomen for 2 months. His general practitioner detected dullness at both lung bases and referred him to a chest physician. On 23 June he was admitted to hospital. Examination revealed an enlarged liver. He had been a heavy drinker. Biochemistry results were:

Date	Bilirubin	ALP	AST	ALT	LDH	GGT
	μmol/L			U/L		
23/6	24	1540	83	98		719
1/7	25	2170	80	107	430	1020

- What is your differential diagnosis in the light of the liver function test results?
- How might alpha-fetoprotein (AFP) be of help in this case?
  Comment in Case history comments.

Want to know more?

Sturgeon CM, Lai LC, Duffy MJ. Serum tumour markers: how to order and interpret them. *BMJ*. 2009;339:b3527. http://www.bmj.com/content/339/bmj.b3527

This authoritative and practical review covers what its title suggests.

73 | Multiple endocrine neoplasia

Multiple endocrine neoplasias (MEN) are inherited tumour predisposition syndromes, characterised by tumours in two or more endocrine glands. Clinical manifestations of these syndromes result either from hormone overproduction by the tumours or from other adverse effects of tumour growth. Inheritance is autosomal dominant.

MEN 1

A clinical diagnosis of MEN 1 can be made if the patient has at least two of the following:

- parathyroid adenoma
- pancreatic endocrine tumour
- pituitary adenoma
- adrenal cortex adenoma
- carcinoid tumour.

The approximate frequencies of these tumours in MEN 1 are shown in Fig. 73.1.

The inactivated gene in MEN 1 is a tumour suppressor gene, the protein product of which (*menin*) normally inhibits genes involved in cell proliferation. MEN 1 gene mutations invariably lead to endocrine tumours, but family members carrying the same MEN 1 gene mutation can have completely different clinical manifestations of the syndrome. Genetic testing for MEN 1 allows earlier recognition and surgical removal of tumours. In the past, patients with MEN 1 died from, for example, peptic ulceration due to gastrinoma or nephrolithiasis resulting from hyperparathyroidism.

Pituitary tumours in MEN 1 most often overproduce prolactin, but sometimes produce adrenocorticotrophic hormone or growth hormone, resulting in Cushing's disease or acromegaly, respectively. The pancreatic tumours can produce gastrin, insulin, vasoactive intestinal polypeptide (VIP), glucagon or somatostatin, resulting in characteristic clinical features. The adrenocortical tumours seen in MEN 1 are often nonfunctional.

MEN 2

In MEN 2 the *RET* (REarrranged during Transfection) gene encodes a tyrosine kinase receptor for a family of growth factors. Unlike MEN 1, different mutations of this gene are associated with specific tumours or tumour combinations. Clinically, MEN 2 presents as several distinct phenotypes.

MEN 2 A

Medullary carcinoma of the thyroid (MCT) is always present, often with phaeochromocytoma or hyperparathyroidism (see Fig. 73.1). Phaeochromocytoma is bilateral in about 50% of affected cases.

MEN 2B

MCT is again always present, along with phaeochromocytomas, but parathyroid adenomas are rare. Additional features specific to MEN 2B include mucosal ganglioneuromas in the gastrointestinal tract and a Marfanoid habitus. MEN 2B presents at an earlier age than MEN 2 A and carries a worse prognosis.

Familial medullary carcinoma of the thyroid

This shares many of the genetic and clinical features of MEN 2, but phaeochromocytomas and parathyroid adenomas occur less frequently.

Screening and treatment

Some of the endocrine tumours associated with MEN, e.g. parathyroid and pituitary adenomas, are common and only rarely part of a wider syndrome. MEN should be suspected where these tumours present early (<35 years) or where there is a family history of a MEN-associated tumour. By contrast, pancreatic endocrine tumours are rare and their diagnosis should prompt routine biochemical screening for, e.g. hyperparathyroidism or prolactinoma. In cases in which MEN is diagnosed, all family members should be screened.

All carriers of MEN mutations will develop one or other of the associated endocrine tumours. Periodic biochemical (phenotypic) screening has an important role to play in the follow-up of identified carriers. However, *definitive confirmation or exclusion of an individual's MEN predisposition requires genetic testing.* In some cases provocation tests may be necessary (Fig. 73.2).

Prophylactic surgical removal of the predisposed gland(s) may be indicated where the certainty of early cancer presentation is high. In particular, thyroidectomy is recommended for children who carry the *RET* mutations with the worst prognosis.

The amine precursor uptake and decarboxylation concept

Carcinoid and pancreatic islet cell tumours are seen in MEN syndromes but also occur

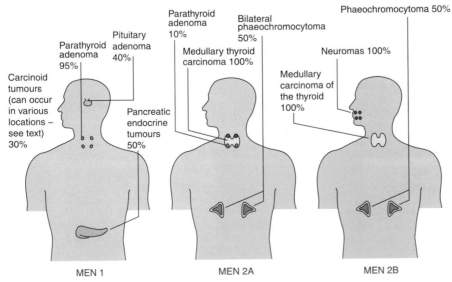

Fig. 73.1 Tumours associated with multiple endocrine neoplasia (MEN) syndromes.
Percentages are approximate.

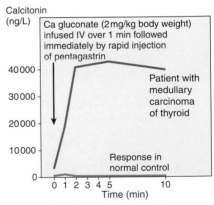

Fig. 73.2 Calcium and pentagastrin provocation test of calcitonin secretion.
There is an exaggerated response to combined calcium and pentagastrin provocation in a patient with medullary carcinoma of the thyroid.

Table 73.1 **Selected molecules which regulate gastrointestinal function**

Substance	Type of Regulator	Major Action
Gastrin	Hormone	Gastric acid and pepsin secretion
Cholecystokinin (CCK)	Hormone	Pancreatic enzyme secretion
Secretin	Hormone	Pancreatic bicarbonate secretion
Gastric inhibitory polypeptide (GIP)	Hormone	Enhances glucose-stimulated insulin release, inhibits gastric acid secretion
Vasoactive intestinal polypeptide (VIP)	Neurotransmitter	Smooth muscle relaxation. Stimulates pancreatic bicarbonate secretion
Motilin	Hormone	Initiates intestinal motility
Somatostatin	Hormone Neurotransmitter Paracrine	Numerous inhibitory effects
Pancreatic polypeptide (PP)	Hormone Paracrine	Inhibits pancreatic bicarbonate and protein secretion
Encephalins	Neurotransmitter	Opiate-like actions
Substance P	Neurotransmitter Paracrine	Contraction of smooth muscle

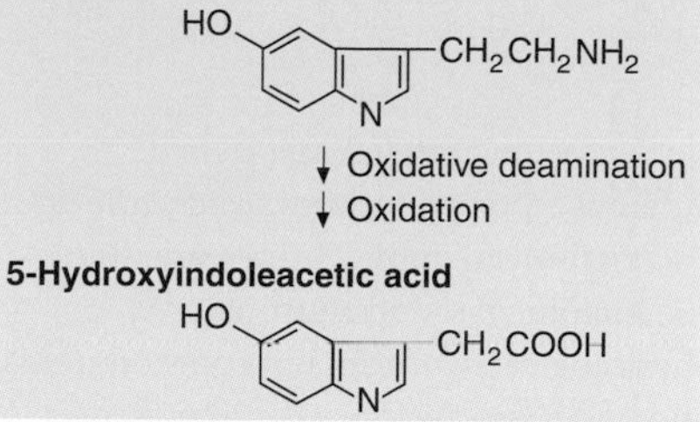

Serotonin

Fig. 73.3 Serotonin and its urinary metabolite 5-hydroxyindoleacetic acid. Certain foodstuffs, e.g. bananas and tomatoes, contain 5-hydroxyindoleacetic acid and may interfere with the urinary determination.

sporadically. They arise from specialised neuroendocrine cells that have the capacity for *amine precursor uptake and decarboxylation* (APUD). Some of the peptides and amines secreted by these cells act like classic hormones, being delivered through the bloodstream, whereas others are local paracrine regulators or neurotransmitters (Table 73.1). Overproduction of peptides or amines by tumours gives rise to associated tumour syndromes.

Carcinoid tumours

These most commonly arise in the appendix and ileocaecal region, where the embryonic foregut and midgut meet. Carcinoid tumours may convert as much as half of the dietary intake of tryptophan into serotonin, secretion of which causes distinctive clinical effects, known as the *carcinoid syndrome*. This is characterised by flushing, diarrhoea and sometimes valvular heart disease. Intestinal carcinoid tumours produce carcinoid syndrome only if they have metastasised to the liver, whereas extraintestinal carcinoids, e.g. bronchial, which do not drain into the portal circulation, may cause it even in the absence of metastasis. Serotonin may be measured directly in plasma or platelets, but the diagnosis is more often made by measurement in urine of its metabolite, 5-hydroxyindoleacetic acid (5HIAA) (Fig. 73.3).

Insulinomas

These are the commonest pancreatic endocrine tumours. They should be suspected particularly when hypoglycaemia is documented. They require specialist investigation.

Others

Gastrinomas, VIPomas, glucagonomas and somatostatinomas are all either rare or very rare.

Clinical note

Proton pump inhibitors (PPIs), such as omeprazole, are widely used to treat peptic ulcers. They may cause an increase in plasma gastrin concentrations to values that might suggest the presence of a gastrinoma. These drugs should be stopped before samples are taken for gastrin measurements.

Multiple endocrine neoplasia

- Multiple endocrine neoplasias (MEN) are inherited cancer predisposition syndromes.
- Diagnosis of MEN should prompt screening of family members.
- Prophylactic surgical removal of endocrine glands may be appropriate.
- The carcinoid syndrome is related to overproduction of serotonin.
- Pancreatic islet cell tumours are rare.

Case history 55

A 50-year-old man was referred to a neurologist after complaining of a 6-month history of severe headache. He was found to be slightly hypertensive. Urea and electrolytes and liver function tests were unremarkable. The only abnormality initially noted was a serum adjusted calcium concentration of 2.80 mmol/L.

- What further investigations are required in this patient?

Comment in Case history comments.

Want to know more?

Thakker RV. Multiple endocrine neoplasia. *Horm Res*. 2001;56(suppl 1):67–72 [review]. http://www.karger.com/Article/Pdf/48138

This quite short article reviews the clinical features, biochemical associations and genetic basis of the main multiple endocrine neoplasia (MEN) syndromes.

74 | Hyperuricaemia

Nucleic acids contain bases of two different types: pyrimidines and purines. The catabolism of the purines, adenine and guanine, produces uric acid. At physiological hydrogen ion concentration, uric acid is mostly ionised and present in plasma as sodium urate (Fig. 74.1). An elevated serum urate concentration is known as *hyperuricaemia*. Uric acid and sodium urate are relatively insoluble molecules that readily precipitate out of aqueous solutions such as urine or synovial fluid (Fig. 74.2). The consequence of this is the medical condition gout.

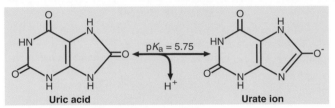

Fig. 74.1 Uric acid and urate.

Urate formation and excretion

Urate is formed in three ways. These are:
- by *de novo* synthesis
- by the metabolism of endogenous DNA, RNA and other purine-containing molecules such as adenosine triphosphate (ATP)
- by the breakdown of dietary nucleic acids.
Urate is excreted in two ways:
- *Via the kidney*. The majority of urate is excreted via the kidney. Renal handling of urate is complex. It is freely filtered at the glomerulus, but 99% is reabsorbed in the proximal tubule. The distal tubules secrete urate, but again much is reabsorbed. The amount of urate excreted in the urine is around 10% of that filtered at the glomerulus.
- *Via the gut*. Smaller amounts of urate are excreted into the gut, where it is broken down by bacteria, into carbon dioxide and ammonia. This process is called uricolysis.

Urate concentrations in serum are higher in males than females. Even within the reference interval, serum urate is near its aqueous solubility limit. The presence of protein helps keep the molecule in solution. A high serum urate concentration may arise from increased urate formation or decreased excretion. The common causes of hyperuricaemia are summarised in Fig. 74.3.

Lesch–Nyhan syndrome

Lesch–Nyhan syndrome is an X-linked disorder caused by deficiency of hypoxanthine-guanine phosphoribosyltransferase, an enzyme that is involved in salvaging purine bases for resynthesis to purine nucleotides. The syndrome is characterised clinically by excessive uric acid production, hyperuricaemia and neurological problems

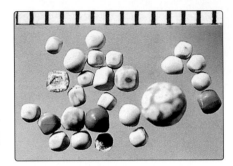

Fig. 74.2 Urate stones from the urinary tract.

that include self-mutilation and profound intellectual disability.

Gout

Gout is a clinical syndrome characterised by hyperuricaemia and recurrent acute arthritis. Whereas all patients who develop gout will have had hyperuricaemia at some point in the development of the disease, only a minority of patients with hyperuricaemia develop gout. Although the exact reason for this is not known, it is accepted that various other factors may contribute to the development of gout. These include genetic predisposition, diet, lifestyle, certain medications and chronic kidney disease.

Acute gout is triggered by the tissue deposition of sodium urate crystals, causing an intense inflammatory response. In the chronic situation, tophaceous deposits of sodium urate may form in the tissues (Fig. 74.4). Gout is exacerbated by alcohol. There are at least two reasons for this. First, ethanol increases the turnover of ATP and urate production. Second, ethanol in excess may cause accumulation of organic acids that compete with the tubular secretion of uric acid, thereby enhancing its retention. For example, ethanol intoxication, diabetic ketoacidosis and starvation lead to elevations of lactic acid, β-hydroxybutyric acid and acetoacetic acid and will cause hyperuricaemia.

Treatment

The symptoms of acute gout respond to nonsteroidal antiinflammatory drugs, but these drugs have no direct effect on the serum urate level. Low-dose aspirin

should be avoided as it inhibits renal urate excretion. Treatment also must be directed at the hyperuricaemia. A diet that is low in purines and alcohol may be prescribed in an effort to reduce the plasma urate concentration. Allopurinol, a specific inhibitor of the enzyme xanthine oxidase that catalyses the oxidation of hypoxanthine to xanthine and uric acid, is prescribed if a patient has recurrent episodes of gout.

A number of other crystalline arthropathies may present as gout but are not associated with hyperuricaemia (so-called *pseudogout*). Most notably, pseudogout is due to the deposition of calcium pyrophosphate crystals.

Renal disease and hyperuricaemia

Renal disease is a common complication of hyperuricaemia. Several types of renal disease have been identified. The most common is urate nephropathy, which is caused by the deposition of urate crystals in renal tissue or the urinary tract to form urate stones. This may be associated with chronic hyperuricaemia. Acute kidney injury can be caused by the rapid precipitation of uric acid crystals that commonly occurs during treatment of patients with leukaemias and lymphomas. In the tumour lysis syndrome (Chapter 71), nucleic acids are released as a result of tumour cell breakdown and are rapidly metabolised to uric acid; this sometimes results in very high concentrations, precipitating gout or nephropathy. In these cases, recombinant urate oxidase (rasburicase) is sometimes administered prophylactically to metabolise the uric acid to allantoin, which is water-soluble and safely excreted by the kidney.

Urate in pregnancy

Serum urate is of value in monitoring maternal well-being in pregnancy-associated hypertension (preeclampsia), alongside other markers such as blood pressure, urine protein excretion and creatinine clearance (see Chapter 77).

NORMAL

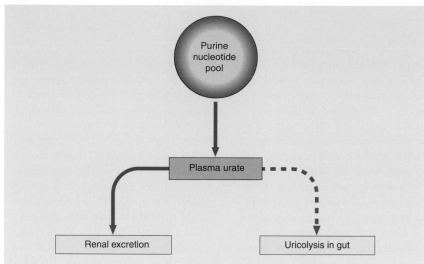

INCREASED PRODUCTION

Primary hyperuricaemia

- Hypoxanthine-guanine phosphoribosyl transferase deficiency (Lesch–Nyhan syndrome)
- Glucose-6-phosphatase deficiency (glycogen storage disease type 1)

Secondary hyperuricaemia

- Increased dietary intake
- Increased nucleic acid turnover
- Increased ATP breakdown

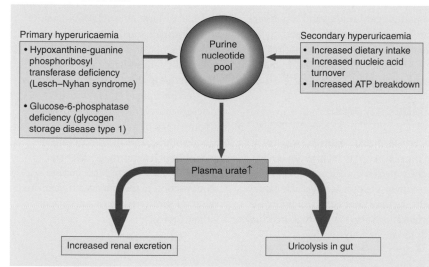

DECREASED EXCRETION

Primary hyperuricaemia

- Idiopathic

Secondary hyperuricaemia

- Renal insufficiency
- Elevated lactic acid or ketones, thiazide diuretics, furosemide and low-dose aspirin cause decreased tubular secretion
- Increased tubular reabsorption

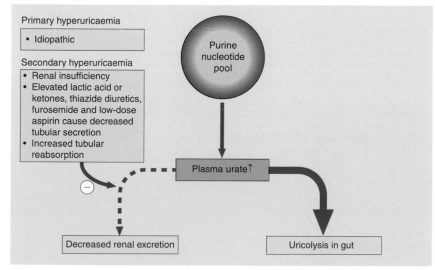

Fig. 74.3 The causes of hyperuricaemia. *ATP,* Adenosine triphosphate.

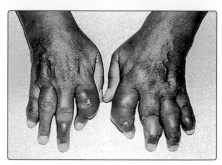

Fig. 74.4 Tophaceous deposits of sodium urate in tissues.

Clinical note

The definitive diagnosis of gout is by examination of synovial fluid from an acutely inflamed joint. Needle-shaped sodium urate crystals will be observed within polymorphonuclear leucocytes viewed under polarising light. However, in practice this is rarely performed.

Hyperuricaemia

- Uric acid is formed from the breakdown of purines.
- Hyperuricaemia may be caused by:
  - an increased rate of purine synthesis
  - an increased rate of turnover of nucleic acids, as in malignancies, tissue damage or starvation
  - a reduced renal excretion.
- Hyperuricaemia is a risk factor for gout which occurs when urate crystals are deposited in tissues.
- Hyperuricaemia is aggravated by a diet high in purines and alcohol.

Case history 56

A 50-year-old man was awakened by a severe pain in his left big toe. He was shivering and feverish, and the pain became so intense that he could not bear the weight of the bedclothes.

- What biochemical tests would help make the diagnosis?
  Comment in Case history comments.

Want to know more?

Hui M, Carr A, Cameron S, et al. The British Society for Rheumatology Guideline for the Management of Gout [published correction appears in Rheumatology (Oxford). 2017;56(7):1246]. *Rheumatology (Oxford).* 2017;56(7):e1–e20.

https://academic.oup.com/rheumatology/article/56/7/e1/3855179

This clinical guideline includes a helpful algorithm outlining management of acute episodes of gout as well as follow-up.

75 | Myopathy

Myopathies are conditions affecting the muscles that lead to weakness and/or atrophy. They may be congenital (as in the muscular dystrophies), caused by infections, e.g. post-viral, or by acute damage due to anoxia, toxins or drugs. Muscle denervation, a lack of energy-producing molecules (from a variety of inborn/metabolic disorders) and severe electrolyte imbalance also result in impaired neuromuscular function (Fig. 75.1).

Normal muscle that is overused will end up weak or in spasm until rested. In severe cases of overuse, especially where movements are strong and erratic as might occur during convulsions, damage to muscle cells may result. Severely damaged muscle cells release their contents, e.g. myoglobin and the enzyme creatine kinase (CK), a condition known as *rhabdomyolysis*.

Investigation

Diagnosis depends on the clinical context, and may include investigation of genetic disorders by enzymatic or chromosomal analysis, endocrine investigations and the search for drug effects. Infective causes may be diagnosed by isolation of the relevant organism or its related antibody, but often no organism is detected.

In all cases of muscle weakness, serum electrolytes should be checked along with CK; muscle weakness sometimes progresses to rhabdomyolysis. A full drug history should be taken to exclude pharmacological and toxicological causes, and a history of alcohol excess should be excluded. Neuromuscular electrophysiological studies may be performed to detect neuropathies. Where a genetic or metabolic cause is suspected (Box 75.1), specialist laboratories should be involved in the investigations at an early stage. These include measurement of plasma (and cerebrospinal fluid (CSF)) lactate and specialist metabolic tests in blood, CSF and urine; muscle biopsy for histopathological studies and sometimes measurement of muscle enzymes. Serum CK may sometimes be normal in myopathic disorders, especially in the chronic setting and severe muscle atrophy.

Rhabdomyolysis

Muscle cells that are damaged will leak CK into the plasma. Very high serum levels may be expected in patients who have been convulsing or have muscular damage due to electrical shock or crush injury. CK concentrations also may be high in acute spells in muscular dystrophy.

The damaged muscle cells will also leak myoglobin. This compound stores oxygen in the muscle cells for release under conditions of hypoxia, as occurs during severe exercise. The dissociation curve of myoglobin is compared with haemoglobin in Fig. 75.2. It delivers up its oxygen only when the PO_2 falls to around 3 kPa. When muscle cells become anoxic or are damaged by trauma, myoglobin is released into the plasma. It is filtered at the glomerulus and excreted in the urine, which appears orange or brown; on urine dipstick testing, myoglobin gives a false-positive reaction for the presence of blood, which can lead to the mistaken diagnosis of haematuria. The damaged muscle cells also release large amounts of potassium and phosphate ions, giving rise to hyperkalaemia and hyperphosphataemia; potentially serious hypocalcaemia may develop due to the binding of calcium by released phosphate and fatty acids.

Severe muscle damage is frequently accompanied by a reduction in the blood volume. This may occur directly as a result of haemorrhage in severe trauma or indirectly because of fluid sequestration in the damaged tissue. The resultant shock frequently causes acute kidney injury.

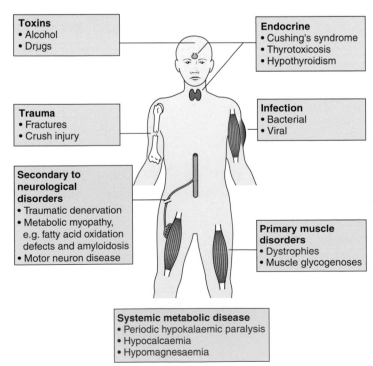

Fig. 75.1 Causes of myopathy.

> **Box 75.1 Metabolic causes of myopathy**
>
> Fatty acid oxidation defects
> Glycogen storage disorders
> Fabry's disease
> Myoadenylate deaminase deficiency
> Carnitine palmitoyl transferase deficiency
> Respiratory chain (electrolyte transport) defects

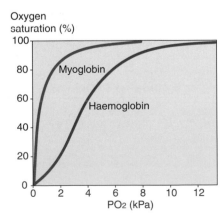

Fig. 75.2 Comparison of oxygen saturation curves for haemoglobin and myoglobin.

Myoglobin *per se* is not nephrotoxic, but the accompanying acidosis, and volume depletion lead to acute tubular necrosis. Additionally, in an acidic cellular environment, myoglobin is converted to ferrihaemate, which produces free radicals and causes direct nephrotoxicity. However, children with muscular dystrophy do not usually develop renal failure despite having increased levels of myoglobin in urine for many years. Additionally, serum creatinine may not be a sensitive marker of declining renal function due to reduced muscle mass.

Investigation and treatment

The biochemistry laboratory has a major role to play in the diagnosis and investigation of rhabdomyolysis (Fig. 75.3). This includes:

- serum total CK, which allows the diagnosis to be made and levels monitored to assess recovery and prognosis
- urea and electrolytes, to look for evidence of resulting renal impairment
- alcohol and drugs of abuse screen, to look for specific causes.

From the previous section, it might be expected that urine or plasma myoglobin would be a sensitive marker of muscle damage. It is, in fact, too sensitive. Even minor degrees of muscle damage that do not warrant investigation or treatment will give rise to myoglobin release. This limits its usefulness.

Treatment is directed towards maintaining tissue perfusion and control of electrolyte imbalances. It includes:

- cardiac monitoring
- control of hyperkalaemia, hyperphosphataemia and hypocalcaemia.

Haemodialysis may be necessary where renal function is severely compromised.

Duchenne muscular dystrophy

This X-linked recessive disorder results from abnormalities in the dystrophin gene. Clinically, it is characterised by progressive muscle weakness, usually in boys, from the age of 5. Very high serum CK may precede the onset of symptoms, but later in the disease the CK levels fall. Approximately 75% of female carriers also have raised CK levels.

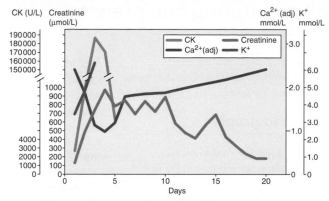

Fig. 75.3 Biochemical results following rhabdomyolysis in a patient who had taken a drug overdose. *CK*, Creatine kinase.

Clinical note

The finding of a marked rise in creatine kinase (CK) (more than five times the upper limit of normal) should prompt renal function to be checked. Peak serum CK of greater than 5000 U/L is a sensitive marker of impending acute kidney injury but may sometimes be a delayed finding. Therefore CK levels, along with other variables, are incorporated in scoring matrices to calculate risk of severe acute kidney injury and mortality in patients presenting to the hospital with rhabdomyolysis.

Skeletal muscle disorders

- Muscle weakness is a common complaint with a wide variety of causes.

- Biochemical investigation of muscle weakness can provide rapid diagnosis and offer effective treatment strategies.

- Intracellular enzyme analysis from muscle biopsies can provide a diagnosis in some inherited disorders.

- Severely damaged muscle cells release potassium, creatine kinase (CK), myoglobin and phosphate.

- Severe rhabdomyolysis, e.g. following injury, is an important cause of acute kidney injury.

Case history 57

A 41-year-old labourer was admitted to hospital. He had collapsed and gave a 4-day history of flu-like illness, with shivering, myalgia, headaches, dyspnoea, vomiting and diarrhoea.

Serum enzymes (on admission)

AST	ALT	LDH	CK
		U/L	
149	88	1330	6000

- What tissues could have contributed to the high serum enzyme activities?
- What tests may help identify the source(s) of enzyme elevation?
  Comment in Case history comments.

Want to know more?

When a patient presents with rhabdomyolysis, it is important to identify the cause. Rarely, patients will have an inherited metabolic disorder. This guideline gives an approach to investigation of the cause of unexplained rhabdomyolysis, with an emphasis on metabolic investigations.

Guidelines for the investigation of rhabdomyolysis for inherited metabolic disorders. Metabolic Biochemistry Network.

Metbionet guidelines on rhabdomyollysis: https://www.smn.scot.nhs.uk/wp-content/uploads/2021/05/Rhabdomyolysis-Management-v1.pdf

76 | Fetal monitoring and prenatal diagnosis

Biochemical tests have limited value in monitoring fetal development, but some components of maternal blood and urine and amniotic fluid may be measured to give evidence of pathology.

Human chorionic gonadotrophin

Human chorionic gonadotrophin (HCG) is a glycoprotein produced by the chorionic cells of the developing embryo that is detectable by sensitive assays within days of conception. Measurement of HCG is used to confirm pregnancy and forms the basis of pregnancy tests. The protein's rapid rate of synthesis in early pregnancy provides systemic evidence of the blastocyst as early as 24 hours after implantation. HCG continues to be secreted by the developing placenta, and serum and urine concentrations increase during the first 9 weeks of pregnancy, then decline gradually until the third trimester (Fig. 76.1). The function of HCG is to maintain the activity of the corpus luteum, sustaining progesterone synthesis. Measurement of HCG is also of value in:

- Assessing fetal viability in threatened abortion (miscarriage).
- Detecting ectopic pregnancy. HCG fails to rise at the expected rate. In the first trimester of a normal pregnancy, it approximately doubles every 48 hours.
- Detecting and monitoring hydatidiform mole and choriocarcinoma. HCG may be used as a tumour marker for diagnosis and monitoring of these rare trophoblastic malignancies (Table 72.1).

Fetoplacental function

Biochemical assessment of fetoplacental function has been superseded by other investigations such as ultrasound and cardiotocography. Human placental lactogen (HPL) and oestriol both reflect placental function and increase in maternal blood during pregnancy until term. Although they can in principle be used to monitor placental function, they are now of historic interest only.

Prenatal diagnosis

Prenatal diagnostic techniques fall into two groups: invasive and noninvasive (Table 76.1). Prenatal diagnosis may be required because of increased risk of inherited disease. Neural tube defects usually cannot be predicted by family history, and pregnant women may be offered a screening test to detect these disorders. For further details on antenatal screening (see Chapter 78).

Alpha-fetoprotein

Alpha-fetoprotein (AFP) is a small glycoprotein synthesised by the yolk sac and fetal liver and is a major fetal plasma protein. Because of its size it appears in fetal urine and hence is present in amniotic fluid and maternal blood. AFP concentrations increase in maternal blood until 32 weeks of gestation in a normal pregnancy (Fig. 76.2).

Detection of higher-than-normal AFP concentrations can suggest central nervous system defects such as anencephaly or spina bifida early in pregnancy, because such malformations of the neural tube are associated with leakage of plasma or cerebrospinal fluid proteins into amniotic fluid, and consequently maternal serum AFP concentrations increase. In some countries all pregnant women in antenatal care are given the opportunity to have their serum AFP measured between 16 and 18 weeks of gestation, with appropriate counselling. When a high result is obtained, the test must be repeated on a fresh sample. Once other possibilities for an elevated AFP, such as wrong dates or multiple pregnancies, have been excluded, an amniocentesis may be offered and AFP determined in amniotic fluid. High levels suggest the presence of a neural tube defect.

Amniotic fluid acetylcholinesterase (an enzyme found in high concentrations in neural tissue) is also used in some centres to detect fetal malformations.

Serum AFP and HCG concentrations and maternal age may be considered together to assess the risk that chromosomal disorders such as Down syndrome are likely to be present. If the risk is high, amniocentesis may be performed to obtain cells for karyotyping (see Chapter 78).

Cells for study of inborn errors may be obtained either by biopsy of the chorionic villus, which is genetically identical to the fetus, or by culture of cells from amniotic fluid. The latter process takes 3 to 4 weeks. Both enzyme studies and DNA analysis may be carried out on these tissue samples.

Table 76.1 **Techniques for prenatal diagnosis**	
Invasive	Amniocentesis
	Chorionic villus sampling
	Cordocentesis
	Fetoscopy
	Fetal skin biopsy
	Fetal liver biopsy
Noninvasive	Ultrasound
	Radiography

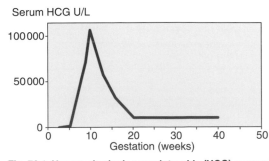

Fig. 76.1 Human chorionic gonadotrophin (HCG) concentration in maternal blood in early pregnancy.

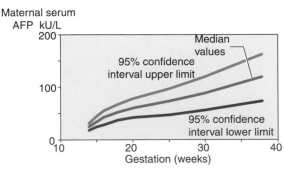

Fig. 76.2 AFP in maternal blood during pregnancy. *AFP,* Alpha-fetoprotein.

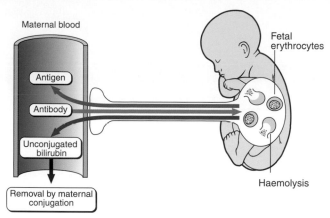

Fig. 76.3 Hyperbilirubinaemia in Rhesus (Rh) incompatibility.

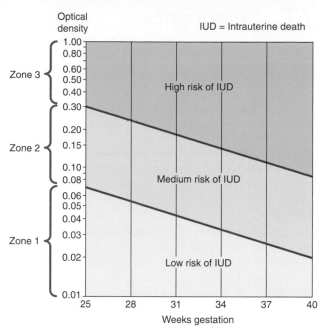

Fig. 76.4 Liley graph. Bilirubin absorbs light at 450 nm. The absorbance is directly related to its concentration and this enables the risk of intrauterine death (IUD) to be estimated.

Bilirubin

Bilirubin is measured in amniotic fluid to assess fetal risk in incompatibility ('incompatibility' here means that the mother's immune system sees the fetal antigens as foreign and reacts accordingly). Incompatible red cell antigens can enter the maternal circulation either from the fetus at the time of delivery or, rarely, because of transfusion of incompatible blood; this stimulates production of specific red cell antibodies in the mother. The best known of these antigens is the Rhesus (Rh) antigen. If a Rh −ve mother has a Rh +ve child, these antibodies may cross the placenta and react with fetal Rh antigens on the red cell membrane, causing haemolysis (Fig. 76.3). This is more likely to happen in subsequent pregnancies where the fetus is Rh +ve. Excess breakdown of fetal red cells leads to anaemia, overproduction of bilirubin and oedema (*hydrops fetalis*).

During fetal life, unconjugated bilirubin (from haemolysis of fetal red cells) crosses the placenta and is removed by the mother, so the baby may not be jaundiced at birth. However, persistence of maternal Rh antibodies in the neonate's circulation leads to haemolysis and jaundice in the first few days postpartum. In utero, the amount of bilirubin in the amniotic fluid can be used to predict the severity of the fetal condition. Amniocentesis is performed on women who have previously had an affected fetus and on women who show a high and rising Rh titre. The severity of the problem can be assessed with reference to a nomogram that relates amniotic bilirubin to gestational age, such as that shown in Fig. 76.4. Fetal exchange blood transfusion or early delivery may be considered.

Rh incompatibility is much less common today, since susceptible women are given an intravenous injection of anti-Rh antibody at the time of delivery to eliminate fetal red blood cells that may have entered the maternal circulation. As a consequence, the fetal red cells do not survive long enough to stimulate the maternal immune response. However, haemolytic disease of the newborn cannot be completely eliminated, because it may be caused by other blood group incompatibilities.

Fetal blood gases

Hydrogen ion concentration, blood gases and serum lactate concentration can be measured in fetal blood. These are requested only when noninvasive investigations have indicated that the fetus is at risk. Fetal blood can be obtained by the technique of cordocentesis, in which the blood is sampled from the umbilical cord through a fine needle inserted through the abdomen under ultrasound guidance.

Hydrogen ion concentration also can be measured in fetal blood to assess fetal distress during labour. Capillary blood samples can be obtained directly from the baby's scalp once the cervix is sufficiently dilated. Fetal hypoxia causes lactic acidosis and elevated hydrogen ion concentration. Measurement of fetal PO_2 can be obtained directly using a transcutaneous oxygen electrode.

Clinical note

Fetal ultrasound scanning, related to time of conception and/or sequential measurements, has become the most widely used way of monitoring fetal growth. This technique has superseded many biochemical tests of fetal well-being that were once commonly performed.

Fetal monitoring and prenatal diagnosis

- Confirmation of pregnancy is by detection of human chorionic gonadotrophin (HCG) in maternal urine.
- Alpha-fetoprotein (AFP) concentrations in maternal blood and amniotic fluid are usually high in neural tube defects and low in Down syndrome.
- Amniotic fluid bilirubin measurements are of value in the detection of risk of Rh incompatibility.

Case history 58

A 30-year-old woman who had previously delivered one live child and had one miscarriage attended for antenatal care. She was known to be Rhesus negative. At 30 weeks gestation she was found to have a high titre of anti-D antibodies.

- What investigations are needed now?
  Comment in Case history comments.

Want to know more?

https://www.nature.com/articles/srep18866

This review examines different approaches to screening for Down syndrome.

77 | Pregnancy

Maternal physiology

Maternal physiology changes so dramatically during pregnancy that the normal reference intervals for biochemical tests in nonpregnant women are often not applicable. Some of the changes may be significant enough to mislead clinicians and suggest pathology, where none exists. Table 77.1 lists the differences observed for some analytes.

Weight gain

Mean weight gain in pregnancy is 12.5 kg, but the standard deviation is large (~4 kg). This is made up of several components:
- *The products of conception*. These include the fetus, placenta and amniotic fluid.
- *Maternal fat stores*. These may account for up to 25% of the weight increase.
- *Maternal water retention*. Total body water increases by about 5 L, mostly in extracellular fluid (ECF). The volume of the intravascular compartment increases by more than 1 L.

Respiratory function

Mild hyperventilation occurs from early pregnancy, probably due to a centrally mediated effect of progesterone, and PCO_2 falls. However, blood hydrogen ion concentration is maintained within nonpregnant limits, since the plasma bicarbonate falls due to a compensatory increase in renal excretion. Oxygen consumption increases by about 20%, but PO_2 is relatively unchanged.

Renal function

Because of increases in plasma volume and cardiac output, renal blood flow increases. Glomerular filtration rate rises early in pregnancy, and may be 150 mL/min or more by 30 weeks. As a result, serum urea and creatinine concentrations fall. Tubular function alters, and, in particular, there is a reduction in the renal threshold for glucose; glycosuria is a common finding in pregnancy. Tubular reabsorption of uric acid and amino acids alters, and their excretion in urine increases.

Glucose

Fasting blood glucose falls early in pregnancy, probably because of substrate utilisation. In late pregnancy, development of insulin resistance favours hyperglycaemia, similar to early diabetes mellitus.

Plasma proteins and enzymes

Serum albumin concentration falls gradually from early pregnancy due to ECF expansion. The concentrations of many other proteins increase, particularly placental alkaline phosphatase, transport proteins such as transferrin and hormone-binding glycoproteins such as thyroxine-binding globulin and fibrinogen.

Hormonal changes

Oestrogens and progesterone are secreted in greater amounts early in pregnancy, and hormones such as human chorionic gonadotrophin (HCG) are produced by the placenta. These hormonal changes form the biochemical basis of the diagnosis of pregnancy. HCG should normally be undetectable in the nonpregnant state. Exceptions to this are HCG production in trophoblastic disease, germ cell tumours, other malignancies and also a small amount of pituitary HCG production after menopause.

Table 77.1 **Reference intervals in the third trimester of pregnancy compared with nonpregnant controls**		
Serum/blood measurement	Pregnant	Nonpregnant
Potassium (mmol/L)	3.2–4.6	3.5–5.3
Chloride (mmol/L)	97–107	95–108
Bicarbonate (mmol/L)	18–28	22–29
Urea (mmol/L)	1.0–3.8	2.5–7.8
Glucose (fasting) (mmol/L)	3.0–5.0	4.0–5.5
Adjusted calcium (mmol/L)	2.2–2.8	2.2–2.6
Magnesium (mmol/L)	0.6–0.8	0.7–1.0
Albumin (g/L)	32–42	35–50
Bilirubin (µmol/L)	<15	<21
Alanine aminotransferase (U/L)	3–28	3–55
Aspartate aminotransferase (U/L)	3–31	12–48
Alkaline phosphatase (U/L)	174–400	30–130
Blood H+ (nmol/L)	34–50	35–45
Blood PCO_2 (kPa)	3.0–5.0	4.4–5.6

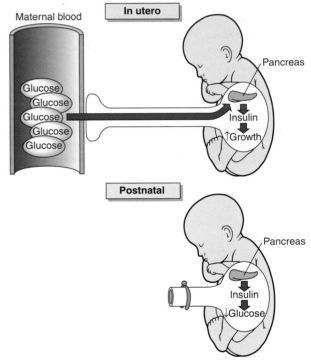

Fig. 77.1 Diabetes mellitus in pregnancy is associated with fetal hyperinsulinaemia. In utero this leads to increased growth, while postnatally the persisting hyperinsulinaemia causes neonatal hypoglycaemia.

Pregnancy-associated pathology

Morbidity during pregnancy may be due to preexisting medical conditions in the mother such as diabetes mellitus, hypertension, renal disease or thyrotoxicosis, or due to new-onset pregnancy-associated conditions.

Gestational diabetes

Gestational diabetes mellitus (GDM) is defined as any degree of glucose intolerance which begins or is first recognised during pregnancy. This definition applies irrespective of treatment modality and regardless of whether the condition persists after pregnancy. It recognises that the glucose intolerance may have been present before the pregnancy. Depending on the population studied, the prevalence of GDM may be as high as 10% of all pregnancies. Maternal glycaemic status should be rechecked 6 weeks after delivery; women with GDM are at increased risk of developing diabetes, usually type 2, after pregnancy. Maternal hyperglycaemia promotes hyperinsulinism in the fetus (Fig. 77.1). Insulin is a growth factor *in utero*, and babies of poorly controlled diabetic patients are often heavier at birth (*macrosomia*). GDM is associated with increased fetal morbidity and mortality. Optimal control of diabetes during pregnancy decreases complications. Risk factors for developing gestational diabetes include a previous personal history of gestational diabetes or delivery of a macrosomic baby, obesity, first-degree relative with diabetes, and ethnicity, e.g. South Asian.

Hypertension

The patient who develops hypertension in pregnancy – a condition described variously as *preeclampsia* or *pregnancy-induced hypertension* – is at increased risk of placental insufficiency and consequent fetal intrauterine growth restriction. Full-blown eclampsia usually occurs in the second half of pregnancy and is characterised by generalised seizures, extreme hypertension and impaired renal function, including proteinuria. It is a significant cause of maternal death, most commonly as a result of cerebral haemorrhage. The features of preeclampsia are shown in Fig. 77.2. There are similarities between preeclampsia and two other conditions seen in pregnancy – namely the *HELLP syndrome* (*h*aemolysis, *e*levated *l*iver enzymes and *l*ow *p*latelets) and acute fatty liver of pregnancy. Blood-borne factors from a poorly perfused placenta may cause maternal endothelial dysfunction and vascular damage. Altered liver metabolism may lead to triglyceride accumulation in the liver (*acute fatty liver of pregnancy*). Decisions on when the baby should be delivered are difficult to make; they may be guided by maternal serum levels of alanine aminotransferase, lactate dehydrogenase, platelets and triglyceride, and urine protein.

Obstetric cholestasis

This multifactorial condition affects about 1% of pregnancies and is characterised by pruritus in the absence of a skin rash, with abnormal liver function tests, neither of which has an alternative cause and both of which resolve after birth. High levels of circulating hormones probably impair normal bile flow and impair bile acid uptake by hepatocytes. It is more common in the third trimester but usually subsides within a few days of delivery. It is important because of the risk to the fetus of preterm birth and intrauterine death. Known risk factors include personal or family history of cholestasis, multiple pregnancy, gallstones, and hepatitis C. Elevated serum bile acid concentration is a sensitive indicator of

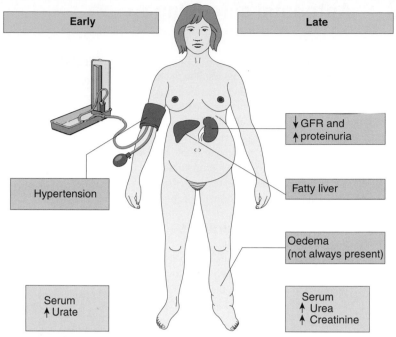

Fig. 77.2 Clinical features of preeclampsia. *GFR*, Glomerular filtration rate.

obstetric cholestasis, but normal levels do not exclude the diagnosis. Other features include pale stools, dark urine, jaundice and elevated liver enzymes. Treatment is directed towards symptomatic relief and includes topical antihistamines and oral ursodeoxycholic acid; supplemental vitamin K is also often prescribed. In severe cases, early elective delivery may be considered.

Drugs in pregnancy

It is necessary for many women to continue to take drugs (medications) during pregnancy. No drugs are without risk to the developing fetus, and drug levels should be kept as low as possible during gestation and thereafter if the mother is breast-feeding, since many drugs are secreted in breast milk. Of particular concern are anticonvulsant drugs. Careful monitoring of levels is necessary to steer between the dangers of maternal seizures and potential fetal damage from the drug.

Clinical note

- Pregnancy is the commonest cause of secondary amenorrhoea in a woman of reproductive age. A pregnancy test should always be performed before other endocrine investigations of the cause of absent menstruation.
- Rarely, in mothers with HELLP syndrome, the underlying cause may be related to an inborn error of fatty acid oxidation in the baby called long-chain 3-hydroxyacyl-CoA dehydrogenase (LCHAD).

Pregnancy

- Physiological changes occur in pregnancy, altering many biochemical reference intervals. They do not per se indicate pathology.
- Diabetes in pregnancy is associated with increased fetal morbidity and mortality. Optimal glycaemic control during pregnancy decreases complications. The baby of a diabetic mother has an increased probability of developing respiratory distress syndrome.
- Hypertension and a rising serum urate concentration are early features in the development of preeclampsia, a rapidly progressing condition that carries considerable risk to mother and fetus.

Case history 59

A 20-year-old woman in her first pregnancy was referred to hospital by her general practitioner when she was 31 weeks pregnant. At 12 weeks pregnant she appeared well, she had no oedema and her blood pressure was 110/70 mmHg. Now, she complained that she was unable to remove her wedding ring and that her vision was blurred. On examination ankle oedema was also observed and her blood pressure was found to be 180/110 mmHg.

- What is the most likely diagnosis?
- What side room test(s) should be performed?
- What biochemical investigations should be performed immediately?
  Comment in Case history comments.

Want to know more?

http://assets.cambridge.org/97805212/68271/excerpt/9780521268271_excerpt.pdf

This article provides a useful summary of key changes that occur to maternal physiology and anatomy during pregnancy.

78 | Antenatal screening

There are approximately 700,000 pregnancies per annum in the UK and 200 to 250 million worldwide. Most result in the birth of a healthy baby, though in a few cases there may be problems affecting delivery or a baby's development. Antenatal screening is a way of assessing whether the fetus could develop, or has developed, an abnormality at conception or during pregnancy. If the risk is high, the mother may be offered prenatal diagnosis to establish the likelihood of developing the abnormality. Prior knowledge of problems can help parents plan how best to deal with them: by preparing for special care or choosing to terminate the pregnancy.

Overview of screening programmes

Most antenatal screening programmes include tests to diagnose various genetic and infectious conditions, including Down syndrome, spina bifida, sickle-cell anaemia, thalassaemia, HIV, hepatitis B, syphilis and rubella. In general they may be considered in four groups:

1. Fetal screening for Down, Edwards and Patau syndromes, and spina bifida.
2. Fetal anomaly screening by ultrasonography, usually at 18 to 20 weeks, to identify developmental abnormalities, including congenital heart defects and cleft lip, and to confirm spina bifida.
3. Sickle-cell and thalassaemia.
4. Infectious disease in pregnancy screening: HIV, hepatitis B, syphilis and rubella.

In addition, pregnant women with existing type 1 and type 2 diabetes should also be offered eye screening at, or soon after, their first antenatal visit and after 28 weeks of pregnancy.

Screening for Down, Edwards and Patau syndromes

In the UK, all pregnant women are offered screening for Down syndrome (trisomy 21), Edwards syndrome (trisomy 18) and Patau syndrome (trisomy 13) simultaneously. The first screening test estimates the probability that the fetus is affected. If it is higher than a predetermined cut-off, a second-line noninvasive prenatal test is offered. If this test also shows a higher probability of the baby having any of these conditions then a definitive diagnostic test will be offered (see later). These tests are optional – women may opt out of the process at any stage. Screening tests are not foolproof; there is a small number of false negative results, and a larger number of false-positive results, where a positive screening test is not confirmed on diagnostic testing. Fig. 78.1 outlines the screening pathway described in the following sections.

First-trimester screening

Screening for Down syndrome can be performed in either the first or second trimester. Second-trimester screening used to be routine, but higher detection and lower false-positive rates are seen when so-called 'combined' screening is performed in the first trimester, and this is now considered best practice. Combined screening includes (1) ultrasound measurement of fetal nuchal translucency, (2) maternal serum human chorionic gonadotrophin (HCG) and (3) maternal serum pregnancy-associated plasma protein A (PAPP-A). (Nuchal translucency (NT) is a measure of the amount of fluid under the skin at the back of the baby's neck – see later). The results are expressed in relation to the values obtained in unaffected pregnancies, as *multiples of the median* (MoMs). MoM is a measure of how far an individual test result deviates from the median; it is commonly used to report the results of medical screening tests.

Each of the three tests, including nuchal translucency, varies with gestation. Thus an accurate measurement of fetal maturity is required for accurate interpretation of results. For first-trimester screening, ultrasound measurement of fetal crown-rump length (CRL; Fig. 78.2), performed at the same time as the NT measurement, is used to calculate gestation.

Nuchal translucency

NT (Fig. 78.3) is the fluid-filled area at the back of the fetal neck and, at 11 to 14 weeks' gestation, measures around 1.0 mm in unaffected pregnancies. It tends to be increased in Down syndrome and can be measured to the nearest 0.1 mm by ultrasound. NT measurement is converted to a multiple of the median NT at the appropriate CRL, and a risk estimated.

NT measurements should be taken only when fetal CRL is between 45 and 84 mm (equivalent to a gestation range of 11 + 2 to 14 + 1 weeks). Before this, the fetus is too small to allow accurate NT measurement; after 14 weeks, the strength of the association between NT and fetal chromosome abnormalities is not strong enough to be used.

Biochemical tests

In Down syndrome, maternal serum HCG is increased to levels approaching twice those in unaffected pregnancies (2.0 MoM), whereas PAPP-A levels are reduced to around half the normal level (0.5 MoM); the magnitude of the deviation is maximum at earlier gestations.

Risk calculation

The MoM of NT, HCG and PAPP-A are used to calculate the risk of Down syndrome. A cut-off probability of 1 in 150 is used to define 'low risk' or 'high risk'. In approximately 2%, the risk of Down

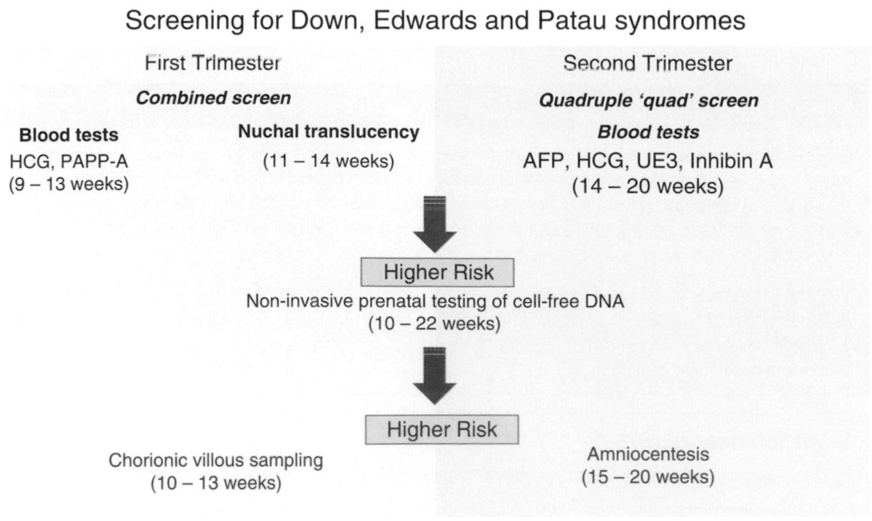

Screening for Down, Edwards and Patau syndromes

First Trimester		Second Trimester
Combined screen		**Quadruple 'quad' screen**

Blood tests	Nuchal translucency	Blood tests
HCG, PAPP-A	(11 – 14 weeks)	AFP, HCG, UE3, Inhibin A
(9 – 13 weeks)		(14 – 20 weeks)

Higher Risk

Non-invasive prenatal testing of cell-free DNA
(10 – 22 weeks)

Higher Risk

Chorionic villous sampling   Amniocentesis
(10 – 13 weeks)   (15 – 20 weeks)

Fig. 78.1 Screening for syndromes associated with trisomies of chromosome 21 (Down), 18 (Edwards) and 13 (Patau) *AFP*, Alpha-fetoprotein; *DNA*, deoxyribonucleic acid; *HCG*, human chorionic gonadotrophin; *PAPP-A*: pregnancy-associated plasma protein A; *UE3*: unconjugated oestriol; 'Weeks' refers to weeks of gestation.

syndrome from combined first-trimester screening is at least 1 in 150 ('high risk'); these women are offered further counselling and next line noninvasive testing. Where the risk is less than 1 in 150 ('low risk'), no further action is usually indicated. Maternal age is a component of the screening risk calculation, and the proportion of positive screening tests is higher in older women.

Diagnostic tests

Women whose first-trimester screening results fall in the high-risk category are offered chorionic villus sampling to test for chromosomal abnormalities. In the first trimester, this procedure carries a miscarriage rate of about 1% to 2%.

Second-trimester screening

Although first-trimester screening is preferred, some women present too late for first-trimester screening. For second-trimester screening, the maternal blood sample should be taken between 14 + 2 weeks and 20 + 0 weeks for measurement of alpha-fetoprotein (AFP), HCG, unconjugated oestriol (UE3) and inhibin A. This is known as the quadruple marker test or simply the 'quad' test. Pregnancies affected by Down syndrome have elevated levels of HCG and inhibin A (2.0 MoM), whereas AFP and UE3 are lower than normal (0.75 MoM). These results, along with maternal age, are used to calculate the risk of Down syndrome. As with first-trimester screening, a cut-off of 1 in 150 is used to define levels of risk. Approximately 3% to 4% of pregnancies are considered to be high risk, and these women are offered further counselling and next line noninvasive testing.

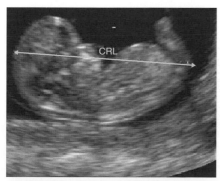

Fig. 78.2 Crown-rump length (CRL) on ultrasound.

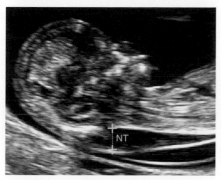

Fig. 78.3 Nuchal translucency (*NT*) on ultrasound.

Noninvasive prenatal testing

Noninvasive prenatal testing, which is also known as cell-free DNA screening, has been available in the UK since 2012, but has only relatively recently been included in the UK screening programme. It is offered to women who have a higher chance of trisomy from the first-line tests. A maternal blood sample is analysed for cell-free DNA material; most of the DNA comes from the mother but a small amount is shed by the baby's placenta. If the test result is reported as high probability of having the condition(s) then a diagnostic test will be offered.

Diagnostic tests

Women whose second-trimester screening results fall in the high-risk category are offered amniocentesis in order to exclude or identify a chromosome abnormality. Amniocentesis is associated with a risk of miscarriage of around 1%.

Other factors affecting interpretation of biochemical markers

Several factors have been identified which affect serum marker concentrations and therefore the risk estimate derived from them. Corrections for these variables may be made to provide a more accurate estimate of risk for individual women.

- *Gestation*. All of the screening tests vary with gestation, and so, as pointed out earlier, results are expressed as multiples of the appropriate *gestational* median level in unaffected pregnancies. However, this means that the accuracy of the gestational estimate is crucial. An ultrasound estimate of gestation is used in preference to that calculated from the last menstrual period.
- *Maternal weight*. Women who weigh more than 65 kg tend to have increased blood volume, resulting in a dilutional lowering of serum concentration of various markers. The opposite effect is found in women of lower than average maternal weight. The effect of maternal weight is particularly marked at the extremes of the weight range, and a correction factor is usually applied. Maternal weight has no effect on NT measurements.
- *Maternal smoking*. Smoking in pregnancy affects placental function, resulting in reduced secretion of PAPP-A, HCG and UE3, and increased secretion of AFP and inhibin A. Correction for smoking status allows for a more accurate risk calculation.
- *Assisted reproduction*. An important practical consideration in in vitro fertilisation pregnancies is that the age of the egg *donor* (if applicable) must be used to derive the maternal age risk, while for frozen embryos, the age at *conception* should be used.
- *Previous affected pregnancy with Down syndrome*. A previous pregnancy with Down syndrome increases the risk in subsequent ones. This is in addition to increased maternal age and significantly increases the probability that a screening result will fall into the high-risk category.
- *Ethnicity*. If this information is available, then the appropriate ethnic median concentration should be used to calculate the MoMs and produce a more accurate risk estimate.

Clinical note

Screening for 11 conditions is offered to all pregnant women as part of the 20-week scan; this includes neural tube defects. The latter may also be suspected when elevated maternal alpha-fetoprotein (AFP) levels are found during second-trimester screening. Elevated maternal AFP is not always due to fetal neural tube defects. Other causes include multiple pregnancy, placental disruption, liver disease or fetal or maternal tumours.

Want to know more?

https://www.gov.uk/government/publications/fetal-anomaly-screening-care-pathways

This describes the screening pathway, including noninvasive prenatal testing, for Down, Edwards, and Patau syndromes.

Antenatal screening

- Antenatal screening includes tests for Down, Edwards and Patau syndromes, spina bifida, sickle-cell anaemia, thalassaemia, HIV, hepatitis B, syphilis and rubella.
- Combined test for first-trimester screening includes ultrasound measurement of nuchal translucency (NT) and maternal serum concentrations of human chorionic gonadotrophin (HCG) and pregnancy-associated plasma protein A (PAPP-A).
- Maternal serum alpha-fetoprotein (AFP), human chorionic gonadotrophin (HCG), unconjugated oestriol (UE3) and inhibin A (quad test) are measured for second-trimester screening.
- Multiples of the median (MoMs) are calculated for each marker and, along with various other factors, used to calculate risk or probability of the baby having a chromosomal abnormality.
- If the risk is greater than or equal to 1 in 150, then the mother is offered chorionic villus sampling or amniocentesis as diagnostic tests to confirm or rule out a chromosomal abnormality. Either procedure carries an approximate 1% risk of fetal loss.

79 | Screening the newborn for disease

Neonatal screening programmes

Many countries have neonatal screening programmes for various diseases. Until recently in the UK, newborns were screened for congenital hypothyroidism, phenylketonuria (PKU), cystic fibrosis, sickle-cell disease and medium-chain acyl-CoA dehydrogenase deficiency. Four additional disorders have now been added to this list: homocystinuria, maple syrup urine disease, glutaric aciduria type 1 and isovaleric acidaemia. A capillary blood sample is collected from every baby around the seventh day of life; this is best performed on the plantar aspect of the foot (Fig. 79.1). 'Blood spots' (i.e. drops of whole blood collected in this way) are applied onto circles on a thick filter paper card known as the *Guthrie card* (Fig. 79.2). This can be sent conveniently by post to a central screening laboratory.

The following questions are usually considered when discussing the cost-effectiveness of a screening programme.

- Does the disease have a relatively high incidence?
- Can the disease be detected within days of birth?
- Can the disease be identified by a biochemical marker which can be easily measured?
- Will the disease be missed clinically, and would this cause irreversible damage to the baby?
- Is the disease treatable, and will the result of the screening test be available before any irreversible damage to the baby has occurred?

Internationally, the list of diseases screened for varies, depending on various factors, including the prevalence of each disease in the screened population. For example, the American state Alaska screens for congenital adrenal hyperplasia, due to its high prevalence in the population. Conversely, the prevalence of PKU is low in Finland and this disease is not screened for there. Other factors that determine whether diseases are included or excluded are public pressure and availability of funding, as well as debates about the benefits and risks of tests. In general, neonatal screening programmes for hypothyroidism and PKU have been established in many countries. Both of these disorders carry the risk of impaired intellectual development, which can be prevented by prompt recognition of the disease.

There is debate in the UK about whether severe combined immunodeficiency syndrome (SCID) should be added to the newborn blood spot screening programme. This is currently the subject of a pilot evaluation. There are implications beyond screening for SCID – live vaccines, e.g. BCG for tuberculosis – can cause severe side-effects in babies with SCID, and may have to be deferred if it is suspected.

Congenital hypothyroidism

Primary hypothyroidism is found in 1 in 4000 births in the UK. There is often no clinical evidence of abnormality at birth, yet if congenital hypothyroidism is unrecognised and untreated, affected children develop irreversible intellectual disability and characteristic features (Fig. 79.3). Many cases of congenital hypothyroidism are due to failure of the thyroid gland to develop properly during early embryonic growth (thyroid gland dysgenesis). The presence of a high blood thyroid-stimulating hormone (TSH) concentration is the basis of the screening

FILL ALL CIRCLES FROM THE BACK.
DO NOT DETACH FOLD OR PLACE IN A POLYTHENE BAG.

Baby Surname _____ Date of Birth _____

Lab use only

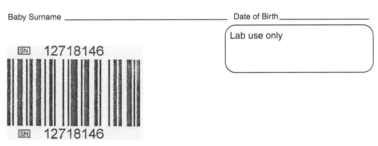

Fig. 79.2 Filter paper card for collection of 'blood spots'.

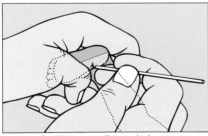

Capillary sampling techniques for neonates

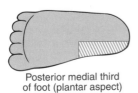

Posterior medial third of foot (plantar aspect)

Fig. 79.1 Capillary blood sampling in neonates.

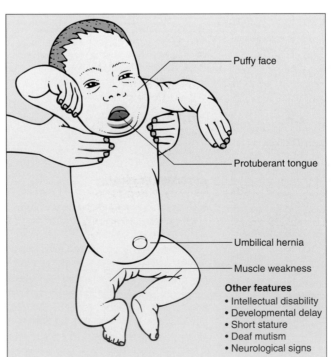

Puffy face

Protuberant tongue

Umbilical hernia

Muscle weakness

Other features
- Intellectual disability
- Developmental delay
- Short stature
- Deaf mutism
- Neurological signs

Fig. 79.3 Features of congenital hypothyroidism.

test (Fig. 79.4). In addition to congenital hypothyroidism, iodine deficiency in the mother and/or the baby may also cause babies to be hypothyroid at birth and have a high TSH on screening. It is important that these babies are not incorrectly labelled as having congenital hypothyroidism and unnecessarily treated with thyroxine for life.

A positive result of a screening test should be confirmed by demonstration of an elevated TSH in a blood sample obtained from the infant. When necessary, thyroxine treatment should be initiated as soon as possible after diagnosis. If a positive screening test is obtained, the mother's thyroid function is usually also assessed; maternal autoantibodies can cross the placenta and block receptor sites on the fetal thyroid. In this rare situation, after initial transient hypothyroidism just after birth, the baby's own thyroid function recovers and develops normally thereafter.

TSH screening does not detect *secondary* hypothyroidism due to pituitary disease, which is due to lack of TSH. However, this is much rarer than primary hypothyroidism (1 in 100,000 births).

Phenylketonuria

Phenylketonuria (PKU) is found in approximately 1 in 10,000 births in the UK. PKU arises from impaired conversion of phenylalanine to tyrosine, usually because of deficiency of phenylalanine hydroxylase. (This enzyme uses tetrahydrobiopterin (BH4) as a cofactor; rarely, deficiency of the cofactor causes the impaired activity of phenylalanine hydroxylase.) Fig. 79.5 shows how phenylalanine, an essential amino acid, is metabolised. In PKU, phenylalanine cannot be converted to tyrosine, accumulates in blood and is excreted in the urine. The main urinary metabolite is phenylpyruvic acid (a 'phenylketone'), which gives the disease its name. The clinical features include:

- irritability, poor feeding, vomiting and fitting in the first weeks of life
- intellectual disability
- eczema
- reduced melanin formation in the skin, resulting in the classic fair-haired, blue-eyed appearance.

The detection of PKU was the first screening programme to be established. The screening test is based on the detection of increased phenylalanine concentration in the blood spot.

Management of PKU

The mainstay of the management of PKU is to reduce the plasma phenylalanine concentration by dietary control. Intellectual disability is not present at birth and can be prevented from occurring if plasma phenylalanine concentrations are kept low in the early years of life. It was thought that dietary control needs to be followed for only 10 years or so, but currently lifelong therapy is advocated.

Women with PKU can have healthy children provided they maintain strict adherence to a low-phenylalanine diet throughout their pregnancy. These women should have counselling and dietary advice before becoming pregnant and should be followed in specialist clinics after conception. Poor maternal control puts the baby at risk of delayed development, intellectual disability, microcephaly, poor somatic growth and congenital defects. In case preganancy is unplanned, ideally they should always remain in good control.

Follow-up of screening tests

A positive or equivocal result in a screening test should be followed up rapidly and efficiently. A clearly positive result requires immediate referral to a paediatrician. Requests for a repeat specimen (because the result was borderline, or there was insufficient sample, or the analysis was unsatisfactory) must be handled tactfully. Parents frequently find it distressing if their child is suspected of a serious disorder, even if subsequently the baby is found to be normal.

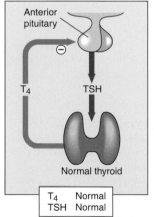
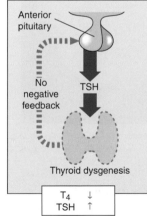

Fig. 79.4 Control of thyroid-stimulating hormone (TSH) secretion. T_4, Thyroxine.

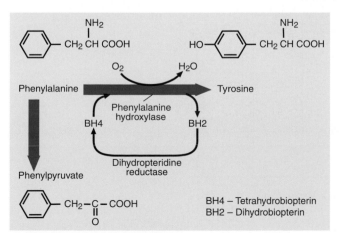

Fig. 79.5 Metabolism of phenylalanine.

BH4 – Tetrahydrobiopterin
BH2 – Dihydrobiopterin

Clinical note

N-Aspartyl phenylalanine methyl ester (aspartame) is a commonly used artificial sweetener. It is broken down in the gut to phenylalanine. Patients with phenylketonuria (PKU) must avoid any food containing this additive. It is particularly important that foodstuffs, including soft drinks, should be clearly labelled with a warning that they contain this artificial sweetener.

Screening the newborn for disease

- In some countries, screening programmes have been established to detect specific diseases in babies.
- Analyses are performed on blood spots obtained around 1 week after birth.
- Diseases commonly tested for in this way include congenital hypothyroidism and phenylketonuria (PKU).
- For it to be worthwhile to screen for a disorder, the disease should have a sufficiently high prevalence, be detectable within days of birth, result in serious consequences if missed clinically, and be treatable.

Case history 60

The 'blood spot' analysis on a 6-day-old baby girl indicated a high thyroid-stimulating hormone (TSH) (28 mU/L). A second blood sample was quickly obtained for a repeat TSH estimation. The laboratory reported a TSH concentration of 6 mU/L.

- What further investigations should be carried out?
  Comment in Case history comments.

Want to know more?

https://www.gov.uk/guidance/newborn-blood-spot-screening-programme-overview

This provides an overview of the newborn screening programme.

80 | Paediatric biochemistry

Paediatric biochemistry differs from adult biochemistry in several respects. First, profound changes in physiological maturity occur from birth through to adulthood, reflected in differences in the results of biochemical measurements. Second, the diseases of childhood are not the same as those of adulthood; genetic and developmental disorders feature much more prominently. Third, the practicalities of sample collection and processing differ significantly and pose specific challenges, e.g. small sample size.

Immaturity

Children are, by definition, immature and in a state of development. After birth, immaturity of organ systems may persist for weeks, months or even years, and accounts for several common clinical presentations (see later).

Jaundice

The liver of a newborn baby may not be capable of conjugating all of the bilirubin presented to it. Many babies become jaundiced during the first week of life. In full-term babies this usually resolves rapidly, but in premature babies it may persist. As a general rule, jaundice during the first 24 hours after birth is always pathological and often indicates increased unconjugated bilirubin resulting from haemolysis due to blood group incompatibility or infection. Similarly, jaundice that lasts more than 10 days after birth always should be investigated. It may indicate any of several clinical conditions, including galactosaemia, congenital hypothyroidism, cystic fibrosis or glucose-6-phosphate dehydrogenase deficiency.

Unconjugated bilirubin is lipophilic and can cross the blood–brain barrier and bind to proteins in the brain, where it is neurotoxic. This happens when albumin (which carries unconjugated bilirubin) becomes saturated. The clinical syndrome of bilirubin-encephalopathy is called *kernicterus*, referring to the yellow discoloration of the basal ganglia (nuclei) in the brain (Fig. 80.1), and may result in death or severe intellectual disability.

Unconjugated hyperbilirubinaemia usually arises by one or more of the following mechanisms:
a) Excess bilirubin production, e.g. increased haemolysis
b) Impaired bilirubin uptake, e.g. reduced hepatic blood flow or some medications
c) Impaired bilirubin conjugation, e.g. Criggler–Najjar syndrome.

Where the excess bilirubin is conjugated, the pathology is different, and kernicterus is not a feature since conjugated bilirubin is water-soluble rather than lipophilic and so cannot cross the blood–brain barrier. Causes include neonatal hepatitis, possibly contracted from the mother at birth; biliary atresia, resulting in severely impaired biliary drainage; and inherited deficiency of α1-antitrypsin, a protease enzyme, the absence of which is associated with liver and lung damage.

Hypoglycaemia

Before birth, the chief source of energy for the fetus is glucose obtained from the mother via the placenta. Any excess

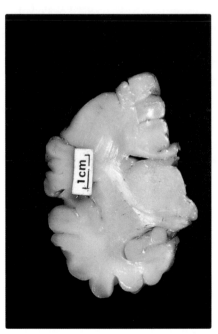

Fig. 80.1 Kernicterus. *(Reproduced with permission from Ellison D, Love S, Chimelli L, et al. Neuropathology: A Reference Text of CNS Pathology. 2nd ed. St. Louis, MO: Mosby; 2004.)*

glucose is stored as liver glycogen. Free fatty acids cross the placenta and are stored in fat tissue. At birth the baby suddenly has to switch to its own homeostatic mechanisms in order to maintain its blood glucose concentration between feeds. These include gluconeogenesis and glycogenolysis. However, glycogen stores are often insufficient, therefore transient hypoglycaemia is not uncommon in neonates. Lipolysis provides another energy source in the form of free fatty acids until feeding is established. Hypoglycaemia, including neonatal hypoglycaemia, is dealt with in Chapter 34.

Dehydration

There are very significant differences in the body composition of preterm and term infants, children, and adults (Fig. 80.2). The total body water of a newborn baby is around 75% of body weight, compared with 60% in the adult. In the first week after birth the extracellular fluid contracts, and this explains why most babies initially lose weight before gaining it back subsequently. Infants are very vulnerable to fluid loss because their renal tubular function is not fully mature. Their ability to concentrate urine (and hence retain water) is poor – the maximum urine osmolality that can be produced is about 600 mmol/kg, compared with more than 1200 mmol/kg in a healthy adult. In addition, reabsorption of bicarbonate and glucose is reduced, leading to low serum bicarbonate and glycosuria, respectively.

In general, dehydrated infants are relatively more water depleted than sodium depleted, partly because of the immature tubular function described previously, but also because their larger ratio of body

Fig. 80.2 Body composition at different stages of development. *(From Lissauer T, Carroll W. Illustrated Textbook of Paediatrics. 6th ed. Elsevier; 2022.)*

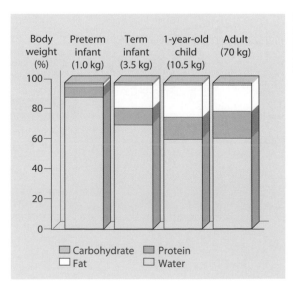

Body weight (%)	Preterm infant (1.0 kg)	Term infant (3.5 kg)	1-year-old child (10.5 kg)	Adult (70 kg)

☐ Carbohydrate ■ Protein
☐ Fat ☐ Water

surface area to body weight renders them more susceptible to insensible water loss. Monitoring of fluid balance requires regular assessment of hydration status. Short of bladder catheterisation, urine output is virtually impossible to assess with any degree of accuracy in infants, and serial body weight measurement is often used instead as a cruder way of monitoring trends in hydration.

Prematurity

Prematurity presents an even more extreme challenge to organ function. A good example of organ failure resulting from prematurity is respiratory distress syndrome. Babies born before 32 weeks gestation cannot make their own pulmonary surfactant, resulting in respiratory distress syndrome due to failure of alveolar expansion. Measurement of the lecithin/sphingomyelin ratio was used in the past to assess fetal lung maturity but has largely been supplanted by the advent of surfactant therapy. Fig. 80.3 illustrates the role of surfactant.

Practical considerations

- *Sampling.* Although venepuncture is preferred in older children, heel-prick sampling is less traumatic for very young children. Heel puncture can, rarely, be complicated by calcaneal osteomyelitis, and other sites of collection may be used instead.
- *Sample volume.* This is a major issue for paediatric biochemistry laboratories. A premature baby weighing less than 1000 g may have as little as 75 mL total blood volume (compared with 5 L in an adult). The sample volume must, therefore, be kept to an absolute minimum. At low sample volumes, e.g. 100 μL, evaporation from uncovered specimens can alter results of analyses by as much as 10% in 1 hour.
- *Plasma or serum.* In most laboratories that process paediatric specimens, plasma is preferred. The turnaround time is reduced because clotting does not have to occur before centrifuging the sample. In addition, there is generally less haemolysis.
- *Interferences.* Haemolysis increases plasma concentrations of potassium and some other analytes that are present in higher concentrations in red blood cells than in extracellular fluid. Hyperbilirubinaemia can interfere with creatinine measurement.
- *Instrumentation.* Automated analysers must be chosen with sample size in

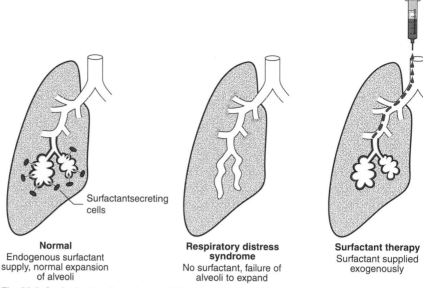

Normal
Endogenous surfactant supply, normal expansion of alveoli

Respiratory distress syndrome
No surfactant, failure of alveoli to expand

Surfactant therapy
Surfactant supplied exogenously

Surfactantsecreting cells

Fig. 80.3 Surfactant and respiratory distress syndrome.

mind, as well as the 'dead volume' (the amount of sample that must remain in the sample cup after the sample has been aspirated for analysis); both of these should be kept to a minimum. Common interferences should, ideally, not affect results. Some analysers make use of dry slide technology to prevent interferences.

Clinical note

Newborn babies have low levels of vitamin K, which is required for synthesis of blood coagulation factors. To minimise the risk of intracerebral haemorrhage, it has been recommended that all newborn babies, particularly those who are breast-fed, be given this vitamin.

Paediatric biochemistry

- Jaundice is common in babies in the first week of life. In term babies, this usually resolves rapidly. Jaundice during the first 24 hours of life is nearly always pathological.
- Neonatal hypoglycaemia is commonly encountered in the premature infant, the 'small-for-dates' baby or the infant of a diabetic mother.
- Relative to adults, babies have increased total body water and extracellular water. Renal function changes with age. Guidelines for fluid and electrolyte replacement therapy in babies are quite different from those in adults.
- Respiratory distress syndrome results from lack of pulmonary surfactant, which prevents expansion and aeration of pulmonary alveoli.

Case history 61

The baby of a diabetic mother weighed 1.64 kg (below 10th centile for weight) when born at gestational age of 32 weeks. The baby was well at birth, but her condition deteriorated within hours, and she had respiratory problems.

- What biochemical determinations should be requested on this baby?
- Why is it important to consider each request carefully?
  Comment in Case history comments.

Want to know more?

https://www.nps.org.au/australian-prescriber/articles/interpreting-paediatric-biochemistry-results
This article is a simple and basic guide to interpreting paediatric biochemistry results.

81 | Inborn errors of metabolism

The spectrum of genetic disorders is enormous. It encompasses *chromosomal* disorders, as well as many *polygenic* diseases in which multiple genes confer susceptibility to the effects of environmental influences. 'Classic' genetic diseases are *monogenic*, resulting from single-gene mutations that result in either reduced synthesis of a particular protein or synthesis of a defective protein. In 1909, Garrod first defined the concept of *inborn errors of metabolism*, in which blocks in specific metabolic pathways result from defects in particular enzymes. Certainly, in most inborn errors, the defective or absent protein is an enzyme; exceptions include familial hypercholesterolaemia, cystinuria and Hartnup disease, in which the affected proteins are either receptors or are otherwise involved in transport processes.

Patterns of inheritance

Inborn errors can be autosomal (involving a chromosome other than X or Y) or X-linked, and the genetic defect can be either dominant or recessive. In dominant disorders, everyone who carries the gene is affected by the disease, so every affected individual has at least one affected parent. If the defective gene is recessive, it will be silent unless both copies (maternal and paternal) of the gene carry the mutation, i.e. affected individuals must be homozygous; parents carrying only one copy of the affected gene are heterozygotes and are not clinically affected (they are *carriers*). These patterns of inheritance are illustrated in Fig. 81.1.

Establishing pedigrees may not be straightforward. One reason for this is that the severity of the disease can vary widely among individuals even within the same family. Sometimes the clinical manifestations may be so mild that the disease cannot be detected, even though the defective gene is present. When this occurs the disease is said to be *nonpenetrant*. Thus, dominant diseases may clinically appear to 'skip' generations.

Mechanisms of disease

Inborn errors of metabolism can manifest clinically through a variety of mechanisms:
- accumulation of substrate of the defective enzyme
- reduced product
- diversion of intermediates
- failure of negative feedback
- failure of transport mechanisms.

These mechanisms are shown in Fig. 81.2.

Clinical diagnosis

Several problems confront the clinician suspecting an inborn error of metabolism. First, the clinical presentation is often nonspecific. In an infant, the symptoms may include poor feeding, lethargy and vomiting, which are seen with any significant illness; in older children, failure to thrive or developmental delay may be the only presentation. Second, the range of specialist tests used to diagnose inborn errors is extensive and, for many, bewildering. Useful clues that should increase the index of suspicion include:
- parents are cousins (so-called *consanguineous mating*)
- history of unexplained premature death in an older sibling
- onset of symptoms following change in feeding regimen
- dysmorphic features
- unusual odour (Table 81.1).

Autosomal dominant

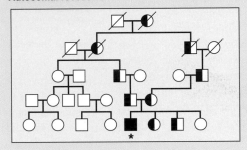

The second copy of the gene on the homologous chromosome cannot compensate for the mutated copy:
- Consecutive generations affected
- Half of offspring affected, male = female
- Unaffected individual cannot transmit disease

Autosomal recessive

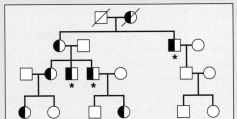

The second copy of the gene on the homologous chromosome compensates for the mutated copy:
- Unaffected carrier individuals transmit disease
- If both parents are carriers, then one-quarter of their offspring are affected, and one-half are carriers
- Usually only one generation is affected – denoted by *
Affected individuals may have two identical mutant copies arising from a common ancestor as shown, or copies of two different mutations in 'compound heterozygotes'

X-linked recessive

A second copy of the gene is only present in females. In X-linked recessive disease:
- Males only are affected - denoted by *
- Unaffected female carriers transmit the disease
- Half of a female carrier's offspring will inherit the mutation - the males who do are affected, and the females who do are carriers.
- Affected males cannot transmit the disease to their sons, but all of their daughters are carriers

Fig. 81.1 Patterns of inheritance.

One useful classification of inborn errors includes both clinical and laboratory features (Table 81.2).

Laboratory diagnosis

Clearly, if there is a clinical basis for suspecting a particular inborn error of metabolism, specific investigations should be requested. For example, the presence of cataracts should make one suspect galactosaemia, for which the appropriate investigation is measurement of galactose-1-phosphate uridyl transferase in red blood cells. More often, however, there are no specific features. Routine laboratory investigations may help point the direction of further investigations by suggesting particular groups of metabolic

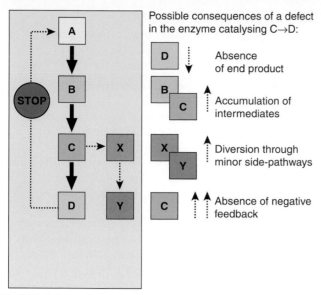

Possible consequences of a defect in the enzyme catalysing C→D:

D ⋯↓ Absence of end product

B / C ⋮↑ Accumulation of intermediates

X / Y ⋮↑ Diversion through minor side-pathways

C ⋮↑↑ Absence of negative feedback

Fig. 81.2 Pathogenic mechanisms resulting from enzyme deficiency.

Table 81.1 Inborn errors of metabolism associated with characteristic smells due to volatile organic intermediates

Inborn error of metabolism	Smell
Maple syrup urine disease	Maple syrup
Phenylketonuria	Musty
Isovaleric acidaemia	Sweaty feet or cheese
Trimethylaminuria	Fish
Hypermethioninaemia	Cabbage

Table 81.2 Classification of inborn errors of metabolism on basis of clinical and laboratory features

Presentation	Most likely diagnoses
'Intoxication', ketoacidosis	Maple syrup urine disease (amino acid disorder)
'Intoxication', ketoacidosis	Organic acid disorders
'Energy deficiency', lactic acidosis	Congenital lactic acidosis
'Intoxication', high ammonia, no ketoacidosis	Urea cycle defects
'Energy deficiency', no metabolic disturbance	Peroxisomal disorders Nonketotic hyperglycinaemia
Storage disorders, no metabolic disturbance	Lysosomal storage diseases
Hypoglycaemia, hepatomegaly, abnormal liver function tests	Glycogen storage diseases

'Intoxication' and 'energy deficiency' are contrasting clinical manifestations of neurological distress in the neonatal period. 'Intoxication' is characterised by a symptom-free interval, then onset of lethargy or coma. 'Energy deficiency' is often associated with hypotonia and dysmorphic features. Lethargy and coma are rarely the initial signs, and often there is no symptom-free interval.

Table 81.3 Biochemical investigations that may help direct further investigations

Test	Comment
Urinalysis	
Reducing substances	Positive for reducing substances but not for glucose: suspect galactosaemia.
Ketones	Strongly positive: suspect hypoglycaemia (see later) Relative hypoketosis, despite hypoglycaemia or fasting: suspect a disorder of fatty acid oxidation.
pH	pH <5.5 excludes renal tubular acidosis as cause of metabolic acidosis and points to an organic acid disorder.
Blood	
High anion gap metabolic acidosis	High anion gap metabolic acidosis (>20 mmol/L): suspect an organic acid disorder.
Hypoglycaemia	Relatively nonspecific – found in normal neonates, and compatible with many inborn errors of metabolism: fatty acid oxidation defects organic acid disorders amino acid disorders glycogen storage disorders galactosaemia.
Hyponatraemia	If found with ambiguous genitalia: suspect congenital adrenal hyperplasia.
Respiratory alkalosis	If found with neurological distress: suspect urea cycle disorder.
Abnormal liver function tests	Relatively nonspecific: consistent with galactosaemia glycogen storage disorders tyrosinaemia α1-antitrypsin deficiency.
Hyperammonaemia	Significantly high plasma ammonia: strongly suspect urea cycle disorders or organic acid disorder.

- *Plasma lactate.* Should be measured especially if there is acidosis, hypoglycaemia or neurological distress. This test is readily available in most laboratories.
- *Galactose-1-phosphate uridyl transferase.* Unusual in this list in being specific to one disorder (galactosaemia). However, this is easily treated by excluding galactose from the diet, is frequently fatal if unrecognised (especially in neonates) and is sufficiently common that it is included in some population screening programmes.

Selected inborn errors of metabolism are listed in Chapter 84.

Clinical note

Making the diagnosis of an inborn error postmortem is not pointless; it may permit genetic counselling and may save the life of a future sibling. Where possible, blood and urine samples should be collected after discussion with a specialist laboratory. Inborn errors are also diagnosed sometimes using samples of skin, liver or vitreous humour.

disorders (Table 81.3). In the acute situation, in the absence of clues, the following investigations always should be considered and performed urgently if indicated:

- *Plasma ammonia.* Indicated particularly when there is neurological distress/intoxication; grossly elevated levels are most frequently due to urea cycle disorders.
- *Organic acids (urine)* and *amino acids (urine and plasma).* Organic and amino acid disorders collectively make up a large group of inborn errors of metabolism.

Want to know more?

http://www.vademetab.org/

The 'Vademecum Metabolicum' contains far more information about inborn errors of metabolism (IEM) than you need at undergraduate level. It is essentially a highly rated IEM handbook. It is available as an application for download.

82 | Methods involving antibodies: immunoassay

This focus of this book has been deliberately clinical, apart from a brief chapter on analytical aspects (Chapter 6) at the end of the first section. In this chapter and the next, we provide a brief introduction to some of the ways in which biochemical analytes are measured. The purpose of these chapters is to provide some insight into how the results of investigations are generated, as well as some of the practical challenges involved.

Immunoassays

In this chapter we describe some of the methods that use antibodies to measure analytes, or *immunoassays*. Immunoassays are used to measure a whole range of analytes; for example, many hormones are routinely measured in this way. The property of antibodies that is exploited for this purpose is their ability to recognise and bind to antigens. The key feature of this recognition is its *specificity*. (The term is used here in essentially the same way as it was in Chapter 6, but in a very different sense from the way it was used in Chapter 3.)

Many of the antibodies used in immunoassay are *polyclonal*. These are not quite identical to each other but share a common specificity. They are raised by injecting the antigen of interest into another species and isolating the antibodies produced in response. Thus, immunoassays may involve antibodies from mice, sheep, goats, etc. Others are *monoclonal*. The ability to engineer the production of antibodies of desired specificity from a single clone of cells was a huge breakthrough in medicine that still resonates today.

The history of immunoassay as we know it goes back to the 1960s, when the first generation of immunoassays were developed. The significance of this cannot be overstated. Several fields of medicine, for example, endocrinology, were transformed, since these new assays allowed hormones to be measured at concentrations that were much smaller than anything that had previously been possible.

An immunoassay that is widely used in the current generation of clinical biochemistry analysers is shown in Fig. 82.1. It is known as a *sandwich chemiluminescent immunoassay*. The term 'sandwich' is used because the analyte of interest (the 'antigen' in Fig. 82.1) is sandwiched between two antibodies. One of these (the 'capture' antibody) is immobilised on a solid phase, where it binds the analyte in proportion to its concentration in the sample. A second antibody (the 'detection' antibody), carrying the chemiluminescent label, and recognising a different part (*epitope*) of the analyte molecule, then binds to the analyte. The label on the second antibody is what is detected at the end of the assay. The key point is that the label is detected *in proportion to the concentration of analyte* in the sample. The solid phase simply acts to facilitate the *separation* of the bound label which will be detected, from the unbound label in the assay solution.

Nephelometry

Nephelometry (Fig. 82.2) represents a specific form of immunoassay, based on the principle that a suspension of small particles will scatter light passed through it rather than simply absorb it. The amount of light scatter can be measured and compared to the amount of scatter from assay mixtures with known concentrations of analyte. The unknown amount of analyte is then read off a *standard curve*. The light source is usually a laser.

Although nephelometry represents a cruder application of the antigen–antibody reaction than the sandwich immunoassay described previously, it is relatively easy to automate, and is widely used. For example, the total levels of each immunoglobulin class (IgG, IgA, IgM) are often measured in this way. (This is a special case where the antigen of interest also happens to be an antibody itself).

Immunoassay interference

Sometimes immunoassay results do not make sense. When this occurs, the possibility of immunoassay interference, leading to false results, should be considered. This can happen when the patient has antibodies that interfere with the assay. Fig. 82.3 illustrates two ways in which interference can occur. Fig. 82.3A shows the kind of sandwich immunoassay illustrated in Fig. 82.1. In Fig. 82.3B, a cross-reacting antibody from the patient manages to act as a sandwich connecting the capture and detection antibodies, in the absence of the antigen of interest (i.e. what is being measured). This causes *positive interference* – the result will be falsely *higher* than the true result. In Fig. 82.3C, an antibody from the patient does the opposite – it blocks the antigen-binding site of the capture

Nephelometry

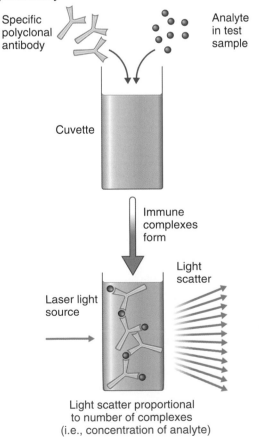

Nephelometry

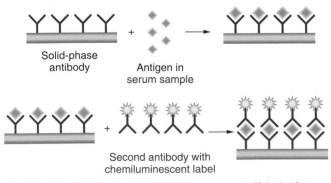

Fig. 82.1 Chemiluminescent sandwich immunoassay. *(Adapted from Jandreski MA. Chemiluminescence technology in immunoassays.* Lab Med. *1998;29(9):555–560.)*

Fig. 82.2 Principles of nephelometry. *(Modified from Turgeon ML.* Immunology and Serology in Laboratory Medicine. *6th ed. Elsevier; 2018.)*

antibody, thereby preventing the antigen of interest from binding. This causes *negative interference* – the result will be falsely *lower* than the true result.

The prevalence of interfering antibodies in patients is unclear. As indicated earlier, immunoassay interference should be considered when results contradict the clinical impression – or indeed each other. For example, the results of analysis of free thyroxine (T_4), and thyroid-stimulating hormone (TSH), are sometimes discrepant. Consider an example: free T_4 result 32 pmol/L (reference interval 10–22 pmol/L), and TSH 7.2 mU/L (reference interval 0.4–4.0 mU/L) on the same sample. The free T_4 result appears to suggest hyperthyroidism, the TSH appears to suggest hypothyroidism. In this situation, immunoassay interference with one or other of the assays might explain the opposing results. In practice, a hospital biochemistry laboratory will usually send the sample for measurement by an immunoassay that uses different antibodies to those used in its own immunoassay.

Immunofixation

We have seen previously in Chapter 26 that in multiple myeloma, there is gross overproduction of a specific immunoglobulin molecule by a single

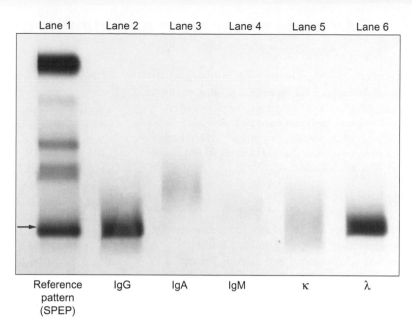

Fig. 82.4 **Immunofixation of an Ig paraprotein.** *(From Clarke W, Marzinke MA, eds. Contemporary Practice in Clinical Chemistry. 4th ed. Elsevier; 2020.)*

clone of cells. One of the key investigations in suspected myeloma is protein electrophoresis, and where the suspicion of immunoglobulin overproduction is confirmed by the finding of a paraprotein band, as shown in Fig. 26.3B, the specific identity of the immunoglobulin is confirmed by *immunofixation*. In this process, antibody to each of the immunoglobulin heavy and light chains, is applied to specific electrophoresis lanes.

In the example of immunofixation shown in Fig. 82.4, the paraprotein band is shown by the arrow. Antibody to IgG is applied in lane 2, antibody to IgA in lane 3, and so on as shown. In this way, the paraprotein is shown to be an IgGλ.

Immunoassay: labels, formats and applications

It is beyond the scope of this chapter to describe the wide range of labels, immunoassay formats and applications.

For example, the chemiluminescent label shown in Fig. 82.1 is just one of many that have been used in immunoassays. In the original immunoassays, the labels were radioactive isotopes (hence *radioimmunoassay*), but these are no longer widely used. The applications are likewise varied, ranging from point of care pregnancy tests and lateral flow covid tests through to measurements of many different hormones and drugs.

Immunoassays and assay interference

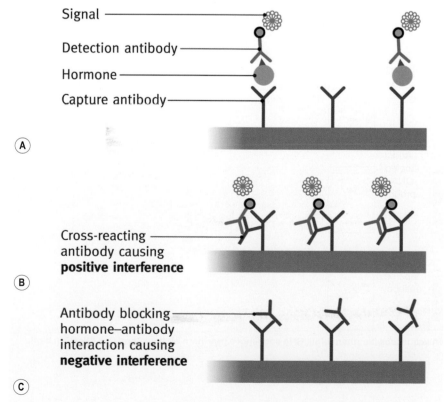

Want to know more?

For the reader who would like to learn more about immunoassay, this short article is a good starting point – short and accessible, and, importantly, lavishly illustrated.

http://booksite.elsevier.com/9780080970370/immunoassay.php

This article, by César Milstein, outlines the development of the ideas that led to the design of monoclonal antibodies:

https://www.jstor.org/stable/pdf/24966435.pdf?refreqid=excelsior%3A3e41a7e7af874851a9bca42f8d63888f&ab_segments=&origin=&acceptTC=1

Fig. 82.3 **Mechanisms of immunoassay interference due to antibodies in patient's blood.** *(From David SC, David JH. The endocrine laboratory. Medicine. 2013;41(9):489–490.)*

83 | Methods to separate and identify molecules

As pointed out at the beginning of this book, the workload of biochemistry departments is conventionally divided into the 'core' repertoire, where high volumes of samples are processed efficiently by automated analysers, and specialised tests, which often require sample processing before they can be analysed. In this chapter we will consider some of the techniques that are widely used to separate and identify molecules.

Electrophoresis

Electrophoresis is widely used in research and routine settings. Fig. 83.1 shows different 'blotting' techniques that use electrophoresis to separate molecules of interest before their identification. Molecules differ in their charge/mass ratio, and so move at different rates in an electric field – this is how they are separated. 'Blotting' denotes the transfer of separated molecules from one medium to another. Southern, Northern and Western blotting were all developed, in that order, within a few years of each other in the 1970s. (Sir Edwin Southern developed and gave his name to the first of these techniques; the 'compass point' nomenclature was an easy way to distinguish very similar techniques, and has stuck.) The key point is that each technique separates and identifies a different class of molecule – DNA, RNA and proteins.

Because they are labour-intensive and time-consuming, blotting techniques are mostly confined to research. In hospital biochemistry laboratories, electrophoresis is most commonly used to investigate protein disorders. For example, we saw in Chapter 26 how it is used to investigate suspected immunoglobulin disorders including multiple myeloma. It can also be used to diagnose deficiency of proteins, e.g. alpha-1-antitrypsin deficiency.

Chromatography

The term *chromatography* derives from the Greek words for 'colour' and 'write'; it was originally used to separate plant pigments, which were identified on the basis of colour. In a wide variety of subsequent adaptations, colour has rarely been used to identify the separated substances, but the label has persisted nevertheless. All forms of chromatography involve a *stationary phase* which is most often a column, and a *mobile phase* which is gas or liquid (hence the terms *gas chromatography* (GC) and *liquid chromatography* (LC)). The sample is dissolved in the mobile phase, which is passed through the stationary phase, and collected at the other end. The substances to be separated have different affinities for the stationary phase and so are retained for different lengths of time before they emerge (*elute*) from the other end of the column.

Different forms of chromatography exploit different properties, e.g. molecular size, in order to separate substances. Some of these are illustrated in Fig. 83.2. The separated substances in the mixture being eluted off the column are then identified by detection systems, which likewise utilise physical properties; sometimes the mixture is physically transformed by, for example, burning or evaporation before detection, e.g. flame photometry.

Mass spectrometry

Mass spectrometry (MS) is one of the most widely used detection systems linked to chromatography. It can be used to quantify known analytes, but also to identify unknown compounds. This makes it a very versatile and powerful tool. It can be linked with GC or LC, further enhancing its versatility. (The abbreviations are GC-MS and LC-MS, respectively.)

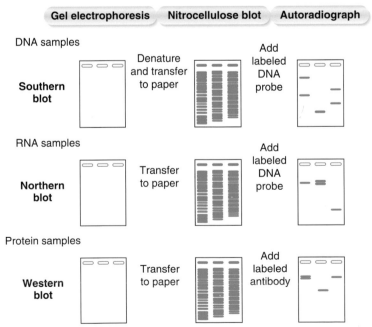

Fig. 83.1 Blotting analysis can detect specific DNA sequences (Southern blot), RNA sequences (Northern blot) and proteins (Western blot). *(From Pelley JW, Goljan EF. Rapid Review Biochemistry. 3rd ed. Mosby Elsevier; 2011.)*

Adsorption chromatography
Separation based on adsorption of
chemicals to the surface of a support

Partition chromatography
Separation based on partitioning of chemicals
into a layer of the stationary phase

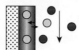

Ion-exchange chromatography
Separation of ions based on their binding to
fixed charges on a support

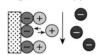

Size-exclusion chromatography
Separation of chemicals based on their size
and ability to enter a porous support

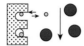

Affinity chromatography
Separation of chemicals based on their interactions
with a biologically related binding agent

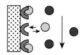

Fig. 83.2 Main types of liquid chromatography based on their separation mechanisms. *(From Hage DS, Rifai N, Wittwer CT, Burnham CAD, Young I, Chiu RWK.* Tietz Textbook of Laboratory Medicine. *7th ed. Elsevier; 2023.)*

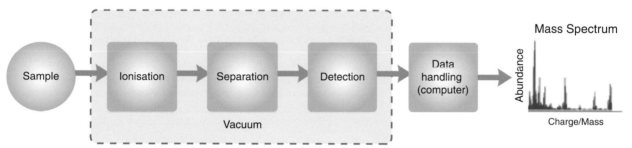

Fig. 83.3 The main elements of mass spectometry.

Fig. 83.3 illustrates the main elements of MS. The first step is the introduction of the sample, in the form of a gas. If LC has been used for the initial separation, the sample (which will have come off the column as a liquid eluate) is made suitable for introduction, by nebulising and/or evaporation.

The second step is the bombardment of the sample with electrons. This has two consequences. First, the molecules of interest in the sample become ionised (indeed this step is usually referred to as the ionisation step). Second, they fragment, and the fragments become ionised too. This step thus generates from each 'parent' molecule a whole series of ionised fragments varying in size and abundance.

The third and fourth steps are the separation and detection of the ionised molecules and molecular fragments. Separation is on the basis of charge/mass ratio, and the molecules and fragments are detected in proportion to their abundance. The final output of the mass spectrometer is a *mass spectrum* of each molecule, which plots the ion abundance against charge/mass ratio. The mass spectrum of each parent molecule is unique.

For some applications, two mass spectrometers are joined together, with an area in between where molecules can be fragmented. The first MS step effectively 'purifies' the molecule(s) of interest, based on their molecular mass. The second then allows a further refinement of separation/identification. This arrangement, called *tandem mass spectrometry*, is used where complex mixtures of similar molecules are being studied.

Clinical note

The first fully functioning mass spectrometer was built in 1919 at the Cavendish Laboratory in Cambridge by Francis Aston.

84 | Selected inherited disorders

Selected inherited disorders are summarised in Table 84.1.

Table 84.1 **Selected inherited disorders**

Disorder	Main Feature
Acute intermittent porphyria	The porphyrias are disorders of haem biosynthesis. The acute porphyrias, which present with abdominal pain and neurological features, all have increased urinary porphobilinogen during an attack, and this is diagnostic.
Adrenoleucodystrophy	This rare neurodegenerative disease is characterised by impaired metabolism and accumulation of very-long-chain fatty acids in plasma and tissues, and adrenal insufficiency.
Agammaglobulinaemia	There is a complete absence of immunoglobulin production. There are variants, e.g. selective immunoglobulin A deficiency – this is more common in children and typically presents as recurrent respiratory infections.
α1-Antitrypsin deficiency	Patients with deficiency of this protease inhibitor may present with liver disease in childhood or with pulmonary emphysema in adults. All patients with genotypes associated with low α-1-antitrypsin in serum are more likely to develop emphysema if they smoke or are exposed to environmental pollutants.
Biotinidase deficiency	A failure of biotin recycling results in an organic aciduria, developmental delay, seizures, alopecia, skin rash, hypotonia and hearing and vision loss.
Cystic fibrosis	This autosomal recessive condition is relatively common (1 : 1600 Caucasian births); approximately 1 : 22 of the population are carriers. The defective protein is cystic fibrosis transmembrane conductance regulator, which regulates the function of a bicarbonate/chloride exchanger. It results in accumulation of thick, sticky mucus in the lungs and gut, leading to frequent respiratory infections and poor growth.
Cystinuria	An increased excretion of the dibasic amino acids cystine, lysine, arginine and ornithine leads to an increased incidence of renal calculi. A defective carrier protein causes impaired renal tubular reabsorption of these amino acids from the glomerular filtrate.
Cystinosis	This is a lysosomal storage disorder in which there is a defect in the membrane transport of cystine. Cystine crystals are deposited in kidney, liver, spleen, bone marrow and cornea.
Fatty acid oxidation defects	The commonest defect is medium chain acyl-CoA dehydrogenase (MCAD) deficiency. It is caused by a defect in β-oxidation of fatty acids in mitochondria and is a major cause of hypoketotic hypoglycaemia, especially after periods of fasting or increased energy expenditure. The enzyme block also results in accumulation of fatty acid intermediates that inhibit gluconeogenesis and cause hepatic dysfunction, metabolic acidosis and hyperammonaemia.
Galactosaemia	This is due to a deficiency of galactose 1-phosphate uridyl transferase. It is present in approximately 1 : 100,000 babies in the UK. The baby cannot utilise the galactose component of the lactose in milk. Such infants may present with failure to thrive, vomiting and diarrhoea and if untreated may die in the neonatal period or go on to develop liver disease, intellectual disability, cataracts and renal tubular damage.
Glucose-6-phosphate dehydrogenase deficiency	This is an X-linked disorder associated with neonatal jaundice on the second or third day of life and drug-induced haemolytic crises.
Glycogen storage disease (Type I: von Gierke's)	(There are several glycogen storage diseases which differ according to which enzyme in glycogen breakdown is affected, and the severity of the deficiency.) Deficiency of glucose-6-phosphatase (von Gierke's) makes the glycogen stores of the body inaccessible. Children with this disorder have hepatomegaly and hypoglycaemia accompanied by hyperlipidaemia and lactic acidosis.
Homocystinuria	A deficiency of the enzyme cystathionine synthase leads to the accumulation of sulphur-containing amino acids. Affected children are normal at birth but develop eye problems, osteoporosis and intellectual disability.
Lesch–Nyhan syndrome	This is a severe form of hypoxanthine–guanine phosphoribosyltransferase deficiency, an enzyme involved in the metabolism of the purine bases resulting in delayed motor development, bizarre sinuous movements and self-mutilation.
Maple syrup urine disease	This defect in the decarboxylation of branched chain amino acids such as leucine, isoleucine and valine leads to severe brain damage and, if untreated, death during the first year of life.
Mucopolysaccharidoses	This group of disorders is characterised by tissue accumulation of glycosaminoglycans such as heparan sulphate and dermatan sulphate. This results in skeletal deformities, organomegaly, intellectual disability and premature death.
Propionic acidaemia	This is a type of organic acidaemia caused by deficiency of enzyme propionyl-CoA carboxylase, resulting in hyperammonaemia and metabolic acidosis, which may be life threatening.
Urea cycle defects	Deficiency of enzymes of the urea cycle results in a build-up of ammonia in the blood, which can rapidly reach very high concentrations and result in irreversible neurological damage and death. Severe cases are often fatal in the first few days after birth.

Case history comments

Case history 1

The delay in transporting the specimen to the laboratory was not known to the laboratory staff, and the pattern of results obtained (serum urea = 11.8 mmol/L, sodium = 130 mmol/L and potassium = 6.7 mmol/L) suggested that the patient may be sodium depleted with prerenal uraemia and hyperkalaemia. This pattern, if correct, is typical of Addison's disease, an endocrine emergency. However, a delay in separating the serum from the clot makes the potassium and sodium concentrations unreliable as these ions move out of and into the erythrocytes along their concentration gradients. Thus, another specimen is required to establish the patient's true electrolyte status.

Case history 2

After 2 days or so, the kidneys would adapt to the decreased input and would conserve sodium, potassium and water. However, he will continue to lose water insensibly and as a result the intracellular fluid (ICF) and extracellular fluid (ECF) will contract in equal proportion. After 3 to 4 days the contraction will become critical, when the ECF may be insufficient to maintain the circulation and, if not corrected, will lead to death.

Many individuals in this situation will also be severely injured, with significant blood loss. This would obviously further compromise the ECF volume and would make survival unlikely.

Case history 3

The clinical history and these urea and electrolyte values are typical of dilutional hyponatraemia. Her normal blood pressure and serum urea and creatinine concentrations make sodium depletion unlikely as the mechanism of her hyponatraemia. The absence of oedema excludes a significant increase in her total body sodium. These results are characteristic of the so-called syndrome of inappropriate antidiuresis (SIAD) and are due to secretion of arginine vasopressin (AVP) in response to nonosmotic stimuli. The ectopic production of AVP is extremely rare even in patients with malignant disease. The urine osmolality signifies less than maximally dilute urine, i.e. impaired water excretion, which is in keeping with SIAD. However, it is equally consistent with sodium depletion (the hypovolaemia resulting from sodium and water loss is a powerful nonosmotic stimulus to AVP secretion). In any case, maximally dilute urine (≤50 mmol/kg) is clinically obvious – it is associated with urine flow rates in excess of 500 mL/hour. Thus, measurement of urine osmolality usually adds little to the diagnosis of hyponatraemia.

Case history 4

This is a classic presentation of severe sodium and water depletion with clinical evidence (hypotension, tachycardia, weakness) and biochemical evidence (prerenal uraemia with a significant increase in the serum urea and a modest increase in serum creatinine) of severe contraction of the ECF volume. It is worth noting that the serum sodium concentration is a very poor guide to the presence, or absence, of sodium depletion. This patient requires both sodium and water as a matter of urgency. In view of his gastrointestinal symptoms, this will need to be given intravenously as a 0.9% sodium chloride solution.

Case history 5

The biochemical results strongly suggest prerenal uraemia, as there is a marked increase in the serum urea with a very modest increase in the serum creatinine. He has severe hypernatraemia, and these two observations would indicate that the patient is primarily suffering from water depletion. The serum potassium is normal, as is his anion gap. These results would, therefore, indicate the presence of profound uncomplicated water depletion.

In cases such as this, it is essential to exclude nonketotic, diabetic, precoma status. His blood glucose was 9.2 mmol/L, which excludes this diagnosis. Ketones were not detected, nor did he have acidosis. It was rapidly established from the clinical history that the man had not eaten or drunk for more than 3 days. A diagnosis of pure water depletion was therefore established on the basis of the history, clinical findings and biochemical features.

Case history 6

It would be unusual for her blood pressure to be this high if she was taking her prescribed medication. The first thing that should be done is to check compliance. Assuming she is compliant, renal artery stenosis should be considered, particularly given the history of vascular disease. This is best detected using imaging (e.g. magnetic resonance angiography), although grossly elevated renin may be helpful in the diagnosis. In this case the hypokalaemia results from the increased mineralocorticoid activity. Causes of this, e.g. Conn's and Cushing's syndromes, must be excluded.

Case history 7

This woman displays features of sodium depletion; she is also likely to have a mild degree of water depletion. The evidence for sodium depletion is her progressive weakness, prerenal uraemia and hyponatraemia. Although her glomerular filtration rate (GFR) has decreased, her tubular function appears satisfactory, as demonstrated by her ability to produce a concentrated urine and conserve urine sodium. This woman received inadequate intravenous fluid therapy postoperatively. Her treatment regimen was especially deficient in sodium, which led to a contraction of her ECF and caused her to develop prerenal uraemia. The contraction in her ECF will also have stimulated AVP secretion, and thus she conserved water and became even more hyponatraemic. The contraction in her ECF also stimulated aldosterone secretion, which caused her renal tubules to conserve sodium (and water).

Ideally, in order to prescribe appropriate fluid therapy for this woman, one needs to estimate her sodium, potassium and water deficits from her fluid balance charts. Particular note must be taken of losses that are relatively rich in sodium, such as drainage fluid, losses from fistulae, stomas or by nasogastric aspiration. Insensible water loss and urinary losses also must be taken into account.

Case history 8

The creatinine clearance is calculated using the following formula in which U is the urine creatinine concentration, V is the urine flow rate and P is the plasma or serum creatinine concentration. Because there are 1440 minutes in a day, in this case the man's urine flow rate, $V = 2160/1440 = 1.5$ mL/min. His urinary creatinine must be in the same units as his serum creatinine. His urinary creatinine concentration:

$U = 7.5$ mmol/L $= 7500$ µmol/L. His serum creatinine: $P = 150$ µmol/L.

Thus,

$$\frac{UV}{P} = \frac{7500 \times 15}{150} = 75\,mL/min$$

This is low for a young male.

When it was discovered that the urine collection was for 17 hours and not 24 hours, his urine flow rate was recalculated (2160/1020):

$$V = 2.1\,mL/min$$

Recalculating his creatinine clearance:

$$\frac{UV}{P} = \frac{7500 \times 2.1}{150} = 105\,mL/min$$

This is in the range one would expect in a young male. One can see, therefore, how errors in the timing and collection of urine significantly influence the calculation of the creatinine clearance. Errors in collection are by far the most common and serious errors encountered when estimating the creatinine clearance. This is one of the reasons why this test is not widely performed any more.

Case history 9

One can make a confident diagnosis of central diabetes insipidus from the history of head trauma and the observation that she was producing large volumes of urine and complaining of thirst. Her blood glucose level excludes diabetes mellitus as a cause of her polyuria, and her hypernatraemia accounts for her thirst. In normal circumstances a serum sodium concentration of 150 mmol/L will stimulate AVP production and cause the urine to be maximally concentrated. This patient's urine is, therefore, inappropriately dilute. It would be unnecessary and even dangerous to attempt to perform a water deprivation test on this patient. Note that her serum urea is not increased. This reflects her high urine flow rate despite her significant water depletion.

Case history 10

The patient is on a low-carbohydrate diet in order to lose weight. His carbohydrate intake is so low that he is having to use up adipose tissue supplies of fatty acids to produce enough energy. Ketone bodies are produced and released as part of this process.

Case history 11

The most useful piece of information here is the finding of pitting oedema, because it considerably narrows the differential diagnosis of proteinuria, which would otherwise be extensive. The combination of proteinuria and pitting oedema could be explained by the nephrotic syndrome, in which protein loss in the urine results in hypoalbuminaemia. However, congestive cardiac failure is the most likely explanation. It is much commoner than nephrotic syndrome and is frequently associated with proteinuria.

Case history 12

The marked increase in the serum urea with the modest increase in the serum creatinine would indicate the presence of prerenal uraemia. Pyrexial patients are frequently hypercatabolic, which will contribute to his high serum urea. His low serum bicarbonate and high anion gap indicates that he has metabolic acidosis. This acidosis will cause the potassium to move from the intracellular to the extracellular compartment. The reduction in his GFR results in his inability to maintain normal serum potassium in the face of this efflux, as both these factors contribute to his hyperkalaemia.

Case history 13

The high urea and creatinine are consistent with the patient's very low GFR. The serum bicarbonate is low, indicating the presence of metabolic acidosis. However, the anion gap is normal and, hence, it is unlikely that this patient's [H+] will be grossly abnormal. The hyperkalaemia, therefore, is likely to be entirely due to the low GFR, with the efflux of potassium from the intracellular to the extracellular compartment being of minor importance. The hyponatraemia in this case reflects impaired water excretion resulting from the inability of the renal tubules to respond to AVP. These results clearly indicate that the patient needs to continue with dialysis. This woman's serum calcium status also should be assessed. Hypocalcaemia should be excluded, and high serum alkaline phosphatase (ALP) would indicate the presence of metabolic bone disease. A raised serum parathyroid hormone (PTH) concentration is another very sensitive marker of metabolic bone disease in patients with renal failure.

Treatment of metabolic bone disease in renal failure is aimed at correcting hypocalcaemia and hyperphosphataemia, e.g. oral calcium salts and calcitriol (active form of vitamin D).

Case history 14

The low [H+] and high bicarbonate concentration confirm that this patient has metabolic alkalosis. The raised PCO_2 indicates partial respiratory compensation for this. The loss of H+ will have been caused by his severe vomiting, which, in view of the history, is likely to be due to pyloric stenosis. Ingestion of bicarbonate would not lead to this degree of metabolic alkalosis, though it will have aggravated the situation. The severe vomiting has led to dehydration, manifested by the presence of prerenal uraemia. The hypokalaemia is due to a combination of potassium loss in the vomitus and the metabolic alkalosis, causing the influx of potassium from the ECF to the ICF.

The urine results are typical of a patient with dehydration and metabolic alkalosis due to vomiting. Aldosterone is being secreted in an attempt to expand his ECF, and the patient is conserving sodium despite his hypernatraemia. The hyperaldosteronism is promoting potassium loss despite hypokalaemia, and hydrogen ion loss, resulting in the classic paradoxical acid urine.

Case history 15

The high [H+] and PCO_2 confirm the presence of respiratory acidosis (and low PO_2, hypoxia), which, from the history, will have been expected. Note that the bicarbonate is not abnormally increased, which indicates this is an acute development, and renal compensation for the respiratory acidosis has not had time to have a significant impact on the respiratory acidosis.

Case history 16

The dominant feature in this patient's acid–base disorder is alkalosis because the [H+] is low. The bicarbonate concentration is increased, indicating metabolic alkalosis. The PCO_2 is increased (respiratory acidosis), and this could be due to partial compensation for the metabolic alkalosis. However, the increase in PCO_2 is too high for this to be the only explanation. The PCO_2 rarely rises above 7.5 kPa in compensation; further increases require significant hypoventilation, compromising oxygenation. The PO_2 indicates that the patient is satisfactorily oxygenating her blood. Therefore she has developed a mixed acid–base disorder: partially compensated metabolic alkalosis with respiratory acidosis. The background history of respiratory disease is also an important clinical pointer towards this conclusion.

This patient's hypokalaemia and metabolic alkalosis can be explained by profound potassium depletion due to the use of a diuretic with an inadequate intake of potassium. The principles of therapy are potassium supplementation and alteration of her drug regimen to one that will ameliorate potassium loss, e.g. use of an angiotensin-converting enzyme inhibitor.

Case history 17

By far, the most likely diagnosis based on the information given is the nephrotic syndrome. In the nephrotic syndrome, you would expect the serum albumin to be low and the urinary albumin to be high. The serum urea and electrolytes are frequently normal. Although the glomerular basement membrane may be damaged, the GFR is usually normal in the early stages of the nephrotic syndrome. Hypercholesterolaemia is a feature of the nephrotic syndrome. The history of recurrent infections suggests a degree of immune deficiency. This patient is likely to be losing immunoglobulin and some of the components of the complement system in her urine, and this could lead to a relative immune deficiency.

Case history 18

This man is suffering from multiple myeloma. He is one of the approximately 20% of patients with myeloma that do not have a paraprotein in the serum but have Bence-Jones proteinuria. His renal function should be tested, and hypercalcaemia should be excluded.

Case history 19

This man's presentation is typical of an acute coronary syndrome, which may be the manifestation of a full-blown myocardial infarction (MI) in this case. He should have an electrocardiogram recorded as soon as possible, which may, in combination with the history, confirm the diagnosis of an MI. His plasma troponin should be measured.

Case history 20

Metastatic breast carcinoma is the most likely diagnosis in this case. The liver function tests indicate that there is little hepatocellular damage present, and that bilirubin excretion is normal. These findings, however, do not exclude the possibility of hepatic metastasis, giving rise to localised areas of intrahepatic obstruction. If this were so, the gamma-glutamyl transpeptidase (GGT) also should be increased. A normal serum calcium does not exclude the possibility of bone metastasis, which is another source of the high ALP activity. This could be confirmed by studying ALP isoenzymes. A third possibility is that there may be a local recurrence, with the tumour itself producing ALP, though this would be very unlikely. A bone scan would be very helpful in this case.

Case history 21

In this case, the most likely diagnosis is carcinoma of the head of the pancreas obstructing the common bile duct. The other major differential would be enlarged lymph nodes at the porta hepatis obstructing the common bile duct, which would explain the clinical picture, as well as pancreatic cancer. This could result from any abdominal or haematological malignancy, e.g. hepatoma (he was a moderate drinker) or lymphoma. Other differentials include cholangiocarcinoma and gallstones, although these are unlikely. Carcinoma of the head of the pancreas classically gives rise to severe, painless, jaundice, which is in keeping with a bilirubin value of 250 µmol/L. This is uncomplicated obstructive jaundice, which is characterised by an ALP activity that is more than three times the upper limit of the reference interval. The aspartate and alanine aminotransferase (AST and ALT) activities do not indicate severe hepatocellular damage. By far the most important further investigations to be performed on this patient would be to image the structures in the vicinity of the head of the pancreas and the common bile duct looking for the cause of the obstruction. This could be done by ultrasound or radiology.

Case history 22

The most striking features of these results are the marked increase in the AST and ALT activities. These indicate the presence of acute hepatocellular damage. There is a degree of cholestasis as indicated by the increase in bilirubin associated with an increase in serum ALP activity. As the increase in ALP is less than twice the upper limit of the reference interval, cholestasis is unlikely to be the dominant cause of the jaundice. The increase in the GGT is to be expected as this enzyme is increased in many forms of liver disease.

The differential diagnosis here includes viral and alcoholic hepatitis. An idiosyncratic drug reaction is also possible.

Case history 23

Repeat the fasting blood glucose. The diagnosis of diabetes mellitus is not confirmed until specimens collected on at least two separate occasions place the patient in the diabetic category.

Case history 24

By far the most likely diagnosis in this case is diabetic ketoacidosis. This may be precipitated by a number of conditions, e.g. infection. This may have caused anorexia, and, thus, the patient may have omitted to take her insulin. Trauma can increase a patient's requirement for insulin, but there is nothing to suggest that in this case. Blood glucose and ketones can both be checked at the bedside. The laboratory tests that may be requested are urea and electrolytes to assess renal function, the presence or absence of hyperkalaemia and the serum sodium concentration. The patient's acid–base status should be assessed to quantitate the severity of the acidosis present, and the blood glucose can be more accurately measured. These results will influence the patient's treatment. It is essential in cases such as this that samples of blood and urine and, if appropriate, sputum are sent to the microbiological laboratory to look for the presence of infection.

Case history 25

Nocturnal hypoglycaemia is the most likely cause of this woman's symptoms. This could readily be established by continuous glucose monitoring. If this is not available, indirect evidence of nocturnal hypoglycaemia may be obtained by measuring her urinary catecholamine excretion or urinary cortisol excretion overnight. A further clue may be obtained if the woman's glycated haemoglobin level indicates good diabetic control in the face of hyperglycaemia during the day. Sometimes the diagnosis of nocturnal hypoglycaemia is inferred if the symptoms are relieved by changing the insulin regimen or getting the patient to eat more food before she goes to bed.

Case history 26

As renal failure is the most common cause of hypocalcaemia, her serum urea and electrolytes should be measured. However, unsuspected renal failure is unlikely as her serum phosphate is normal. Her plasma PTH should be measured, and if high (appropriate to the low calcium), then vitamin D deficiency is the most likely diagnosis, and the cause should be sought. In particular, a detailed dietary history should be taken. An increased serum ALP would be compatible with vitamin D deficiency. The bone pain is due to the underlying osteomalacia.

A low PTH would indicate hypoparathyroidism. Other causes of hypocalcaemia would be unlikely in this case.

Case history 27

The two most likely diagnoses in this case are primary hyperparathyroidism and hypercalaemia of malignancy. The most important biochemical investigation to be performed at this stage would be plasma PTH measurement, which will be high in primary hyperparathyroidism and suppressed in hypercalcaemia of malignancy. In patients with hypercalcaemia of malignancy, the underlying disease is usually detectable by a careful clinical history and examination. There are, however, notable exceptions, multiple myeloma being one, and therefore a sample of serum and urine should be sent for protein electrophoresis to see if a paraprotein band can be identified. A 'fishing expedition' request for tumour markers such as carcinoembryonic antigen (CEA) or alpha-fetoprotein (AFP) should not be requested unless there is a clear clinical indication for doing so. The patient's ALP activity should be measured, and ALP isoenzyme studies may be indicated, especially if the plasma PTH concentration is suppressed.

The patient shows evidence of dehydration and has severe hypercalcaemia, which should be treated by rehydration in the first instance.

Case history 28

Though this patient is hypocalcaemic, the expected compensatory rise in PTH may not occur in view of the severe hypo-magnesaemia. Thus the PTH may be low.

This patient needs magnesium supplements. As magnesium salts cause diarrhoea, they need to be given parenterally, especially in this case in which there is established diarrhoea and malabsorption. It is likely that once the patient is magnesium replete, her original vitamin D and calcium supplements will be sufficient to maintain her in a normocalcaemic state. However, she may require regular 'top-ups' of intravenous magnesium in the future.

Case history 29

As Paget's disease can be considered a disorder of bone remodelling, the serum ALP, which is a good marker of osteoblastic activity, can be used to monitor the disease

activity. It cannot, however, be used to demonstrate the involvement of a specific bone or deformity; this has to be done radiologically. Although zoledronic acid can reduce serum calcium, clinically significant hypocalcaemia is unusual. Routine monitoring of serum calcium is not required.

Case history 30

If panhypopituitarism is suspected, a lower dose of insulin should be used. This is because the relative deficiency of glucocorticoids and growth hormone is associated with an increase in insulin sensitivity.

The basal prolactin was so high in this case that prolactinoma was the diagnosis until proven otherwise. Imaging of his pituitary confirmed the diagnosis.

The hypoglycaemic stress induced in this patient did not cause the expected rise in serum cortisol. It is essential, therefore, that he is commenced on steroid replacement before surgery. His low free thyroxine (T_4) combined with the abnormal response in his thyroid-stimulating hormone (TSH) (i.e. the 60-minute level being greater than the 30-minute level) would support a diagnosis of central hypothyroidism. He should, therefore, also be commenced on thyroxine replacement. As prolactinomas frequently shrink dramatically in response to dopamine agonists, he should be commenced preoperatively on either bromocriptine or cabergoline to reduce the size of the tumour.

Case history 31

Growth hormone (GH) deficiency should be suspected, particularly in view of the documented fall-off in the patient's growth rate over the previous year. Random GH measurement is potentially misleading – false-positive and false-negative results are frequent. Many endocrinologists measure stimulated GH; a result greater than 6 µg/L excludes GH deficiency.

Case history 32

This patient has primary hypothyroidism. The thyroid gland is not secreting enough thyroid hormone, and as a result the anterior pituitary has increased secretion of thyroid-stimulating hormone (TSH) in an attempt to stimulate the thyroid gland to produce more thyroid hormone. In hypothyroidism, down-regulation of low-density lipoprotein (LDL) receptors on hepatocytes results in reduced clearance of LDL cholesterol. Once the patient has been established on adequate thyroxine

treatment, the lipid profile should be rechecked.

Case history 33

The low free T_4 and markedly elevated TSH results indicate primary hypothyroidism. Skeletal and cardiac muscles are affected in hypothyroidism, causing the release of creatine kinase (CK) into the circulation. This, combined with a decrease in the catabolic rate of CK, will be sufficient to cause the CK to increase to the levels observed in this case. The AST is mildly elevated, and this will fall along with the CK and cholesterol after a few weeks' treatment with thyroxine. In view of the evidence of myocardial ischaemia, it is prudent to introduce thyroxine replacement cautiously (initially 25 µg daily). High initial doses can precipitate myocardial ischaemia, and where the hypothyroidism is severe, as in this case, pericardial effusions and impaired ventricular function.

Case history 34

It is likely that this patient has suffered a relapse of her thyrotoxicosis. The severity of the derangement in her thyroid biochemistry (free T_4 66 pmol/L) makes it likely that she will be clinically thyrotoxic and symptomatic.

Repeated failure of medical therapy may warrant consideration of alternative treatment options, namely radioactive iodine and surgery. The former ablates the production of thyroid hormones irreversibly, and the patient would need to take replacement thyroxine therapy permanently thereafter.

Case history 35

Whenever one encounters the combination of hyponatraemia with hyperkalaemia, adrenocortical failure must be excluded. There is a modest increase in the serum creatinine with a normal serum urea that is not typical of Addison's disease. (In adrenal failure the patient usually has prerenal uraemia, which causes the serum urea to rise more than the creatinine – 'the biochemistry of dehydration'.) The low serum bicarbonate is a feature of adrenal insufficiency and may reflect both the lack of mineralocorticoid activity and lactic acidosis, the latter resulting from hypovolaemia and associated reduced tissue perfusion.

It is essential that, at the very least, a timed random cortisol is requested on this patient. Unless the result is grossly elevated, thus excluding adrenal insufficiency, a Synacthen test is warranted. As the patient has severe skeletal muscle pain, the CK should be measured because the hyperkalaemia may be due to potassium released from damaged muscle. If rhabdomyolysis were detected, it would be important to monitor renal function and calcium status carefully.

Case history 36

This presentation is classic of acute adrenal failure with characteristic symptoms, physical findings and electrolyte pattern. The diagnosis is confirmed by the Synacthen test.

On presentation, this woman was sodium depleted with prerenal uraemia. As her ECF was expanded with 0.9% sodium chloride, this improved her GFR, which is sufficient, even in the absence of aldosterone, to correct the hyperkalaemia by increasing her urinary potassium excretion. The reduction in this patient's blood volume will stimulate vasopressin secretion, giving rise to the hyponatraemia. The sodium chloride infusion by restoring her blood volume will inhibit AVP secretion, enabling her to correct the hyponatraemia.

Case history 37

Cushing's syndrome is the most likely diagnosis in this case. One can be confident of the diagnosis in view of the increased urinary cortisol/creatinine ratio and failure to suppress with low-dose dexamethasone.

Establishing a diagnosis of Cushing's syndrome is insufficient as it is essential to discover the underlying cause to enable the correct treatment to be given. This patient should have a high-dose dexamethasone suppression test with measurement of serum cortisol and adrenocorticotrophic hormone (ACTH). Suppression of the cortisol would point to the pituitary-dependent Cushing's syndrome, as would an abnormally increased ACTH concentration. An adenoma should be actively sought in her pituitary and adrenal glands by computed tomography or magnetic resonance imaging. If her ACTH is abnormally increased, she may undergo selective venous catheterisation to locate the source, which may be due to a carcinoid tumour of the lung.

Case history 38

This clinical presentation combined with biochemical findings of increased testosterone, reduced sex hormone-binding globulin (SHBG) and increased luteinising hormone/follicle-stimulating hormone (LH/FSH) ratio are characteristic of the polycystic ovarian syndrome (PCOS). Ultrasound examination of her ovaries would confirm the diagnosis. Patients with obesity and/or PCOS are insulin-resistant. This stimulates compensatory hyperinsulinaemia. In many insulin-resistant women, the ovaries remain relatively more insulin sensitive than other tissues, and the hyperinsulinaemia stimulates ovarian androgen production.

Case history 39

An accurate measurement of height and serial measurements of weight are the most important means of monitoring the nutritional progress of such a patient. Patients are at risk of developing micronutrient deficiency if they experience difficulty in swallowing and, as a consequence, alter their diet to one that may be deficient in one or more components. For example, fresh fruit and vegetables may be sacrificed in favour of highly processed foods, thus causing vitamin C deficiency. Another alternative that has to be considered in these patients is that because of the relentless, incurable, nature of their disease they may ingest excessive amounts of vitamin and trace element supplements in the vain attempt to halt the progression of their disease. A careful dietary assessment should be made in this man and, if suspected, vitamin or trace element deficiencies or excesses tested for biochemically.

Case history 40

Measuring the serum vitamin B_{12} concentration is inappropriate in patients on parenteral treatment. A routine full blood count is much more valuable. In a patient with pernicious anaemia feeling 'run down', other autoimmune diseases should be suspected. It would be reasonable to request glucose and thyroid function tests. The incidence of carcinoma of the stomach is increased among patients with pernicious anaemia, and this diagnosis also should be borne in mind.

Case history 41

This patient has insufficient small bowel to enable him to be fed enterally. He will, therefore, require long-term parenteral nutrition. It is important that he is encouraged to take some oral fluids and nutrients to maintain the integrity of his remaining bowel.

The caloric and nitrogen requirements for restoration and maintenance of his skeletal muscle and body mass should be assessed.

It is important to assess his baseline micronutrient status so any deficiencies can be corrected. As he will receive the bulk of his nutrition parenterally in the future, his micronutrient status will need to be monitored. Once he is stable this should be formally checked at 6-monthly intervals, along with his weight, skin-fold thickness and skeletal muscle mass.

Case history 42

In a patient such as this in the intensive care unit, the biochemical measurements that are most frequently helpful are:

- *Serum urea and electrolytes* to monitor renal function and *serum potassium* as he may become hyperkalaemic as a result of tissue damage.
- *Pulse oximetry* to assess tissue oxygenation.
- *Blood gas analysis and plasma lactate*, to detect and quantify acid–base disorders that may arise.
- *Serum muscle enzymes*, such as CK, may help detect a compartment syndrome or monitor rhabdomyolysis.

Case history 43

Recurrence or metastatic spread of the breast cancer would need to be excluded in this woman by imaging her liver and skeleton. Measurement of GGT and ALP isoenzyme studies may help localise the source of the ALP. However, increased bone ALP does not necessarily signify bony metastases. In view of the history and symptoms, osteomalacia due to malnutrition or malabsorption might equally explain the raised ALP. If the patient has malabsorption or malnutrition, she may have a macrocytic anaemia due to folate or vitamin B_{12} deficiency and may be deficient in other vitamins or other micronutrients, e.g. zinc. Malabsorption is often difficult to detect clinically, and she should undergo tests for malabsorption.

Case history 44

The clinical history is strongly suggestive of peptic ulcer disease. Accompanying chronic diarrhoea and weight loss points towards possible Zollinger–Ellison syndrome. This is due to a gastrinoma (gastrin-producing neuroendocrine tumour) which usually arise in the stomach, pancreas or duodenum. Excess uncontrolled gastrin production leads to excess gastric acid production. Endoscopy reveals multiple peptic ulcers. The diagnosis may be confirmed by measuring blood gastrin levels after an overnight fast. Elevated blood levels of chromogranin A also point towards neuroendocrine origin. Gastrin is very unstable and must be sent promptly on ice after arrangement with the biochemistry laboratory. Secretin stimulation test for stimulated gastrin levels is rarely required nowadays.

Case history 45

This patient has the classic symptoms and signs of iron-deficiency anaemia. The finding of low serum ferritin with low serum iron and per cent transferrin saturation are typical of this condition. However, if iron-deficiency anaemia is suspected, the most important and usually the only investigation required is to demonstrate the presence of a hypochromic microcytic anaemia by examining the blood film, along with low haemoglobin.

Case history 46

The finding of a high liver copper concentration would indicate that the patient died from Wilson's disease, which is an autosomal recessive disorder. The patient's sister (and brothers, if any) should be screened for Wilson's disease. Serum copper, caeruloplasmin and urinary copper excretion may indicate if any of them has the disease. A liver biopsy may be indicated to confirm the diagnosis and allow treatment to be initiated. Molecular genetic testing is becoming available to assist in the diagnosis. Due to the very large number of mutations, this is only of value within families to detect affected members and identify carriers.

Case history 47

Clarithromycin may increase the plasma concentration of theophylline. Since the clarithromycin treatment was still required, her theophylline was stopped for 2 days and restarted at a lower dose. Once the infection was clear, she was recommenced on her original dose of theophylline.

Case history 48

These results would indicate that the man has taken an overdose of salicylate. The serum salicylate of 635 mg/L will contribute to his relatively high anion gap of 18 mmol/L. Salicylate poisoning is associated with metabolic acidosis due to uncoupling of oxidative phosphorylation, and respiratory alkalosis, due to direct stimulation by salicylate of the respiratory centre. The $[H^+]$ and PCO_2 indicate that the respiratory alkalosis is dominant at this stage.

In all cases of salicylate overdose the serum paracetamol should be measured, as many proprietary analgesics contain aspirin and paracetamol. In the early stages of paracetamol poisoning, and when treatment is effective, patients will not display any specific signs or symptoms.

Case history 49

Some imported cosmetic agents contain lead. Occasionally, children will ingest these agents accidentally and may develop lead poisoning. It is, therefore, appropriate to measure the whole blood lead and, if elevated, erythrocyte zinc protoporphyrin.

Case history 50

A high serum GGT is not diagnostic of alcohol abuse. GGT is induced by a number of enzyme-inducing agents such as phenytoin and phenobarbital, which this boy was taking. Currently, there is no definitive biochemical test to confirm alcohol abuse. However, the combination of an increased serum GGT and urate with a macrocytosis is strongly suggestive of alcohol abuse.

The ALP of 520 U/L is entirely appropriate for a teenager during his pubertal growth spurt. It should not be taken as indicative of liver disease.

Case history 51

This boy's calculated osmolality is approximately 206 mmol/kg. Thus the osmolal gap is approximately 76 mmol/kg. This has arisen because of his severe hyperlipidaemia, which causes pseudohyponatraemia. In severe hyperlipidaemia the increased lipids occupy a larger fraction of the plasma volume than usual, and the water a smaller fraction. Sodium is distributed in the water fraction only, and, in reality, these patients have a normal plasma sodium concentration. However, many of the instruments used to measure sodium take no account of this and thus produce artefactually low sodium results.

Severe hypertriglyceridaemia in a child may be caused by a decrease in lipoprotein lipase activity. This may result from genetic defects in the enzyme itself or in the enzyme's cofactor, apolipoprotein CII. Lipoprotein lipase is essential for the normal catabolism of chylomicrons and very-low-density lipoprotein.

Two further notable points about very high triglycerides are that (1) they are a risk factor for developing acute pancreatitis, and (2) lipaemic samples cause analytical

interference in measurement of various common analytes, including amylase (and thus may preclude accurate laboratory confirmation of acute pancreatitis).

Case history 52

This man has diabetes mellitus, which is the most likely cause of his hyperlipidaemia. His GGT is high, which may be due to the presence of a fatty liver, a common finding on presentation in patients with type 2 diabetes. The high GGT also may be due to high alcohol intake, which may contribute to his hypertension. However, the combination of diabetes mellitus with central obesity and hypertension would suggest insulin resistance or the so-called metabolic syndrome.

Details of his family history with respect to coronary heart disease should be obtained. Palmar or tuberous xanthomas should be looked for and, if present, would suggest type III hyperlipidaemia. His Apo E genotype should then be established.

This patient should be treated with dietary measures. Particular attention should be paid to his alcohol intake. Optimising his diabetes control is likely to lead to a reduction in his serum triglycerides. However, statin treatment will be required (unless contraindicated) to lower his overall cardiovascular risk.

Case history 53

The concern would be that this patient has Cushing's syndrome due to ectopic (malignant) production of ACTH. This is most frequently seen with carcinoma of the lung. As this disease is usually very aggressive, patients tend to develop florid metabolic features of the disease compared with the physical signs, which may be minimal. His serum urea and electrolytes indicate that he has developed profound hypokalaemia, metabolic alkalosis and glucose intolerance. These all can be attributed to hypercortisolism. Cortisol will also cause muscle wasting that, combined with hypokalaemia, will lead to weakness. The nocturia and polyuria can cause profound potassium depletion.

Cushing's syndrome should be confirmed by performing a dexamethasone suppression test. If the suspicion of malignant ectopic ACTH production is high, the low- and high-dose suppression tests should be performed sequentially. Measurement of urinary cortisol output will confirm cortisol overproduction. His plasma ACTH concentration will be grossly elevated. In such cases, if carcinoma of the lung is demonstrated radiologically and/or by bronchoscopy, the diagnosis of ectopic ACTH production is made without necessarily confirming it biochemically. Conn's syndrome and other conditions that may give rise to hypokalaemia with hypernatraemia are much rarer.

Case history 54

Though he is not clinically jaundiced, the high ALP and GGT with modest increases in the AST and ALT would suggest cholestasis. This may be due to liver cirrhosis or malignant disease affecting the liver, both of which would be likely diagnoses in this case. Liver congestion resulting from cardiac failure would explain the clinical findings, but the biochemistry of congestion is classically dominated by raised transaminases.

An AFP level may be helpful as it is a relatively sensitive tumour marker for hepatocellular carcinoma, which is also a possible diagnosis in this case. The most common predisposing factors to the development of hepatocellular carcinoma are alcoholic cirrhosis in Western countries and hepatitis B in the developing world.

Case history 55

The patient's plasma PTH should be measured, and, if increased, a diagnosis of primary hyperparathyroidism can be made. However, hyperparathyroidism with a serum calcium of 2.8 mmol/L is usually asymptomatic and thus another cause for his hypertension, headaches and anxiety should be sought. If the symptoms were episodic, this would suggest the possibility of a phaeochromocytoma, which is associated with hyperparathyroidism in families with multiple endocrine neoplasia (MEN). The patient should have his urinary catecholamines measured, and, if the diagnosis is made, it is important that other members of his family be screened for hyperparathyroidism and phaeochromocytoma.

Case history 56

Acute severe pain in the metatarsophalangeal joint is the classic presentation of gout. The serum urate level is usually high in gout, but only a minority of patients with hyperuricaemia develop gout and frequently patients with acute gout may have a normal serum urate level. The presence of fever would be compatible with septic arthritis. The joint should be aspirated and, in addition to looking for urate crystals that would confirm a diagnosis of gout, some of the aspirate should be sent for microbiological studies to exclude the possibility of infection.

Case history 57

The large increase in the CK and lactate dehydrogenase (LDH) relative to the AST and ALT would indicate that muscle is the major tissue contributing to the increase in serum enzyme activities. However, muscle cells contain only a small amount of ALT; AST and LDH are found in muscle, liver and erythrocytes. Thus, the tissues that could have contributed to the serum enzyme activities include muscle (either skeletal or cardiac), the liver or erythrocytes.

By measuring troponin T or I, one can determine whether cardiac muscle is involved. If the liver is involved, then the serum GGT should be increased, as this is one of the most sensitive indicators of liver disease. Although LDH isoenzyme studies might in theory help identify erythrocyte damage as a possible source of LDH and AST, in practice it is much more useful to look for other evidence of haemolysis, e.g. reticulocytosis and absent or low haptoglobin.

Case history 58

This woman should be offered amniocentesis, with bilirubin measured in her amniotic fluid. In Rhesus incompatibility, the amniotic fluid bilirubin concentration will be high because of the destruction of fetal red cells by maternal antibodies.

Case history 59

Preeclampsia is the most likely diagnosis. The most appropriate side-room test to perform would be to dipstick the urine for protein. Biochemical investigations that should be performed on this woman are:

- *Serum urate*, as this is a sensitive indicator for preeclampsia.
- *Serum urea and electrolytes* should be measured as she may be developing renal failure.
- *Serum liver function* tests should be performed to detect liver disease.

Case history 60

No other investigations should be performed, but the parents should be reassured that their daughter does not have congenital hypothyroidism.

Over 99% of all 6-day-old children will have a TSH of less than 10 mU/L, whereas the majority of patients with congenital hypothyroidism will have a TSH greater than 100 mU/L. Babies with a blood TSH between 15 and 40 mU/L on their first test are considered to have an equivocal result. If, in a second sample, a normal result is obtained, as is usually the case, no further investigation need be made.

Case history 61

This baby's blood gas status should be assessed as she is at risk of developing respiratory distress syndrome. In view of her maternal history, weight and gestational age, she may be hypoglycaemic and her blood glucose should be measured. Hypocalcaemia is another possibility that should be considered, so her serum calcium should be measured.

The total blood volume in neonates is small and is likely to be less than 100 mL in this baby. It is, therefore, very important to collect the minimum amount of blood required as neonates can become anaemic if excessive investigations are performed.

Index

Note: Page numbers followed by '*f*' indicate figures, '*t*' indicate tables and '*b*' indicate boxes.

Tubular phosphate reabsorption, congenital defects of, 74
Tubular proteinuria, 36
Tubulopathies, hypokalaemia and, 27
Tumour lysis syndrome
 acute, 148
 hyperkalaemia, 24
Tumour markers, 144, 145b. *See also* Cancer; Tumours
 in ascitic fluid, 129
 case history in, 145b
 for diagnosis, 144
 with established clinical value, 145, 145t
 for follow-up, assessing, 144
 in the future, 145
 for monitoring treatment, 144
 practical application of, 144–145
 prognosis and, 144
 for screening for the presence of disease, 144
 use of, 144f
Tumours. *See also* Cancer
 adrenocortical, 98–99
 biochemical effects of growth, 142f
 carcinoid, 147
 in female sex hormones, 100
 germ cell, 145
 markers. *See* Tumour markers
 mucosal associated lymphoid, 113
 multiple endocrine neoplasia and, 146f
 pituitary, 84–85, 146
T-waves, 'tented', 24
Type 1 diabetes mellitus, 62, 63t
Type 2 diabetes mellitus, 62, 63t

U

Ulcerative colitis, 113
Ultrasound, antenatal screening and, 157f

Urate
 formation and excretion of, 148
 serum, 148
 sodium, tophaceous deposits of, 148, 149f
 uric acid and, 148f
Urate stones, 148f
Urea cycle defects, 168t
Urea, in acute kidney injury, 38
Uric acid
 renal stones, 33
 urate and, 148f
Urinalysis, 34, 35b. *See also* Proteinuria; Urine
 bilirubin in, 34
 biochemical testing in, 34, 34f
 blood in, 35
 case history in, 35b
 glucose in, 34
 ketones in, 35
 leucocytes in, 35
 Multistix testing in, 35f
 nitrite in, 35
 procedure for, 34
 protein in, 35
 specific gravity in, 35
 urobilinogen in, 34–35
Urinary copper, 119
Urinary free cortisol, 98
Urinary system, potassium losses in, 26
Urinary tract infection, 33, 35
Urinary tract, urate stones from, 148f
Urine. *See also* Urinalysis
 concentration, 33b
 contamination of drain fluids with, 135
 creatinine in, 135f
 ketones in, 64–65, 65b
 microbiological testing of, 35b
 osmolality measurements in, 32
 pH, 32, 35
 protein excretion, 37

Urine (*Continued*)
 specimen collection, 4
 urinary losses, 18
Urobilinogen, 57
 in urine, 34–35

V

Venepuncture, prolonged stasis during, 4
Vertebral fractures, steroid-induced, 78f
Virilism, 100
Vitamin D
 deficiency, 70
 metabolism of, 77f
 metabolites, hydroxylated, 41
Vitamin D-dependent rickets, 77
Vitamin K, 161
Vitamins, 104–105
 average adult daily requirements of, 105f
 classification of, 105t
 in nutritional support, 107
VLDL (very-low-density lipoprotein), 136, 136t
Volatile organic intermediates, characteristic smells, 163t
Vomiting
 hypokalaemia and, 26
 sodium losses, 18–19
 water loss, 16

W

Waldenström's macroglobulinaemia, 53
Water, 16, 16f, 17b
 deprivation test, 32
 intake, 16
 for intravenous fluid therapy, 28
 loss, 16, 22
 in body fluid compartments, 14f
 metabolism, 40
 volume regulation, 17

Water retention, 18
 maternal, 152
Water supplies, aluminium levels in, 125
Water tank model, 19f
Weight, maternal, 157
WHO. *See* World Health Organisation
Wilson's disease, 119
 biochemistry determinations in patients with, 119t
 case history in, 119b
Women
 androgen screen in, 100–101
 elevated testosterone concentration in, 101f
 subfertility in
  diagnostic approach to, 102f
  endocrine investigations in, 102
World Health Organisation (WHO)
 diabetes classification, 64
 hypertension classification, 140
 on iodine intake, 88
 osteoporosis definition, 78

X

Xanthelasmas, in hypercholesterolaemia, 138f
Xanthochromia, 132
Xanthomas
 eruptive, 138f
 tendon, 139f

Z

Zinc, 118, 119b. *See also* Copper
 balance, 118f
 deficiency, 118, 118f
 laboratory assessment for, 118
 physiology of, 118
 prolonged supplementation of, 119b
 toxicity, 118
Zinc protoporphyrin (ZPP), 116